Developmental Neuropathology of Schizophrenia

NATO ASI Series

Advanced Science Institutes Series

A series presenting the results of activities sponsored by the NATO Science Committee, which aims at the dissemination of advanced scientific and technological knowledge, with a view to strengthening links between scientific communities.

The series is published by an international board of publishers in conjunction with the NATO Scientific Affairs Division

A	**Life Sciences**	Plenum Publishing Corporation
B	**Physics**	New York and London
C	**Mathematical and Physical Sciences**	Kluwer Academic Publishers
D	**Behavioral and Social Sciences**	Dordrecht, Boston, and London
E	**Applied Sciences**	
F	**Computer and Systems Sciences**	Springer-Verlag
G	**Ecological Sciences**	Berlin, Heidelberg, New York, London,
H	**Cell Biology**	Paris, Tokyo, Hong Kong, and Barcelona
I	**Global Environmental Change**	

Recent Volumes in this Series

Volume 217—Developmental Neuropathology of Schizophrenia
edited by Sarnoff A. Mednick, Tyrone D. Cannon, Christopher E. Barr, and José M. LaFosse.

Volume 218—Pharmaceutical Applications of Cell and Tissue Culture to Drug Transport
edited by Glynn Wilson, S. S. Davis, L. Illum, and Alain Zweibaum

Volume 219—Atherosclerotic Plaques: Advances in Imaging for Sequential Quantitative Evaluation
edited by Robert W. Wissler

Volume 220—The Superfamily of *ras*-Related Genes
edited by Demetrios A. Spandidos

Volume 221—New Trends in Pharmacokinetics
edited by Aldo Rescigno and Ajit K. Thakur

Volume 222—The Changing Visual System: Maturation and Aging in the Central Nervous System
edited by P. Bagnoli and W. Hodos

Volume 223—Mechanisms in Fibre Carcinogenesis
edited by Robert C. Brown, John A. Hoskins, and Neil F. Johnson

Series A: Life Sciences

Developmental Neuropathology of Schizophrenia

Edited by

Sarnoff A. Mednick, Tyrone D. Cannon, Christopher E. Barr, and José M. LaFosse

University of Southern California
Los Angeles, California

Plenum Press
New York and London
Published in cooperation with NATO Scientific Affairs Division

Proceedings of a NATO Advanced Research Workshop on Developmental Neuropathology of Schizophrenia, held August 28-September 1, 1989, in Castelvecchio, Pascoli, Italy

Library of Congress Cataloging-in-Publication Data

NATO Advanced Research Workshop on Developmental Neuropathology of Schizophrenia (1989 : Castelvecchio Pascoli, Italy)
Developmental neuropathology of schizophrenia / edited by Sarnoff A. Mednick ... [et al.].
p. cm. -- (NATO ASI series. Series A, Life sciences ; v. 217)
"Proceedings of a NATO Advanced Research Workshop on Developmental Neuropathology of Schizophrenia, held August 28-September 1, 1989, in Castelvecchio Pascoli, Italy"--T.p. verso.
"Published in cooperation with NATO Scientific Affairs Division."
Includes bibliographical references and index.
ISBN 0-306-44081-4 (hardbound)
1. Schizophrenia--Pathophysiology--Congresses. 2. Schizophrenia--Etiology--Congresses. I. Mednick, Sarnoff A. II. North Atlantic Treaty Organization. Scientific Affairs Division. III. Title. IV. Series.
[DNLM: 1. Brain--embryology--congresses. 2. Brain--physiopathology. 3. Nervous System--embryology--congresses. 4. Nervous System--physiopathology--congresses. 5. Schizophrenia--etiology--congresses. 6. Schizophrenia--physiopathology--congresses. WM 203 N279d 1989]
RC514.N27 1989
616.89'82071--dc20
DNLM/DLC
for Library of Congress 91-44812
CIP

ISBN 0-306-44081-4

A Division of Plenum Publishing Corporation
233 Spring Street, New York, N.Y. 10013

Printed in the United States of America

PREFACE

This volume reports the proceedings of a NATO Advanced Workshop held in Castelvecchio Pascoli, Italy, from August 28 - September 1, 1989. An important inspiration for this Workshop came from our studies in Helsinki and Denmark, which have found that exposure to an influenza epidemic during the second trimester of fetal development increases the risk of adult schizophrenia. This finding has stimulated an important new hypothesis in the study of the etiology of schizophrenia. It has suggested the possiblity that disturbances of brain development during gestation may contribute to the risk of adult schizophrenia. We determined that it would be of value to bring together schizophrenia researchers and those doing basic studies of the development of the brain. Both groups of researchers were encouraged to communicate at a level that would help other scientists to integrate their knowledge and techniques into their own discipline.

For this reason, perhaps, the papers of this volume are remarkably clear and not difficult to understand. The first four chapters describe the neurochemical and structural aspects of brain development. The chapter by Dziegielewska and Saunders discusses transport mechanisms and the properties of endogenous and exogenous substances that control the internal environment of the developing brain. In the second chapter, Nowakowski reports on his studies of the development of the hippocampus in mice genetically inbred to exhibit disruptions of neural migration. In these genetically inbred mice he observes abnormally positioned cells; he reports on how these cells make and receive connections with normally positioned targets in other parts of the brain.

The chapter by Janas, Moos, and Mollgard discusses differing regional distribution of plasma proteins between human archicortex and neocortex and their possible relevance to disruptions of neuronal proliferation, migration, and cellular damage or death, which have been implicated as potential predispositional factors for schizophrenia. Berger's chapter discusses some functional implications of cortical dopaminergic innervation for the understanding of schizophrenia.

Bogerts and Falkai review the clinical-anatomical relationships of a number of different brain regions that have been studied in schizophrenics and consider the etiological basis of structural brain abnormalities in schizophrenia.

The Dykes, Mednick, Cannon, and Barr chapter discusses the possible importance of obstetric complications as an etiological factor in schizophrenia, particularly schizophrenia characterized by predominantly negative symptoms.

The Nasrallah, Schwarzkopf, and Olson chapter and the Cannon chapter both examine the potential contribution of genetic and perinatal factors to the presence of structural brain abnormalities in schizophrenia.

Bilder and Degreef present three hypothetical constructs, each of which represents different pathological processes, as a heuristic for understanding the heterogeneity of the cerebral morphological, neuropsychological, and clinical features of schizophrenia.

Jones, Goodman, Owen, Lewis, and Murray discuss a number of research findings in the schizophrenia literature and conclude that they point toward the process of neural development as an important factor in the onset of schizophrenia.

The chapter by LaFosse and Mednick concludes by providing an overview of various lines of research that together have led a growing number of investigators to consider that at least some forms of schizophrenia have a neurodevelopmental origin.

The editors wish to thank NATO for their sponsorship, and also for assisting with the expenses of the Danish scientists who attended the meeting. The Letten Saugstad Scientific Foundation was very generous in its support of the participation expenses of young schizophrenia researchers.

We join with all the conference participants in expressing our enthusiastic thanks to the staff of Il Ciocco for their friendly, helpful, and attentive service. Our special compliments to the chef. The manager of Il Ciocco, Mr. Bruno Giannasi, was always there, being supportive constructive and intelligent. We are proud to count him as a personal friend.

June 1991

Sarnoff A. Mednick
Christopher Barr
Tyrone Cannon
Jose LaFosse

CONTENTS

THE DEVELOPING BRAIN

NEUROCHEMICAL ASPECTS OF THE DEVELOPING BRAIN

NEUROPATHOLOGICAL INDICANTS OF NEURODEVELOPMENTAL ANOMALIES IN SCHIZOPHRENICS

PERINATAL COMPLICATIONS IN SCHIZOPHRENICS

STRUCTURAL IMAGING AND NEUROPSYCHOLOGICAL EVIDENCE OF NEURODEVELOPMENTAL ANOMALIES

FACTS ABOUT SCHIZOPHRENIA AND NEURODEVELOPMENT

THE INTERNAL ENVIRONMENT OF THE DEVELOPING BRAIN

Katarzyna M. Dziegielewska and Norman R. Saunders

Clinical Neurological Sciences Group (Developmental)
Southampton General Hospital
Southampton, England

INTRODUCTION

The internal environment of the brain in the adult is remarkably stable, much more so than the general internal environment of the organism as a whole. A series of different mechanisms contributes to this stable internal environment and such mechanisms are no doubt important for the normal functioning of the brain. They are often referred to collectively, if somewhat misleadingly as "the blood-brain barrier." The origin of this term stems from experiments carried out at the end of the last Century involving the injection of dyes into animals (Ehrlich,1885). It was observed that certain dyes did not stain the brain although they did stain almost every other tissue in the body. Ehrlich's own interpretation of this result was that brain has a much lower affinity for dye than other tissues. However Biedl and Kraus (1898) showed subsequently that this was not the case and proposed that there was a "barrier" preventing the penetration of the dye into brain. It was shown much later that the "barrier" was to protein rather than dye and that dyes which do not penetrate into brain do not do so because they are bound to plasma proteins, probably mainly albumin (Tschirgi, 1951). Brightman and Reese (1969) demonstrated the ultrastructural nature of this barrier to protein. It resides in the presence of tight junctions between adjacent cerebral endothelial cells which occlude the intercellular space thus preventing the passage of molecules such as protein from blood to brain extracellular space. In addition they demonstrated a similar diffusion restraint between blood and cerebrospinal fluid (csf) (the blood-csf barrier) which consisted of tight junctions between the epithelial cells of the choroid plexus.

It is perhaps not at first apparent why a mechanism that excludes foreign substances, namely certain dyes, from the brain should be of much biological

Developmental Neuropathology of Schizophrenia
Edited by S.A. Mednick *et al.*, Plenum Press, New York, 1991

interest. However the original dye experiments did lead to the concept that the brain was in some way "protected" from materials circulating in the rest of the body and it was supposed that some of such substances might be harmful or influence brain function in a deleterious manner.

The term <u>the</u> blood-brain <u>barrier</u> is perhaps misleading since, as will be outlined below, many mechanisms contribute to the control of the internal environment of the adult brain and many of these involve more than mere exclusion of materials from the brain. However the tight junctions between cerebral endothelial cells and between choroid plexus epithelial cells can perhaps be justifiably referred to as "the" barrier since they provide an underlying diffusion restraint upon which all the other mechanisms involving ion transfer, transmitter and metabolite transfer must work (see Table 1).

The factors which control the internal environment of the adult brain are a combination of structural properties, biological transport mechanisms and the physico-chemical properties of materials that may pass into or out of the brain. These factors are summarized in Table 1. They have been described and discussed in considerable detail elsewhere (e.g. Bradbury, 1979; Davson et al., 1987). The importance of these factors in the developing brain and the extent to which the

Table 1. Important factors in the control of the internal environment of the brain.

1. Morphological

    Cerebral endothelial cells: tight junctions
    Choroid plexus epithelial cells: tight junctions
    Ependyma: gap junctions
    (Neuroependyma: strap junctions and gap junctions developing brain only)

2. Passive properties

    Lipid solubility
    Molecular size
    Charge, pH

3. Csf secretion - sink effect

4. Facilitated/active transfer mechanisms

    Electrolytes
    Glucose
    Amino acids
    Trace metals, vitamins, hormones
    Proteins (into csf, probably developing brain only)

internal environment of the developing brain is distinct from and controlled separately from that of the rest of the fetus is the subject of this paper. If deleterious materials such as infectious agents or heavy (toxic) metals have access to the fetus via the placenta then it is important to know whether or not such substances may also reach the developing brain. Access of such agents to the immature brain may account for a number of congenital defects of brain development and in the case of viruses this has been suggested to be a much underestimated cause of subsequent brain damage (Volpe, 1987).

It has generally been held that the blood-brain barrier in the fetus and newborn is immature (e.g. Ganong, 1989). This belief seems to stem partly from experimental observations involving a repeat of Ehrlich's dye experiments in immature animals (e.g. Behnsen, 1927) and partly from the teleological argument that the placenta will provide a substantial degree of stability in the internal environment of the fetus as a whole and therefore the fetus would not "need" a blood-brain barrier to protect the brain (e.g. Barcroft, 1938). No doubt it has also seemed a matter of common sense that any mechanism in a developing organism would necessarily be immature. However teleology and common sense can often be misleading and much of the experimental work usually cited in support of the proposition that the blood-brain barrier in the fetus is immature, is not much less misleading. The matter is further confused by a frequent failure to take proper account of the very different stages of brain development at which different species are born.

Stern carried out a large series of barrier experiments in the 1920s that seem to be little known, perhaps because her conclusions were the opposite of the received wisdom of the day. Stern (e.g. Stern et al., 1929) showed that dyes that she referred to as "colloids" did not penetrate into the brains of young animals however immature, providing that the amounts of dye injected were similar to those used in adult experiments, with due allowance for the size of the animals:

"Ces recherches avaient en outre établi que, si la résistance de la barrière chez le nouveau-né etait considerablement plus faible vis-a-vis des substances cristalloides telles que le ferrocyanure ou l'iodure, sa résistance a l'egard des colloides tels que le bleu trypan et le rouge Congo ne differait pas de celle de l'adulte ... Ainsi, chez le Lapin nouveau-né, le passage du bleu trypan ne s'observe que lorsque la quantite injectée depasse 3 a 4 gr. par kilogramme d'animal; le passage du rouge Congo ne se manifeste que lorsque la quantite injectée depasse 3 gr. par kilograme d'animal ... Il faut atteindre des doses massives depassant de 30 a 40 fois les doses utilisees normalement dans nos experiences, pour provoquer l'apparition de ces colorants dans le liquide céphalorachidien. Il faut tenir compte des doses lorsqu'il s'agit d'apprecier les resultats obtenus par les divers auteurs", L. Stern, J.-L. Rapoport and E.-S. Lokschina (1929).

Modern barrier experiments usually involve the use of horseradish peroxidase

(HRP), a plant protein of comparable molecular weight to that of many plasma proteins to which the more traditionally used dyes bind. HRP has the advantage that its enzymic reaction product can be visualized in the electron microscope. Unfortunately, like many of the earlier dye experiments, the more recent ones involving the use of HRP have generally paid no attention to the physiological state of the experimental preparation and have involved the use of literally brain-blowing volumes of fluid or concentrations of protein. For example Risau et al. (1986) used an intracardiac injection of HRP solution that was up to the equivalent of a quarter of the total body volume in the fetal mice studied. In the experiments of Wakai and Hirokawa (1978, 1981) on chick embryos it was only when the HRP amount injected would have more than doubled what can be estimated to have been the likely plasma protein concentration, that HRP could be detected within the central nervous system.

In fact, it seems to have been overlooked until recently that Nature performs its own barrier experiment. Extracellular proteins that circulate within the embryo and fetus are synthesized initially in the yolk sac and subsequently in the liver. One can take sections from fixed brain of an embryo or fetus from even the earliest stages of nervous system development and stain the sections for plasma proteins using immunohistochemical techniques (e.g. Sternberger, 1979). The circulating plasma proteins e.g. albumin, α-fetoprotein, transferrin, are confined to the lumen of the vessels within the brain and spinal cord; no extracellular plasma protein is demonstrable in normal embryonic or fetal brains nor in the newborn of marsupial species which are born at a very early stage of their brain development, particularly the forebrain (Dziegielewska et al., 1988, 1989a; Møllgård et al., 1988). Although there is no detectable plasma protein around the vessels in the brains of developing mammals, there is, rather unexpectedly evidence of such proteins within cells in the developing brain (see section 6 on Brain-liver proteins).

BARRIER MECHANISMS IN THE DEVELOPING BRAIN

If we examine the list of mechanisms in Table 1 that are thought to be important for the stability of the internal environment of the adult brain then we can consider the extent to which these mechanisms function in the developing brain; we should also consider the possibility that the developing brain might possess mechanisms that are not present in the adult.

The physicochemical factors listed are of course as applicable in the developing brain as in the adult. Thus if a material, e.g. drug, is lipid soluble it will penetrate into the brain regardless of the state of maturity or otherwise of any barrier mechanisms, unless it is so firmly bound to proteins in plasma that there is effectively no free ligand to pass into the brain.

Tight Junctions

It was argued above, that although the term blood-brain barrier is now used to describe a whole series of mechanisms that control the internal environment of the brain (Table 1), it can be considered to describe the fundamental barrier mechanism, the tight junctions between cerebral endothelial cells that provide the diffusion restraint that allows the many other mechanisms to be effective. It is therefore important to consider the state of development of tight junctions in the immature brain. Early studies (e.g. Delorme et al., 1970; Doolin and Birge, 1969) using section transmission electronmicroscopy suggest that tight junctions both between cerebral endothelial cells and between choroid plexus epithelial cells were incomplete. These observations were supported by studies using HRP injected into the fetuses and showed HRP on the csf and brain side of the barrier. Unfortunately the amounts of HRP used in such experiments were generally large or unspecified (cf Introduction); also the observation of HRP in csf could be explained by transcellular transfer across the choroid plexus (see Møllgård and Saunders 1975, 1977 and Section 2d). Later studies using both thin section, EM and freeze fracture have shown that tight junctions at both barrier sites (cerebral vessels and choroid plexuses) appear to be complete from as early as these interfaces develop (see Tauc et al., 1984, Saunders & Møllgård, 1984 and Møllgård and Saunders, 1986). Unfortunately it is not possible to examine every tight junction in the developing brain so it may be that incomplete junctions have been missed even with the freeze fracture technique. A more general, if indirect indication that tight junctions within the developing brain are indeed tight comes from experiments involving more modest amounts of injected HRP (e.g. Tauc et al., 1984; Dziegielewska et al., 1988) which did not penetrate into the brain and was not found within incomplete tight junctions. Also the lack of immunocytochemical staining for plasma proteins around vessels in the developing brain (see Introduction and Mollgard et al., 1988) suggests that cerebral endothelial tight junctions are indeed effective early in brain development.

Low Molecular Weight Lipid-insoluble Compounds

Just as Stern was the first to show clearly that "colloid dyes" (subsequently shown to be dyes bound to plasma proteins) did not penetrate into the developing brain providing that reasonable amounts of dye were used, she was also the first to show that the immature brain is more permeable to low molecular weight compounds. Stern used substances such as sodium ferrocyanide that she could visualize by color reaction under the microscope. Stern showed that such low molecular weight substances (mw of sodium ferrocyanide is 304) injected into fetal and newborn animals, e.g. rats, rabbits, penetrated into the brain but not in older animals. A quantitative version of this experiment was carried out by Ferguson and Woodbury (1969) using radioactively labelled inulin and sucrose. They showed that the younger the animal (rat) the more the markers penetrated into brain and csf.

However there was no information given about the physiological state of the animals used and from subsequent work it seems likely that the markers were not at a steady state in the plasma - an essential prerequisite for accurate determination of csf/plasma or brain/plasma ratios. These experiments have been repeated recently under more controlled conditions (Habgood, 1989) and it has been shown that Ferguson and Woodbury's values were too high, although the general conclusion that the immature brain is more permeable to low molecular weight compounds was confirmed.

A more extensive study (Dziegielewska et al., 1979) was carried out in our laboratory using fetal sheep in which it is possible to control the physiological state of the fetus and obtain serial samples of plasma so that the plasma level of markers injected can be estimated and controlled. The results from these experiments at 60 days gestation and 125 days gestation (term is 150 days in a species that is born at a time when its central nervous system is well developed compared with more commonly used laboratory animals such as the rat) are shown in Fig. 1.

These results show that smaller molecular weight compounds penetrate into brain and csf to a greater extent than do larger molecular weight compounds. The level of penetration is much greater in the less mature fetuses. These results also confirm, as indicated in the Introduction, that exogenous proteins when injected into animals in amounts that do not raise the circulating plasma protein concentration substantially, do not penetrate into brain. However it is clear that they do penetrate into csf (see section 2(d) on Protein permeability) especially early in gestation.

Sink-effect of CSF secretion

CSF is secreted by the choroid plexuses and there is probably a contribution to its volume from the brain tissue itself (Davson et al., 1987; Milhorhat, 1976). Davson has proposed that the continuous turnover of csf acts as a "sink" to keep the steady state level of substances penetrating into the brain and csf at a lower level than would otherwise be the case; Davson proposed this in order to explain the experimental observation that extracellular markers such as sucrose never achieve the distribution volume in brain that one would expect if the brain had an extracellular space volume similar to that in other tissues (as appears to be the case providing precautions are taken to prevent shrinkage (e.g. Van Harreveld and Steiner, 1970). This sink effect would be expected to be greater for more slowly penetrating molecules. It would be less if, for example in the immature brain, the turnover of csf is less. The absolute rate of secretion of csf in the immature brain is undoubtedly less than in the adult. This has been shown both in the rat (Johanson and Woodbury, 1974) and in the sheep (Fossan et al., 1985). However it is difficult to know on which basis one can compare the csf secretion rates for different sizes and stages of brain development. Table 2 illustrates data for sheep

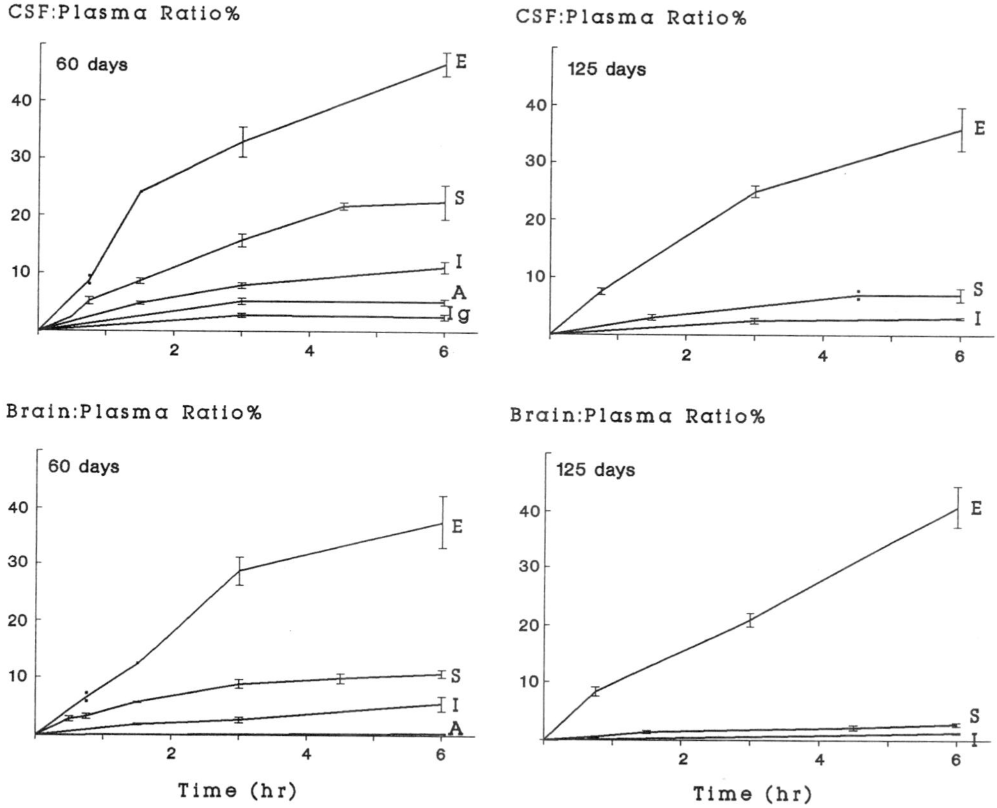

Figure 1. Permeability of blood-brain and blood-csf barriers in anaesthetized fetal sheep at 60 and 125 days gestation (term is 150 days from conception). Fetuses were given i.v. infusions or intermittent injections to maintain approximately constant blood levels of a wide range of molecular size markers: erythritol mol. radius [E, 0.35 nm], sucrose [S, 0.51 nm], inulin [I, 1.3 nm], human albumin [A, 3.5 nm], human IgG [Ig, 5.3 nm]. Experiments were run for 20 min to 6 hr. Three to six experiments were performed for each time point except where individual points are shown. Bars are ± standard error of mean. Results are expressed as the concentration ratio csf: plasma X100 or brain to plasma X100. The ratios for erythritol at both ages and for csf and brain are similar probably because erythritol is small enough to pass through cell membranes. The ratios for brain are smaller than for csf at each age because the markers are distibuted in brain within the extracellular space. Note the decline in ratios with age, which is thought to reflect a decline in passive permeability with age. The values for human albumin in 60 day fetal brain are not significantly above background blood contamination of the brain samples i.e., the blood-brain barrier to protein is well formed even this early in gestation. Redrawn from Dziegielewska et al. (1979).

Table 2. Csf secretion in fetal and adult sheep

Age (days from conception)	Brain wt. (g)	Csf secretion (ul/min)	Csf vol. (ml)	Turnover (%/min)	"sink" (%/min/g brain wt.)
60	1.91	2.8	0.45	0.62	0.32
125	36.70	62.5	7.12	0.88	0.02
Adult	78.40	118.0	14.20	0.83	0.01

Note that the turnover of csf does not change very much in spite of very large changes in brain growth. Secretion rate and volume of csf. Data from Evans et al., 1974 and Fossan et al., 1985.

fetuses. In terms of simple turnover (secretion rate expressed as proportion of total volume of csf) there is surprisingly little difference between the two very different stages of brain development at 60 and 125 days gestation. If we attempt to take account of brain size by expressing the turnover in terms of brain weight we obtain the unexpected result that this estimate of "sink effect" is much higher in the immature fetus than in the mature fetus. Thus it seems unlikely that a reduced sink effect could account for any of the developmental change in permeability illustrated in Fig. 1 for sheep fetuses of 60 and 125 days. A reduced sink-effect may of course be important still earlier in development, but this has so far not been investigated apart from a few measurements in late stage rat fetuses (Johanson and Woodbury, 1974).

Protein Permeability

As indicated above (Introduction), the cerebral vessels themselves in the immature brain do not appear to be permeable to protein in the sense of passively "leaking" protein through intercellular junctions. However csf in the fetus (including the human) contains very high concentrations of proteins that all appear to be immunologically identical to plasma proteins (see Dziegielewska and Saunders, 1988 for review). This is illustrated in Fig. 2 for total protein in several species and in Table 3 for individual proteins in the sheep fetus for which we have the most comprehensive data. A limited amount of data are available on the human fetus (Table 4, data from Adinolfi and Haddad, 1977) although there is necessarily some doubt about how normal such samples can be expected to be.

Permeability experiments in fetal sheep have shown that at least at the beginning of the second trimester of gestation (60 days, term is 150 days) most if not all of the protein in cisternal csf can be accounted for by penetration from blood (Fig. 3). These experiments involved the injection of either heterologous plasma

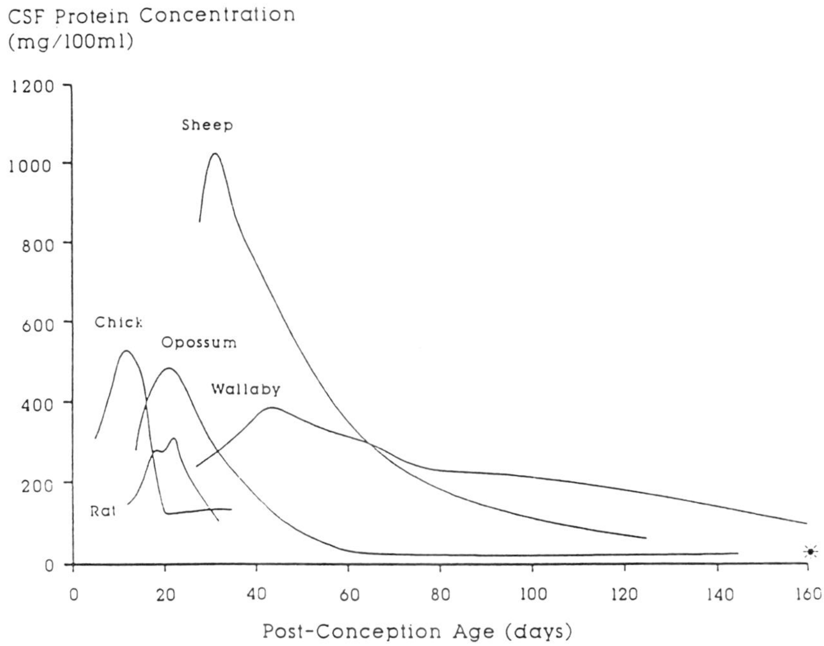

Figure 2. Total protein concentration (mg/100 ml) in csf of various species. Csf obtained from cisterna magna. Protein estimated by Lowry or Bradford method, indicates adult value in mammalian species. Birth occurs in: opossum, 14 days (weaned 60 days); chicken and rat, 21 days; wallaby, 28 days (final pouch exit 250 days); sheep, 150 days.

proteins that could be distinguished from the sheep's own protein by using appropriate antisera, or injection of radioactively labelled proteins, intravenously into fetuses of anaesthetized sheep (Dziegielewska et al., 1980). The results showed that the natural steady states of several of the main proteins in csf at 60 days gestation were approached by 3 to 6 hours after injection of the marker proteins (Fig. 3). Unexpectedly, proteins of rather similar molecular size had significantly different steady states and even more surprisingly the steady state for a "foreign" albumin (human) was only about half that of the sheep's own albumin. This observation is currently under further investigation in our laboratory and preliminary findings have been published (Dziegielewska et al., 1989b). We are studying the penetration of different species of albumin from blood into csf. In addition to sampling cisternal csf we have also sampled csf from the lateral ventricles. In the adult it is known that there is a gradient of protein concentration from a low value in the lateral ventricles, through an intermediate value in the cisterna magna to the highest concentration in the lumbar space (Davson et al., 1987). Although there is

Table 3. Concentration (mg/100 ml) of proteins in CSF of fetal sheep of different gestational ages and in the adult

Fetal age (days)	n	Albumin	α-Fetoprotein	Fetuin	Transferrin	α_1-Antitrypsin	Σ	Total protein
28 (25-28)	4-7	82 ± 9	394 ± 72	253 ± 36	152 ± 12	384 ± 36	1265[a]	850 ± 51
31 (30-33)	5-7	121 ± 16	569 ± 58	229 ± 29	51 ± 11	427 ± 41	1348 ± 98	1143 ± 83
35 (35-36)	6-9	204 ± 22	189 ± 23	271 ± 23	137 ± 28	349 ± 32	1200 ± 49	853 ± 49
40 (37-43)	15-17	212 ± 13	203 ± 23	206 ± 15	163 ± 14	270 ± 19	1066 ± 68	773 ± 52
59 (57-60)	8-12	112 ± 10	61 ± 11	61 ± 5	50 ± 9	63 ± 4	373 ± 30	274 ± 10
87 (85-90)	6-8	56 ± 3	1.3 ± 1.5	22 ± 3	12 ± 2	26 ± 4	124 ± 5	123 ± 7
125 (123-128)	4-7	29 ± 3	0.9 ± 0.3	5.7 ± 0.4	6.1 ± 0.7	12 ± 2	55 ± 4	60 ± 10
Adult	6-7	11 ± 1	ND	(0.5 ± 0.2)[b]	1.1 ± 0.4	1.7 ± 0.4	---	26 ± 2

n = number of fetuses; mean ± SE of mean; age is in days from conception; Σ = sum of all five proteins: total proteins (L) = total protein estimated by Lowry et al. (1951) method; ND = not detectable. The Lowry method underestimates the concentration of mixtures of different proteins especially if they contain large proportions of carbohydrate, e.g, fetuin.

a Calculated from mean values, as some individual protein values were not obtained.
b Approximate value only, near threshold of assay.

Data are from Dziegielewska (1982)

Table 4. Concentrations (mg/100) of proteins in human fetal CSF

Age (weeks)	n	Total Protein	Albumin	α-Fetoprotein	IgG	Prealbumin	Transferrin
15	4	118 (2)	58 ± 19 (3)	76 ± 17	3.7 (2)	6.7 (1)	
19	3	240 (2)	104 (2)	69 ± 18	6.8 (2)	5 (1)	22 (2)
22	10	535 ± 31	249 ± 27	30 ± 6	9.8 ± 1.4	5.7 ± 0.8	10.3 ± 2.6
25	4	339 ± 29	117 ± 28	5.7 ± 0.6	11.4 ± 2.2	1.8 (2)	1.8 (2)

Mean ± SE of mean was calculated from data of Adinolfi and Haddad (1979). n = number of fetal samples (given in parentheses after mean if less than n).

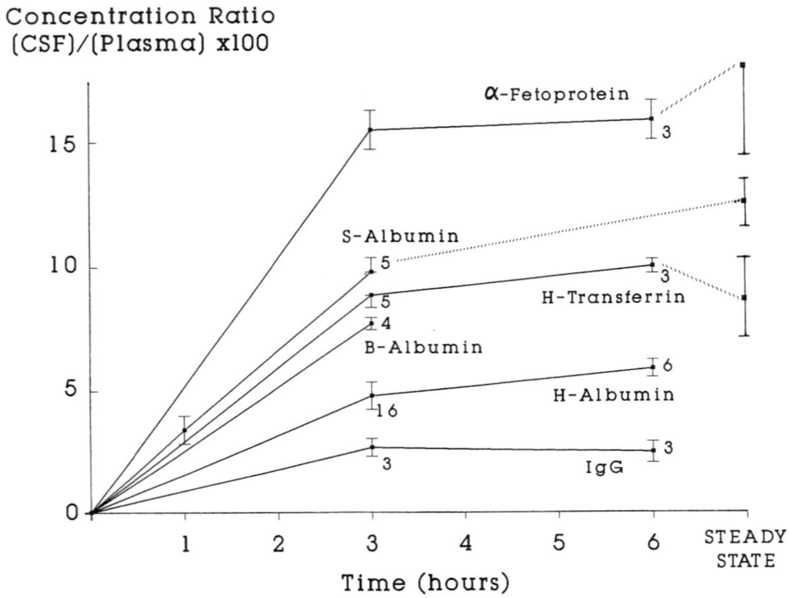

Figure 3. Blood-csf transfer of proteins in anaesthetized 60 day fetal sheep compared with steady state csf/plasma ratios of naturally occurring proteins in csf.

Note: (1) that there is some relation between molecular weight and permeability (the largest molecule IgG has the smallest ratio and the smallest molecule AFP has the largest ratio); (2) proteins of similar size can have significantly different ratios; and (3) albumins from different animal species have different ratios. This suggests that there is a highly selective mechanism that transfers proteins from plasma to csf in addition to the greater passive permeability illustrated in Fig. 1. This specific protein transfer mechanism is not present after about 70 days gestation. Values are mean ± SEM. S= sheep, B = bovine, H = human.

such a gradient, the absolute values of protein concentrations are very low when compared with either adult plasma or fetal csf. Such a protein concentration gradient is also present in the fetus although the absolute values are at a much higher level than in the adult (Table 5 and see also Cavanagh et al., 1983). In our current experiments as in the earlier ones, human albumin only penetrated from blood into csf to less than half the level expected for the natural steady state of sheep albumin. This was also the case into lateral ventricular csf although at an overall level that was about 20% of that in cisternal csf. Chicken albumin gave similar results. However the more closely related bovine albumin penetrated into both csf compartments to a greater extent than human and chicken albumins although still not to the full steady state level of sheep albumin. These results suggest that there is a transfer mechanism present Table 3. Concentrations (mg/100ml) of proteins in CSF of fetal sheep of different gestational ages and in the adult in the immature sheep fetus that is able to distinguish between different species of albumin. This mechanism is not present later in gestation when the concentration of csf protein is much lower and the level of protein penetration from blood into csf is much reduced (Dziegielewska et al., 1980). The differential permeability of different species of albumin in the immature sheep fetus implies that there is a mechanism that is able to distinguish between the different albumins, presumably at a molecular level. The amino acid sequences of human albumin and bovine albumin (Brown, 1977) are known. We have recently determined the deduced amino acid sequence of sheep albumin from the nucleotide sequence (Brown et al., 1989). X-ray crystallographic data on human albumin have been published recently (Carter et al., 1989). Thus it may be possible to make structural predictions about the features of the albumin molecule that are important for this specific protein transport system in the immature fetus (Dziegielewska et al., 1991). We have recently obtained evidence for a similar mechanism that is able to distinguish between different species of albumin in their transfer from blood to csf in the neonatal rat (Dziegielewska et al., 1990).

The route of transfer of albumin and other proteins into csf in the fetus is being studied in collaboration with Professor K. Møllgård and his colleagues in the University of Copenhagen. We have immunocytochemical evidence, both at the light microscopical and electronmicroscopical level, that the route is likely to be across cells in the choroid plexuses. Thus using antisera that are specific for the different albumins (and avoiding cross-reactivity by pre-absorption with the appropriate albumin) we have been able to stain cells in the choroid plexus both for endogenous sheep albumin and for the exogenous foreign albumin (Dziegielewska et al., 1991).

As well as being of fundamental interest, this albumin specific carrier mechanism in the immature fetus may be of considerable importance in relation to the topic of this meeting. Albumin is a well-known carrier protein. If it is transported from plasma into csf in early stages of brain development then a whole

Table 5. Comparison of proteins in CSF from lateral ventricle and IVth ventricle during early brain development (30-60 days gestation) in fetal sheep

LATERAL VENTRICLE

Age (days)	n	Albumin	α-Fetoprotein	Fetuin	Transferrin	α_1-Antitrypsin	Σ
31 (30-33)	n = 4-5	145 ± 6	679[2]	219 ± 49	66 ± 77	388 ± 81	1533[2]
40 (38-43)	n = 5	77 ± 9	77 ± 29	42 ± 14	81 ± 15	130 ± 44	373[4] ± 72
60	n = 3	43 ± 9	21 ± 3	12 ± 2	17 ± 8	23 ± 4	116 ± 11

IVth VENTRICLE

Age (days)	n	Albumin	α-Fetoprotein	Fetuin	Transferrin	α_1-Antitrypsin	Σ
31 (30-33)	n = 4-5	101 ± 24	481 ± 38	219 ± 50	45 ± 51	385 ± 51	1284[3] ± 105
40 (38-43)	n = 5	240 ± 15	189 ± 42	243 ± 19	195 ± 24	322 ± 41	1184[4] ± 133
60	n = 3	152 ± 15	104 ± 24	71 ± 14	68 ± 2	67 ± 5	464 ± 3

Protein concentration in mg/100 ml (mean ± S.E.M.). Age in days from conception (mean and range). Samples at 40 and 60 days were paired ventricular and hindbrain samples from same fetus. Σ = sum of all 5 proteins, taken as 'total protein', this exceeded the "Lowry" value indicating that most if not all of the protein in fetal sheep csf is accounted for by these 5 proteins. [2]n = 2 [3]n = 3 [4]n = 4
From Cavanagh et al. (1983).

range of other materials both endogenous e.g. ions, vitamins, hormones, trace metals and exogenous e.g. drugs and heavy metals will be carried into the csf. Although albumin and other plasma proteins do not appear to penetrate passively across immature vessels in the brain (see Sections 1 and 2(d)) there is evidence that proteins including albumin in the csf are taken up into neuroependymal cells that line the cerebral ventricles (e.g. Cavanagh and Warren, 1975 and see Section 2(e) on Protein uptake from csf, below). Thus a whole range of materials including potentially damaging exogenous materials may have access to particularly immature (i.e. ventricular zone cells) regions of the developing brain (see also sections 4-6).

CSF-brain Barrier and Uptake of Proteins from CSF into Neuroependymal Cells in the Fetus

It has been shown in a number of different species that foreign proteins such as albumin when injected into the cerebral ventricles of the immature brain are taken up by the neuroependymal cells lining the cerebral ventricles (e.g. Cavanagh and Warren, 1985) and there are some indications that different proteins may be taken up at different times in brain development. Thus the uptake mechanism may be both protein-and age-specific. As mentioned in the previous section, such an uptake mechanism when combined with a transchoroidal protein transfer system may allow access of a number of protein-bound materials to the ventricular zone cells of the developing brain (see also Section 5).

In view of the high concentration of protein in fetal csf (see previous section) it seems, at first sight, surprising that this protein has not been demonstrable within the extracellular space of the developing brain (eg Dziegielewska et al., 1988; Møllgård et al., 1988). However we have shown that exogenous protein such as HRP when perfused through the ventricular system of the immature brain is prevented from passing between the adjacent cells of the ventricular zone by the presence of a membrane specialization, the "strap junction" (Fossan et al., 1985; Møllgård et al., 1987). These junctions are present in the neuroependyma early in brain development and disappear during the course of brain growth. In the fetal sheep they are reduced in number by 60 days gestation although still effective in preventing access of HRP to the brain extracellular space (Fossan et al., 1985). They are largely gone by 80 days gestation and the neuroependyma has been shown to be freely permeable to HRP by 125 days gestation in the sheep fetus (Fossan et al., 1985). Neurogenesis in the sheep ceases by around 60 days gestation and is followed by gliogenesis (Astrom, 1968). The strap junctions appear to exclude protein from the extracellular space of the brain at a stage of brain development when the ventricular zone (neuroependyma) is predominantly producing presumptive neurons. In addition to preventing access of protein into the general internal environment of cells in the brain, the strap junctions may also provide some structural stability in a brain region that is undergoing a high rate of mitosis and cell migration. It may be important that these junctions have largely disappeared at a stage of brain development when the brain is particularly vulnerable to a specific type of hemorrhage within the ventricular zone or germinal matrix that may extend into the cerebral ventricles (intraventricular hemorrhage, see Reynolds et al. (1979) and Section 3 on Fragility of vessels in the developing brain, below).

At the time of gliogenesis, the protein concentration in csf is still high compared with the adult, although much less than earlier in development (see Fig. 2). At this stage of brain development the strap junctions have largely disappeared; thus the presumptive glial cells in the ventricular zone are exposed to a relatively high concentration of protein in their extracellular environment whereas earlier in brain development the presumptive neurons are exposed to protein only on the apical surfaces that are in contact with csf. It may be relevant that glial cells in culture are usually successfully grown in the presence of high concentrations of protein whereas for neurons a lesser concentration is generally used (e.g. Coon and Sinback, 1982).

Electrolytes in the Internal Environment of the Developing Brain

One of the notable features of the internal environment of the adult brain is the stability of the concentrations of many functionally important electrolytes in csf and brain extracellular fluid. There are important differences in the ionic composition of csf (and by implication of brain extracellular fluid) when compared with plasma as an indicator of composition of the general extracellular fluid (see Davson et al., 1987). Even in the face of major fluctuations in the concentration of ions such as K^+ and Ca^{++} in plasma, their concentrations in csf remain largely unchanged (see Bradbury, 1979; Davson et al., 1987). This stability presumably reflects the importance of ionic gradients in neuronal function. Glial cells probably have an important role in controlling the local microenvironment within the brain. But the blood-brain extracellular fluid and blood-csf interfaces are thought to be important in the overall control of the composition of electrolytes within the adult brain.

In the developing brain the presence of a gradient of electrolyte concentration between csf and plasma would imply firstly that an adequate ionic "pump" was functioning and secondly that an effective diffusion restraint (i.e. tight junctions between cerebral endothelial cells and between choroid plexus epithelial cells) was present. The absence of any ionic gradients would indicate that no "pumps" had yet become active and possibly that tight junctions were not yet effective. However the evidence from EM studies and from the protein distribution and permeability studies described earlier, makes this last point unlikely (see section 2(d)) even in the immature brain.

The presence of even one ionic gradient would suggest strongly that there was an efficient diffusion restraint between blood and csf (and between blood and brain, since small molecules seem to pass unhindered between csf and brain in the developing brain, Fossan et al., 1985, although electrolyte transfer has not been specifically studied). The time in gestation when ionic gradients are first apparent varies both with the animal species and type of ion, but the data available are rather incomplete so that it is only possible to give examples rather than a comprehensive statement. Thus in the pig a csf:plasma gradient for chloride ions is first apparent at about 40 days gestation (Flexner, 1938; term in the pig is after about 120 days gestation); the adult ratio is acquired well before term. A similar time course for the development of the chloride gradient in fetal sheep was described by Bradbury et al. (1972). The gradients for Na+, K+, Mg++ and Ca++ developed later and apparently independently. Although the gradients (csf: plasma) tended to change over a substantial part of gestation before reaching adult values, for some electrolytes e.g. Mg++ this seems to have been more due to a continued change in plasma concentration rather than in csf concentration, suggesting that once an initial gradient is present, the mechanisms that provides for stability of the ionic composition within the brain's internal environment are functional from an early stage.

In species that are born more precociously than sheep or pigs, for example rats (gestational period 21-22 days) and rabbits (gestational period 32 days) the ion gradients between csf and plasma appear towards the end of gestation and continue to develop in the neonatal period. Once the gradient for a particular ion is established the absolute csf concentration remains rather constant in spite of further changes in plasma concentration (e.g. Amtorp & Sorensen, 1974). However the ability of the control mechanisms to withstand serious perturbations in plasma ion concentrations may take some days to develop. For example Jones and Keep (1987) have shown that the adult csf/plasma K+ ratio is established by E19 but control in the face of acute hyperkalemia was not fully established until P30. The same authors (Jones and Keep, 1988) showed that stability of csf [Ca^{++}] in the face of acute plasma changes was achieved earlier, by 1-5 days postnatal.

Studies in developing animals (mainly rat) using radioactive anions and cations have recently been reviewed by Johanson (1989). The 36Cl uptake into brain declines during the first few weeks of life in the rat. But concomitant changes in sink effect and brain extracellular fluid volume make this change difficult to interpret. Iodide transport (which occurs from csf to blood in the adult) increases during the neonatal period in the rat (Woodbury, 1967) and in present at least as early as 60 days gestation in the 60 day fetal sheep (unpublished observation). The kinetics of distribution of 22Na in neonatal rats were similar to those of 36Cl (Smith et al., 1982).

FRAGILITY OF BLOOD VESSELS IN THE DEVELOPING BRAIN

The conventional wisdom that the blood-brain barrier (to protein) in the fetal and newborn brain is immature is probably misplaced as has been discussed above. However it does seem that the vessels in the developing brain may be considerably more fragile than those in the adult. This may explain some of the experiments that purport to demonstrate barrier immaturity to HRP or to protein-bound dye. It is not clear whether even adult brains would withstand some of the extraordinary conditions that have frequently been imposed in experiments on fetal and newborn animals (see Section 1). In our own experiments in fetal sheep, more modest increases in plasma protein concentrations (e.g. +20%) or circulating blood volume (e.g. +10-20%) especially if induced acutely over 1-2 minutes may result in leakage of some vessels (unpublished observations and Plate 3). There are known pathological hemorrhages that occur in the immature human brain that may have very serious consequences for survival or subsequent brain development if survival occurs. The best known of these hemorrhages is "Subependymal" or "Intraventricular hemorrhage" (IVH) which occurs in prematurely born infants of gestational age 24 to 34 weeks (see Volpe, 1987) and is still probably the main cause of death in such infants.

The advent of non-invasive methods (computerized axial tomography and ultrasound) for the examination of brains in neonates has uncovered a remarkably high incidence of subependymal hemorrhages in prematurely born infants -- as high as over 80% in some series (Bejar et al., 1980). Many of these hemorrhages are "silent" and do not give rise to immediate clinical manifestations, although it is less clear whether they result in subsequent brain malfunction. A proportion of the subependymal hemorrhages progress to intraventricular hemorrhages, some of which have catastrophic effects on the infant. IVH is still the major cause of death and disablement in prematurely born infants. The hemorrhages begin in a characteristic part of the brain, within the ventricular zone or subependymal layer particularly within the ganglionic eminence. This region is a germinal zone within which precursor cells are dividing and migrating into the developing neocortex. At the stage when most hemorrhages occur neurogenesis is largely over and the precursor cells are mainly destined to become glial cells. The vessels within this germinal zone are rather thin walled and of large diameter, with characteristics of immature blood vessels (Pinar et al., 1985). Once gliogenesis is over the ventricular and subventricular zones have disappeared (by 34-36 weeks gestation) and the region is no longer prone to hemorrhage. IVH is much less common in infants born at term and its pathogenesis may be different since bleeding usually originates from the choroid plexus (Volpe, 1987).

The mechanism of subependymal hemorrhage and IVH is unknown. Innumerable descriptive clinical studies of infants with intracranial hemorrhage have been published but relatively few studies on experimental models have been carried out.

The first such model was the mid-gestation fetal sheep which has a ventricular zone similar to that of 28-32 week human fetuses. IVH and subependymal bleeding occurred following various combinations of asphyxia and elevation of systemic arterial or cerebral venous pressure (Reynolds et al., 1979). Using a similar model Ting et al. (1984) did not produce any IVH although following acute asphyxia they did find widespread cerebral necrosis with focal damage in white matter; however these experiments involved different manipulations of vascular pressures than those of Reynolds et al. (1979). Also Ting et al. (1984) did not measure jugular or cerebral venous pressure and it is likely that their withdrawal and re-infusion of blood did not produce the changes in venous pressure that they assumed would have occurred. Experimental IVH has also been induced in newborn beagles in which PCO2 was increased acutely (with associated increases in arterial and jugular venous pressure) (Goddard et al., 1980). Ment et al. (1982) induced IVH in the same model by the production of hemorrhagic hypotension followed by volume re-expansion.

The pathogenesis of IVH and subependymal hemorrhage in prematurely born infants remains obscure but it seems likely that important contributions to their occurrence are wide-swings in vascular pressures, on either the arterial or the venous side of the cerebral circulation, in association with asphyxia. Pneumothorax and sudden expansion of the circulating blood volume associated with exchange transfusion or rapid i.v. infusions appear to be common precipitating events. These and other possible factors contribution to the occurrence of IVH are discussed by Volpe (1987). The brain damage associated with these hemorrhages if not fatal may well be associated with subsequent neurological deficit and psychological impairment.

VIRUS PENETRATION INTO THE CENTRAL NERVOUS SYSTEM

There are three routes by which viruses are thought to enter the central nervous system (Johnson, 1982).

<u>Via the choroid plexus</u> by direct infection of choroid plexus epithelial cells or by transfer across the choroid plexus epithelial cells into the brain. This latter route appears to be particularly important for mumps virus and certain arboviruses.

<u>Via cerebral vascular endothelial cells</u> either by direct infection of these cells or by transfer across the vascular wall of virus-infected leucocytes.

<u>Uptake of viruses by nerve fibers</u> that project from the central nervous system to beyond the blood-brain barrier. The virus particles are transported retrogradely within axons to reach the cell bodies of neurons within the nervous system e.g. Poliovirus, rabies virus and herpes simplex virus. Different viruses may show a

predilection for specific areas of the nervous system e.g. poliovirus for anterior horn cells or cranial nerve motor nuclei; herpes simplex virus involves particularly the medial temporal lobes or orbitofrontal cortex. This may imply a similarity between virus structure and receptor structure in the exposed neuronal surface membrane.

There are well known examples of congenital viral infections leading to subsequent maldevelopment of the brain. The best known and commonest examples of such intrauterine infections are cytomegalovirus and rubella, which may result in characteristic brain defects (see Volpe, 1987).

There is evidence that some viruses are found particularly in germinal zones in the developing brain, for example in the subventricular zone of the forebrain and germinal zone of the cerebellum (Johnson, 1982). Apart from chronic infections such as rubella or cytomegalovirus, viruses have not generally been isolated from fetuses or neonates thought to have been infected in utero. It is therefore possible that the incidence of virus infection in utero is higher than is generally supposed. This is suggested by the studies of Thompson and Glasgow (1980) who used immunological methods to detect early intrauterine exposure to virus in eight of 23 human infants. The transport of specific proteins from blood into csf and uptake from csf into ventricular zone cells described in Sections 2(d),(e) presumably involves a carrier recognition site on the protein molecule. If it were shared with specific viruses then this fetal protein transport system, which does not appear to be present later in development or in the adult, might render the immature fetus particularly susceptible to infection by some viruses.

Some epidemiological studies have suggested that mid trimester infection with influenza virus or some other disruption of fetal brain development at this critical stage may be associated with subsequent development of schizophrenia (Cannon and Mednick, 1989; Lyon et al., 1989; La Fosse and Mednick, this volume). There appears to be evidence that fetal tissues are highly susceptible to influenza virus if infected, but it is much less clear to what extent influenza virus can reach the fetus from an infected mother (see Smith and Sweet, 1988, for review).

TRACE AND HEAVY METALS IN THE DEVELOPING BRAIN

Some trace metals, notably zinc are essential for normal brain development. It is well established that zinc deprivation in pregnant animals at a critical stage in gestation may result in severe congenital malfunctions of the neural tube (Hurley, 21981). Later in gestation zinc deprivation is thought to have profound effects on subsequent brain development and behavior (Sandstead, 1985). There may be important dietary effects on zinc uptake in the gut or availability within the plasma that could have a profound effect on the delivery of zinc to the developing brain. Thus phytate-containing vegetables bind zinc and prevent absorption in the gut.

Some amino acids, especially histidine bind zinc in the plasma and may therefore reduce the availability of zinc for uptake into brain. Zinc binds to a number of proteins in plasma but it is not clear whether zinc uptake into brain depends on uptake of the Zn-protein complex or ionic zinc or zinc bound to amino acids. This problem is currently under study in our laboratory. But it is clear that there are numerous possible ways in which the zinc uptake into the developing brain might be interfered with.

Heavy metal (e.g. lead, cadmium) uptake into developing brain has been associated with developmental brain and behavioral defects. That such uptake can occur has been demonstrated experimentally by Dencker and his colleagues (e.g. Dencker et al., 1983). The mechanism of uptake into fetal brain is not clear but it may well be that the protein transfer system described in Section 2(d) is important. Several of the proteins that we have found to be transported from blood into csf in the immature fetus also bind heavy metals. The presence of similar metal-binding proteins not only in csf (which may be taken up to neuroependymal cells) but also synthesized within cells in the developing brain (see section 6) may determine the brain distribution of heavy metals penetrating into the developing brain.

BRAIN-LIVER (GLYCO)-PROTEINS

Immunocytochemical studies of the distribution of plasma proteins in fetal choroid plexus were carried out as part of an investigation to determine the route by which proteins pass from the blood to csf. This approach led to the unexpected finding that many plasma proteins are also present within cells in the fetal brain at some stages of its development (e.g. Møllgård et al., 1979, 1988). The first observation of immunocytochemical staining of a plasma protein (AFP) in fetal rat brain was published by Benno and Williams (1978). Several plasma proteins have now been demonstrated in a wide range of species: human e.g. Møllgård et al., 1988; sheep, Reynolds and Møllgård, 1985; pig, Cavanagh and Møllgård, 1985; tammar wallaby, Dziegielewska et al., 1988. For the reasons outlined in Section 2(d) and discussed elsewhere (see Møllgård et al., 1988) these proteins probably do not originate from the circulating blood plasma proteins by passage through the intercellular clefts of cerebral endothelial cells, because their tight junctions appear to be well formed very early in brain development (see also Møllgård and Saunders, 1986). Cerebral endothelial cells do stain immunocytochemically for some plasma proteins (e.g. transferrin and $\alpha 2$ macroglobulin) so that it is possible that there is some vascular uptake with subsequent transfer to cells within the brain. However the general pattern of cellular staining is not particularly associated around blood vessels. Thus other origins for these proteins seem more likely:

<u>Uptake from csf into ventricular zone cells</u> as considered inspection 2(e). If such protein has a long half-life then it might still be apparent within cells that

have detached from the ventricular surface and migrated into the wall of the developing cerebrum. Preliminary evidence indicates that this is probably not the case: human albumin injected into lateral ventricles of late fetal and neonatal mice was taken up into ventricular zone cells but was not found in the cortical plate 24-48 hours later (Cavanagh and Warren, 1985). In addition fetuin staining of cortical plate cells in fetal sheep, cattle and pigs is prominent in the early stages of cortical plate formation, but fetuin is also found in ventricular zone cells which have probably taken up the protein from csf (Cavanagh and Møllgård, 1985; Reynolds and Møllgård, 1985; Reynolds et al., 1987).

Uptake of proteins may occur in the terminals of axons projecting beyond the blood-brain barrier. This protein may then be transported retrogradely to the neuronal cell body, thus accounting for the plasma protein staining of some cranial nerve nuclei that project beyond the blood brain barrier e.g. hypoglossal nucleus (see Møllgård et al., 1988).

In situ synthesis of plasma proteins: There is now substantial evidence in a number of species including the human, that mRNAs for a large number of plasma proteins are present in developing brain. Several different techniques have been used: isolation and translation of mRNAs with immunological identification of the translation produce (Dziegielewska et al., 1985, 1986; Møllgård, 1988, hybridization with cDNA for the specific protein e.g. transferrin (Bloch et al., 1985) and fetuin (Jones et al., 1989, in preparation).

The functions of these proteins within the developing brain are not known. But they may include the binding and carrier functions that are described for proteins such as transferrin and ceruloplasmin when they are present in plasma. Since some of these proteins also bind toxic heavy metals, their presence in the developing brain may render the immature brain particularly susceptible to their effects should they gain access to the fetus.

CONCLUSION

Evidence in this paper has been reviewed which suggests that the brain develops within an internal environment that is distinct in some important respects from that of the rest of the fetus. Some specialized mechanisms eg protein transfer between blood and csf, are present early in gestation that are not present in later life. Although such mechanisms are presumably of fundamental importance for the normal development of the brain, their very presence may render the brain more susceptible to exogenous materials such as heavy metals, drugs or viruses that gain entry to the fetus. More detailed considerations of most of the above aspect of blood brain barrier mechanisms are considered in other reviews (Saunders, 1991, 1992).

Much of the data described are from animal experiments, often from species with very different periods of gestation and stages of brain development at the time of birth. Some information from observations on human fetal material has been discussed that suggests that the mechanisms described in experimental animals are likely to be present in the human fetus. A clear definition of when these specialized fetal mechanisms are present in the human fetus would help to delineate periods of particular susceptibility to external agents that might be related to the subsequent development of schizophrenia in predisposed individuals.

REFERENCES

Adinolfi, M. and Haddad, S. A., 1977, Levels of plasma proteins in human and rat fetal csf and the development of the blood-csf barrier, Neuropaediatrie, 8:345-353.

Amtorp, O. and Sorensen, S. C., 1974, The ontogenetic development of concentration differences for protein and ions between plasma and cerebrospinal fluid in rabbits and rats, J. Physiol. 243:387-400.

Åström, K. -E., 1967, On the early development of the isocortex in fetal sheep, pp 1-59 in: "Progress in Brain Research" vol. 26 "Developmental Neurology", C. G. Bernhard and J. P. Schade, ed., Elsevier, Amsterdam, London, New York.

Barcroft, J., 1938, "The brain and its environment", Yale University Press, New Haven.

Behnsen, G., 1927, Uber die Farbstoffspeicherung im Zentralnervensystem der weissen Maus in verschiedenen Alterzustanden, Z Zellforsch, 4:515-572.

Bejar, R., Curbelo, V., Coen, R. W., Leopold, G., James, H., Saunders, B., Porreco, R., Gluck, L., 1980, Early diagnosis of intraventricular and germinal layer hemorrhage (IVH/GLH) by ultrasound, Padiat.Res., 14: 629.

Benno, R.H. and Williams, T.H., 1978, Evidence for intracellular localization of alpha-fetoprotein in the developing rat brain, Brain Res., 142: 182-186.

Biedl, A. and Kraus, R., 1898, Uber eine bisher unbekannte toxische Wirkung der Gallensaure auf das Zentralnervensystem, Zentralblatt fur innere Medizin, 19: 1185-1200.

Bloch, B. Popovici, T., Levin, M. J., Tuil, D. and Kahn, A., 1985, Transferrin gene expression visualized in oligodendrocytes of the rat brain by using in situ hybridization and immunohistochemistry, Proc. Natl. Acad. Sci. USA, 82: 6706-6710.

Bradbury, M. W. B., 1979, "The Concept of a Blood-Brain Barrier", Wiley, Chichester.

Bradbury, M. W. B., Crowder, J., Desai, S., Reynolds, J. M., Reynolds, M. and Saunders, N. R., 1972, Electrolytes and water in the brain and cerebrospinal fluid of the foetal sheep and guinea-pig, J. Physiol., 227: 591-610.

Brightman, M. W. and Reese, T. S., 1969, Junctions between intimately apposed cell membranes in the vertebrate brain, J. Cell Biol., 40: 648-677.

Brown, J. R., 1977, Serum albumin: amino acid sequence, in: "Albumin Structure, Function and Uses", pp 27-51, V. M. Rosenoer, M. Oratz and M.A. Rothschild, eds., Pergamon, Oxford.

Brown, W.M., Christie, D.L., Dziegielewska, K.M., Saunders, N.R. and Yang, F., 1991, The rat protein encoded by clone pp63 is a fetuin/α_2HS glycoprotein-like molecule, but is it the tyrosine kinase inhibitor PP^{63}? Cell, in press.

Cannon, T.D. and Mednick, S.A., 1989, Genetic and perinatal determinants of structural brain deficits in schizophrenia, Arch. Gen. Psych., 46: 883-889.

Carter, D. C., He, X-M, Munson, S. H., Twigg, P. D., Genert, K. M., Broom, M. B. and Miller, T. Y., 1989, Three-dimensional structure of human serum albumin, Science, 244: 1195-1198.

Cavanagh, M. E., Cornelis, M. E. P., Dziegielewska, K. M., Evans, C. A. N., Lorscheider, F. L., Møllgård, K., Reynolds, M. L. and Saunders, N. R. 1983, Comparison of proteins in csf of forebrain and hindbrain during early development of fetal sheep, Dev. Brain Res., 11:159-167.

Cavanagh, M. E. and Møllgård, K., 1985, An immunocytochemical study of the distribution of some plasma proteins within the developing forebrain of the pig with special reference to the neocortex, Dev. Brain Res., 18: 183-194.

Cavanagh, M. E. and Warren, A., 1985, The distribution of native albumin and foreign albumin injected into lateral ventricles of prenatal and neonatal rat forebrain, Anat. & Emryol., 172: 345-351.

Coon, H. G. and Sinback, C. N., 1982, pp 1007-1016, in "Growth of Cells in Hormonally Defined Media" Book B, Sirbasku, D.A. et al., eds., Cold Spring Harbor, N.Y.

Davson, H. Welch, K. and Segal, M. B., 1987, "The Physiology and Pathophysiology of the Cerebrospinal Fluid", Churchill Livingstone, Edinburgh.

Delorme, P. Gayet, J. and Grignon, G., 1970, Ultrastructural study on transcapillary exchanges in the developing telencephalon of the chicken, Brain Res., 22: 269-283.

Dencker, L., Danielsson, B, Khayat, A. and Lindgren, A., 1983, Disposition of metals in the embryo and fetus, in: "Reproductive and Developmental Toxicity of Metals", ed. T. W. Clarkson, G. G. Nordberg and P. R. Sager, Plenum Publishing Corporation.

Doolin, P. F. and Birge, W. J., 1969, Ultrastructural differentiation of the junctional complex of the avian choroidal epithelium, J. Comp. Neur., 136: 253-268.

Dziegielewska, K. M., 1982, p54 in Proteins in fetal csf and plasma. PhD thesis, University of London.

Dziegielewska, K. M., Evans, C. A. N., Malinowska, D. H., Møllgård, K., Reynolds, J. M., Reynolds, M. L. and Saunders, N. R., 1979, Studies of the development of brain barrier system to lipid insoluble molecules in fetal sheep, J. Physiol., 292: 207-231.

Dziegielewska, K. M., Evans, C. A. N., Malinowska, D. H., Møllgård, K., Reynolds, M. L. and Saunders, N. R., 1980, Blood-cerebrospinal fluid transfer of plasma proteins during fetal development in the sheep, J. Physiol., 300: 457-465.

Dziegielewska, K. M., Saunders, N. R. and Soreq, H., 1985, Messenger Ribonucleic Acid (mRNA) from developing rat cerebellum directs in vitro synthesis of plasma proteins, Dev. Brain Res., 23: 259-267.

Dziegielewska, K. M., Saunders, N. R., Schejter, E. J., Zakut, H., Zevin-Sonkin, D., Zisling, R. and Soreq, H., 1986, Synthesis of plasma proteins in fetal, adult and neoplastic human brain tissue, Dev. Biol., 115: 93-104.

Dziegielewska, K. M., Hinds, L. A., Møllgård, K., Reynolds, M. L. and Saunders, N. R., 1988, Blood-brain, blood-cerebrospinal fluid and cerebrospinal fluid-brain barriers in a marsupial (Macropus eugenii) during development, J. Physiol., 403: 367-388.

Dziegielewska, K. M. and Saunders, N. R., 1988, The development of the blood-brain barrier: proteins in fetal and neonatal csf, their nature and origins, pp 169-191 in: "Handbook of Human Growth and Developmental Biology" vol. 1, "Neural Sensory, Motor and Integrative Development", Part A: Developmental Neurobiology, E. Meisami and P. S. Timiras, ed., CRC Press, Boca Raton, Florida.

Dziegielewska, K. M., Habgood, M., Jones, S. E., Reader, M. and Saunders, N. R., 1989a, Proteins in cerebrospinal fluid and plasma of postnatal Monodelphis domestica (grey short-tailed opossum), Comp. Biochem. Physiol. 92B, 569-576.

Dziegielewska, K. M., Habgood, M. and Saunders, N. R., 1989b, Species-specific blood-CSF transfer of albumin in anaesthetized immature fetal sheep, J. Physiol., 415: 99P.

Dziegielewska, K. M., Habgood, M. D., Saunders, N. R. and Sedgwick, J. E., 1990, A specific albumin transfer mechanism at the blood-CSF barrier, J. Physiol.

Dziegielewska, K.M., Habgood, M.D., Møllgård, K., Stagaard, M. and Saunders, N.R. (1991). Species specific transfer of plasma albumin from blood into different cerebrospinal fluid compartments in the immature fetal sheep. J. Physiol. 439, 215-237.

Ehrlich, P., 1885, pp 69-72, "Das Sauerstoff Bedurfnis des Organimus. Eine Farbanalytisch Studie", Hirschwald, Berlin.

Ferguson, R. K. and Woodbury, D. M., 1969, Penetration of inulin and sucrose into brain, cerebrospinal fluid and skeletal muscle of developing rats, Exp. Brain Res., 7: 181-194.

Flexner, L. B., 1938, Changes in the chemistry and nature of the cerebrospinal fluid during fetal life in the pig, Am. J. Physiol., 124: 131-135.

Fossan, G., Cavanagh, M. E., Evans, C. A. N., Malinowska, D. H., Mollgard, K., Reynolds, M. L. and Saunders, N. R., 1985, CSF-brain permeability in the immature sheep fetus: a CSF-brain barrier, Dev. Brain Res., 18, 113-124.

Ganong, W. F., 1989, "Review of Medical Physiology" 14th Ed. P. 452 and P. 518, Lange Medical Publications, Los Altos.

Goddard, J., Lewis, R. M., Alcala, H. and Zeller, R. S., 1980, Intraventricular haemorrhage - an animal model, Biol. Neonate., 37: 39-52.

Habgood, M. D., 1989, Blood-CSF barrier permeability in very immature rats, J. Physiol., 417, 31P.

Hurley, L. S., 1981, Teratogenic aspects of manganese, zinc and copper nutrition, Physiol. Rev. 61: 249-295.

Johanson, C. E., 1989, Ontogeny and phylogeny of the blood-brain barrier, pp 157-198 in: "Implications of the Blood-brain Barrier and its Manipulation", Vol. 1, E. A. Neuwelt, ed., Plenum, New York.

Johanson, C. E. and Woodbury, D. M., 1974, Changes in CSF flow and extracellular space in the developing rat, in: "Drugs and the Developing Brains", pp. 281-7, A. Vernadakis and N. Weiner eds., Plenum Press, New York.

Johnson, R. T., 1982, "Viral Infections of the Nervous System", Raven, New York.

Jones, H. C. and Keep, R. F., 1987, The control of potassium concentration in the cerebrospinal fluid and brain interstitial fluid of developing rats, J. Physiol., 383, 441-453.

Jones, H. C. and Keep, R. F., 1988, Brain fluid calcium concentration and response to acute hypercalcaemia during development in the rat, J. Physiol., 402: 579-593.

Lyon, M., Barr, C.E., Cannon, T.D. and Mednick, S.A., 1989, Fetal neural development and schizophrenia, Schiz. Bull., 15: 149-161.

Ment, L. R., Stewart, W. B., Duncan, C. C. and Lambrecht, R., 1982, Beagle puppy model of intraventricular hemorrhage, J. Neurosurg., 57: 219-223.

Milhorat, T. H., 1976, Structure and function of the choroid plexus and other sites of cerebrospinal fluid formation, Int. Rev. Cytol., 47: 225-288.

Mollgard, K. and Saunders, N. R., 1975, Complex tight junctions of epithelial and of endothelial cells in early foetal brain, J. Neurocytol., 4:453-468.

Mollgard, K., Jacobsen, M., Krag Jacobsen, G., Praetorius Clausen, P. and Saunders, N. R., 1979, Immunohistochemical evidence for an intracellular localization of plasma proteins in human foetal choroid plexus and brain, Neurosci. Let., 14: 85-90.

Mollgard, K. and Saunders, N. R., 1977, A possible transepithelial pathway via endoplasmic reticulum in foetal sheep choroid plexus, Proc. Royal Soc. London. B199: 321-326.

Mollgard, K. and Saunders, N. R., 1986, The development of the human bloodbrain and blood-csf barriers, Neuropath. & App. Neurobiol., 12: 337-358.

Mollgard, K., Balslev, Y., Lauritzen, B. and Saunders, N. R., 1987, Cell junctions and membrane specializations in the ventricular zone (germinal matrix) of the developing sheep brain: a CSF-brain barrier, J. Neurocytol., 16: 433-444.

Mollgard, K., Dziegielewska, K. M., Saunders, N. R., Zakut, H. and Soreq, H., 1988, Synthesis and localization of plasma proteins in the developing human brain. Integrity of the fetal blood-brain barrier to endogenous proteins of hepatic origin, Dev. Biol., 128: 207-221.

Pinar, M. H., Edwards, W. H., Fratkin, J., Marin-Padilla, M., 1985, A transmission electron microscopy study of human cerebral cortical and germinal matrix (GM) blood vessels in premature neonates, Ped. Res.., 19: 394.

Reynolds, M. L., Evans, C. A. N., Reynolds, E. O. R., Saunders, N. R., Durbin, G. M. and Wigglesworth, J. S., 1979, Intracranial haemorrhage in the preterm sheep fetus, Early Human Dev., 3: 163-186.

Reynolds, M. L. and Møllgård, K., 1985, The distribution of plasma proteins in the neocortex and early allocortex of the developing sheep brain, Anat. Embryol., 171: 41-60.

Reynolds, M. L., Sarantis, M. E. P., Lorscheider, F. L. and Saunders, N. R., 1987, Fetuin as a marker of cortical plate cells in the fetal cow neocortex: a comparison of the distribution of fetuin, α2HS-glycoprotein, α-fetoprotein and albumin during early development, Anat. Embryol., 185: 355-363.

Risau, W., Hallman, R. and Albrecht, U., 1986, Differentiation-dependent expression of proteins in brain endothelium during development of the blood-brain barrier, Dev. Biol., 117: 537-545.

Sandstead, H. S., 1985, Zinc: essentiality for brain development and function, Nutr. Rev., 43: 129-137.

Saunders, N. R. and Møllgård, K., 1984, Development of the blood-brain barrier, J. Dev. Physiol., 6: 45-57.

Saunders, N.R., 1990, The development of the blood-brain barrier to macromolecules in The Fluids and Barriers of the Eye and Brain. Ed. M.B. Segal MacMillan.

Saunders, N.R., 1991, Ontogenetic development in Physiology and Pharmacology of the Blood Brain-Barrier. Handbook Exper. Pharm. Ed. M.W.B. Bradbury, Springer Verlag. In press.

Smith, H. and Sweet, C., 1988, Lessons for human influenza from pathogenicity studies with ferrets, Rev. Infect. Dis., 10: 56-75.

Smith, W. R., Woodbury, D. M. and Johanson, C. E., 1982, Kinetic analysis of Cl-36, Na-22 and H-3 mannitol uptake into the in vivo choroid plexus-cerebrospinal fluid system: Evidence for active chloride transport by the choroidal epithelium, J. Neurochem., 37: 107-116.

Stern, L., Rapoport, J.-L. and Lokschina, E.-S., 1929, Le fonctionnement de la barriere hemato-encephalique chez les nouveau-nes, Comptes Rendus Soc. Biol. Paris, 100: 231-233.

Sternberger, L. A., 1979, "Immunocytochemistry", 2nd edn, pp 89-92, John Wiley and Sons, New York.

Tauc, M., Vignon, X. and Bouchaud, C., 1984, Evidence for the effectiveness of the blood-csf barrier in the fetal rat choroid plexus. A freeze-fracture and peroxidase diffusion study, Tiss. Cell., 16: 65-74.

Thompson, J. A. and Glasgow, L. A., 1980, Intrauterine viral infection and the cell-mediated immune response, Neurology, 30-212.

Ting, P., Yamaguchi, S., Bacher, J. D., Killens, R. H. and Myers, R. E., 1984, Failure to produce germinal matrix or intraventricular hemorrhage by hypoxia, hypo- or hypervolemia, Exp. Neurol., 83: 449-460.

Tschirgi, R. D., 1950, Protein complexes and the impermeability of the blood-brain barrier to dyes, Am. J. Physiol., 163: 756P.

Van Harreveld, A. and Steiner, J., 1970, The magnitude of the extracellular space in electron micrographs of superficial and deep regions of the cerebral cortex, J. Cell. Sci., 6:793-805.

Volpe, J. J., 1987, "Neurology of the Newborn" 2nd Ed, Saunders, Philadelphia.

Wakai, S. and Hirokawa, N., 1978, Development of the blood-brain barrier to horseradish peroxidase in the chick embryo, Cell Tiss. Res., 195: 195-203.

Wakai, S. and Hirokawa, N., 1981, Development of blood-cerebrospinal fluid barrier to horseradish peroxidase in the avian choroidal epithelium, Cell Tiss. Res., 214: 271-273.

Woodbury, D. M., 1967, Distribution of non electrolytes and electrolytes in the brain as affected by alterations in cerebrospinal fluid secretion, Progr. Brain Res., 29: 297-313.

NEURONAL MIGRATION AND DIFFERENTIATION DURING NORMAL AND GENETICALLY PERTURBED DEVELOPMENT OF THE HIPPOCAMPAL FORMATION

Richard S. Nowakowski

Department of Neuroscience and Cell Biology
University of Medicine and Dentistry of New Jersey
Robert Wood Johnson Medical School
Piscataway, New Jersey

INTRODUCTION

In order to understand the development of the various laminar organizational schemes which exist in the different parts of the adult CNS, it is necessary to understand three distinctly different cellular processes: cell proliferation, cell migration, and cell differentiation. Together these three steps can be considered to comprise "the life history" of a single neuron or glial cell; each cell must pass successively through all three of these steps in order to become a mature component of the CNS. Cell proliferation, cell migration, and cell differentiation occur simultaneously within every division and subdivision of the developing CNS, but for a single cell these steps represent a cascade of developmental events. Cells which pass through the cascade early can influence the fate of those cells which subsequently pass through the cascade. In other words, through intercellular interactions cells present in the same part of the nervous system, in the same or even in different states of maturation, can interact and affect each other's fate. (For reviews see Nowakowski, 1987, 1991a).

It appears that all of the neurons of the primate (including the human) CNS are produced during the developmental period, which probably extends to only about three to six months after birth. [There have, however, been reports of neuron production in the adult canary (Goldman and Nottebohm, 1983; Nottebohm, 1985) and also in the adult rat (Bayer, 1982; Bayer et al., 1982; Kaplan, 1977; Kaplan and Hinds, 1977).] There is essentially no proliferation of neurons in

Developmental Neuropathology of Schizophrenia
Edited by S.A. Mednick *et al.*, Plenum Press, New York, 1991

the adult primate CNS (Nowakowski and Rakic, 1981; Rakic, 1982, 1985, 1988). In the developing CNS cell proliferation occurs, for the most part, in two specialized zones which line the ventricular system (Figure 1). The first of these two zones to appear is the ventricular zone (Boulder Committee, 1970), which is a pseudostratified, columnar epithelium. All parts of the developing CNS have a ventricular zone, and in some parts, the ventricular zone is the only proliferative zone to appear. In other parts of the developing CNS a second proliferative zone appears. This zone, known as the subventricular zone, differs in a number of ways from the ventricular zone. For example, the cells of the ventricular zone and subventricular zone differ from one another in their mode of proliferation (see legend for Figure 1 for details). It has been speculated (see Nowakowski, 1987; Nowakowski and Rakic, 1981) that the subventricular zone is a phylogenetically "newer" feature. For example, all of the neurons of the major subdivisions (areas CA1, CA2, and CA3) of the hippocampus, which is classified as an archicortical or "old" cortical structure, are derived from the ventricular zone (Nowakowski and Rakic, 1981). In contrast, a substantial subventricular zone is present in the developing neocortex, and is believed to contribute large numbers of neurons to that phylogenetically newer cortex, (Nowakowski and Rakic, 1981). A similar developmental scheme seems to exist in the developing diencephalon (Rakic, 1977). These differences in the distribution of the two proliferative zones along the ventricular surface appear early, just as the first neurons are being produced (Nowakowski and Rakic, 1981); this indicates that the ventricular surface of the developing nervous system is a mosaic (Rakic, 1988) and that the development of major subdivisions of the CNS follows distinctly different patterns even at early stages.

While cell proliferation occurs in areas adjacent to the ventricular surface, in many portions of the adult nervous system neurons are located at quite a distance from the ventricular surface. Therefore, a mechanism for the movement of cells from their site of proliferation to their ultimate position is necessary. There are two basic but very different ways that neurons make this movement. The first does not seem to require active locomotory movement by the post-mitotic neuron. In this case a post-mitotic neuron leaves the proliferative population (influenced to do so by some unknown signal or signals) and is displaced only a very short distance from the border of the proliferative zone. Shortly thereafter, as the next post-mitotic neurons are similarly displaced outwardly from the proliferative zone, the original cells are displaced slightly further. This type of cell movement is generally considered to be passive cell displacement (Figure 2). In those parts of the CNS in which passive cell displacement occurs, neurons that leave the proliferative population the earliest are, in general, those that ultimately are located farthest from the proliferative zone. The subsequently generated neurons are found at levels progressively closer to the proliferative zone (Figure 2). Thus, there is a correlation between the final position of a neuron and its time of origin. For areas in which there is passive cell displacement, this correlation is referred to as an "outside-to-inside" spatiotemporal gradient. Outside and inside are both defined with respect to the position of

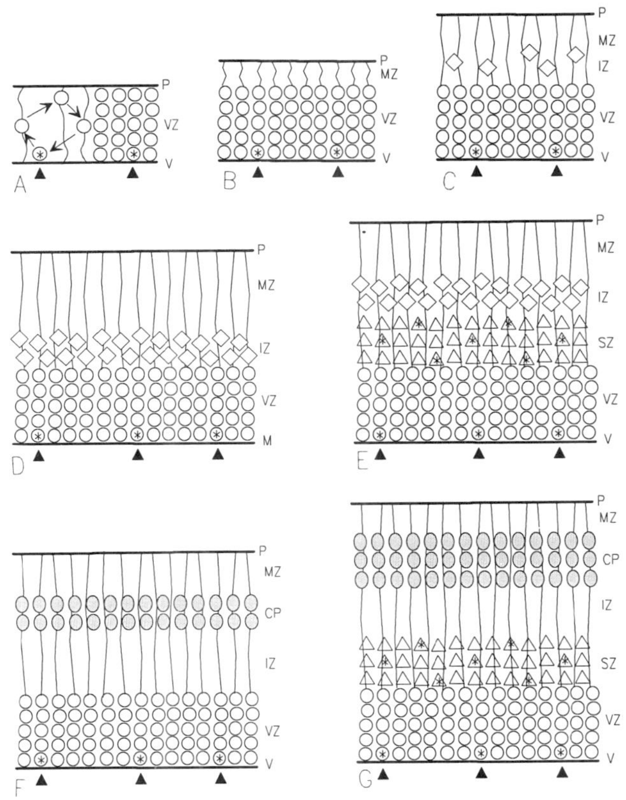

Figure 1. A, B and C illustrate the early stages of the differentiation of the neural tube. All parts of the early developing CNS have a ventricular zone (VZ) and eventually develop a marginal zone (MZ) just subjacent to the pial surface (P). In the ventricular zone the nuclei of the cells are stratified, but each cell has contact that reach both the ventricular (V) and pial surface (P) of the neural tube. The left side of drawing A illustrates the movement of a single cell as it passes through the various phases of the cell cycle; DNA synthesis occurs in the outer half of the ventricular zone and mitosis (i.e., cell division) occurs adjacent to the ventricular surface. This movement of the cell's nucleus is known as interkinetic nuclear migration. The next zone to appear (B) is the marginal zone, which is an almost cell-free zone just subjacent to the pial surface. Shortly after the formation of the marginal zone, an intermediate zone (IZ) forms; this zone contains the first post-mitotic cells of the nervous system. The IZ is located between the VZ and MZ. D, E, F and G illustrate various alternatives for the subsequent radial development of the CNS. D: In some parts of the neural tube the only proliferative zone present is the ventricular zone. The post-mitotic cells derived from the VZ aggregate and mature in the IZ, just adjacent to the VZ. One portion of the nervous system which has this pattern of radial differentiation is the spinal cord. E: In other portions of the nervous system, post-mitotic cells also aggregate in the IZ and differentiate there, but some of these cells are derived from the subventricular zone (SZ). The dorsal thalamus ia an example of a portion of the nervous system which follows this pattern of development. F and G: Examples of cortical regions. In the hippocampus (F) all of the post-mitotic cells are derived from the VZ. They migrate across the sparsely populated IZ and form a cortical plate (CP). In the neocortex (G) both a VZ and an SZ are present. Again the derivatives of these two proliferative zones migrate across the IZ and form a cortical plate. Abbreviations: V, ventricular surface; VZ, ventricular zone; SZ, subventricular zone; IZ, intermediate zone; CP, cortical plate; MZ, marginal zone; P, pial surface.

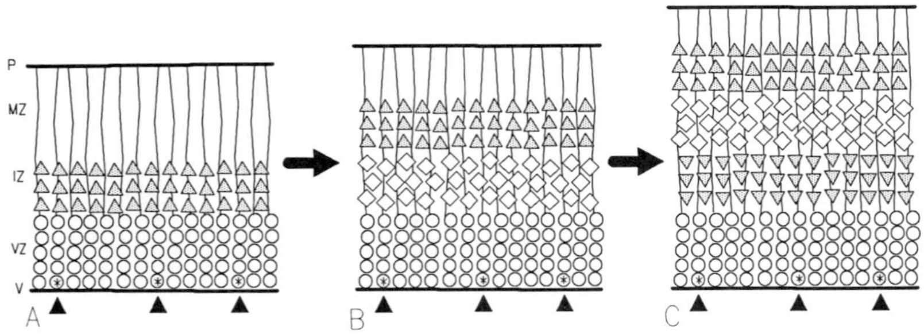

Figure 2. In some areas of the developing nervous system cell movement is by passive displacement. Some cells leave the proliferative zone and take up a position only a short distance from the proliferative zone. Later, as other cells are produced by the proliferative zone, the earlier produced cells are displaced outwardly. Diagrams A through C illustrate the progressive passive displacement of previously generated neurons away from the ventricular surface by subsequently later generated neurons. A: The earliest generated neurons which leave the ventricular zone are shown as triangles. B: The next group of neurons to be generated are represented by diamonds. Their movement out of the ventricular zone displaces the earlier generated neurons toward the pial surface. C: The last neurons generated, represented by inverted triangles, displace both of the earlier generated populations of neurons. This sequence of events produces a specific distribution of neurons known as an outside-to-inside aptiotemporal gradient. Abbreviations: V, ventricular surface; VZ, ventricular zone; IZ, intermediate zone; MZ, marginal zone; P, pial surface.

the cells relative to the proliferative zone; for the most part, outside refers to the pial surface, and inside refers to the ventricular surface. Areas of the nervous system in which the outside-to-inside spatiotemporal gradient is manifest include the thalamus (Altman and Bayer, 1979; Angevine, 1970; Rakic, 1977), the hypothalamus (Ifft, 1972), spinal cord (Nornes and Das, 1974), many regions of the brainstem (Altman and Bayer, 1981; Taber-Pierce, 1972), the retina (Sidman, 1961; Walsh et al., 1983), and the dentate gyrus of the hippocampal formation (Angevine, 1965; Bayer, 1982; Bayer, et al., 1982; Nowakowski and Rakic, 1981; Wyss and Sripanidkulchai, 1985).

The second way that young neurons move from the proliferative zone to their ultimate positions requires the active participation of the post-mitotic neurons in producing their own displacement. In this case, neurons leave the proliferative zone and move a great distance through the intermediate zone with progressively later generated neurons in many instances bypassing neurons produced earlier (Figure 3). This active process of cell movement is generally referred to as neuronal migration (for review see Sidman and Rakic, 1973) and takes place in the cerebral cortex (both archicortex and neocortex). In those parts of the developing CNS in which the migrating young neurons actively contribute to their own

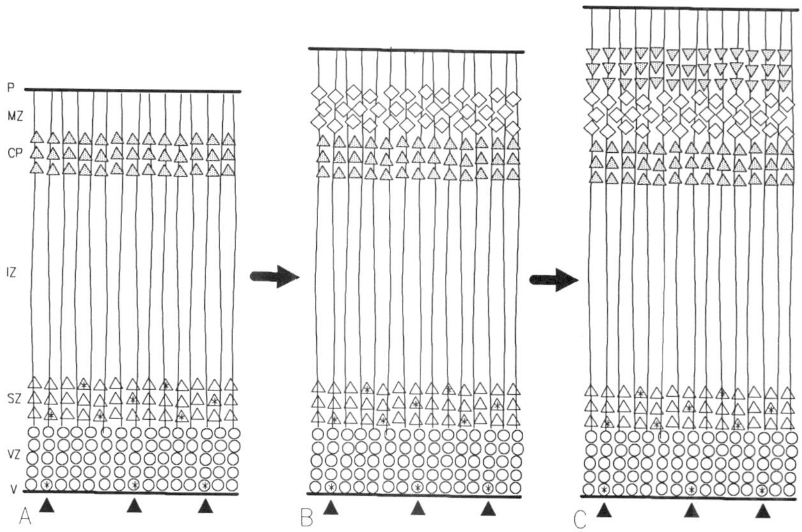

Figure 3. The sequence of events associated with active neuronal migration. In some parts of the developing CNS, neurons leaving the proliferative zone move a great distance before taking up their final position. The sequence of events involved in this process is illustrated in A, B and C. A: The first neurons to leave the proliferative zone (triangles) assemble in a formation known as a cortical plate, which is situated between the intermediate and marginal zones. B: The next group of neurons to be generated (diamonds) leaves the proliferative population and moves across the intermediate zone and past the earlier generated cells to take up a position on the top of the cortical plate. C: The last generated neurons (inverted triangles) migrate across the intermediate zone and past both groups of earlier generated cells to take up residence at the top of the cortical plate. This type of distribution of neurons is known as an inside-to-outside spatiotemporal gradient. Abbreviations: V, ventricular surface; VZ, ventricular zone; IZ, intermediate zone; CP, cortical plate; MZ, marginal zone; P, pial surface.

displacement away from the proliferative zones the result is an "inside-to-outside" spatiotemporal gradient. In this pattern the earliest generated cells remain closest to the proliferative zone and comprise the deepest layers, while the latest generated cells move farthest from the proliferative zone and occupy the most superficial layers. Inside-to-outside spatiotemporal gradients are found in most portions of the cerebral cortex (Angevine, 1965; Angevine and Sidman, 1961; Caviness, 1982; Caviness and Sidman, 1973b; Hinds, 1968; Miller, 1985, 1987; Rakic, 1975b; Rakic and Nowakowski, 1981; Wyss and Sripanidkulchai, 1985) and in several subcortical areas (Cooper and Rakic, 1981; Hickey and Hitchcock, 1968). Areas in which spatiotemporal gradients of the inside-to-outside type occur are, in general, well-laminated structures in that they have tangentially oriented layers that run parallel with the surface of the proliferative zones. During their migration many neurons are guided to their final position by radial glial fibers (Rakic, 1971, 1972), which provide the scaffolding for the future adult neocortex and for other cortical and non-cortical structures as well (Nowakowski and Rakic, 1979; Rakic, 1971, 1978,

1982; Rakic et al., 1974; Eckenhoff and Rakic, 1984). It has also been speculated that radial glial fibers provide the scaffolding for the columnar organization of the adult cortex (Eckenhoff and Rakic, 1984; Mountcastle, 1978; Rakic, 1978, 1982, 1988; Smart and McSherry, 1982). The process of neuronal migration (Figure 4) is a complicated one and consists of at least three phases (for review see Nowakowski, 1985, 1987, 1991a,b). The three phases are: initiation of migration, a locomotory phase, and a termination phase. In the initiation phase a young neuron starts its migration by leaving the proliferative population; during this phase a cell in the proliferating population makes the transition from neuroblast (i.e., a proliferating cell) to young neuron (i.e., a non-proliferating, permanently post-mitotic cell). The young neuron becomes apposed to a radial glial fiber and establishes an axis of polarity away from the ventricular surface. Once aligned with the radial glial fiber the second, or locomotory, phase of migration begins. During this phase a young neuron moves actively along the surface of a radial glial cell, retaining its apposition to the radial glial fiber and its axis of polarity directed away from the proliferative zone. In the cerebral cortex the locomotory phase can be very long, and a migrating neuron can move along a radial glial fiber which may be tens of millimeters long. Once it reaches the vicinity of its final position, a migrating young neuron must stop its migration and become detached from the radial glial fiber. At this point the young neuron can continue its differentiation process by growing dendrites and sending out axons that eventually make contacts with other neurons.

The final phase in the life history of a neuron is its differentiation. This is an extraordinarily complex process which is responsible for a large proportion of the diversity, in all its many aspects, of the adult CNS. During the differentiation of a neuron, axonal and dendritic processes are elaborated, and neurotransmitter phenotypes are expressed. In many cases, the axon grows a long distance over a complicated terrain until it reaches its final target. The dendrites grow out and form a characteristic arborization pattern for each particular cell class. The specific neurotransmitter enzymes which are characteristic of that cell class are also produced; in addition to elaborating the specific enzymes to produce neurotransmitters, neurons must also produce at each post-synaptic site the specific receptors it needs to receive input from its various pre-synaptic partners. Also, some neurons will elaborate a signal which causes their axon to become myelinated; others will not. As neurons acquire their mature properties, glial cells also differentiate into various forms; some become oligodendrocytes that produce myelin, others become astrocytes that perform other functions (Temple and Raff, 1986; ffrench-Constant and Raff, 1986). In humans, it is known that the myelination of most pathways in the CNS continues long after birth (for review see Richardson, 1982). In fact, Flechsig (1920) in his classical work on myelination in the developing human cerebral cortex, established the basis of the traditional classification of neocortical areas into primary, secondary and association cortices. The complexity of the process of cell differentiation in the CNS, as outlined briefly above, is beyond the

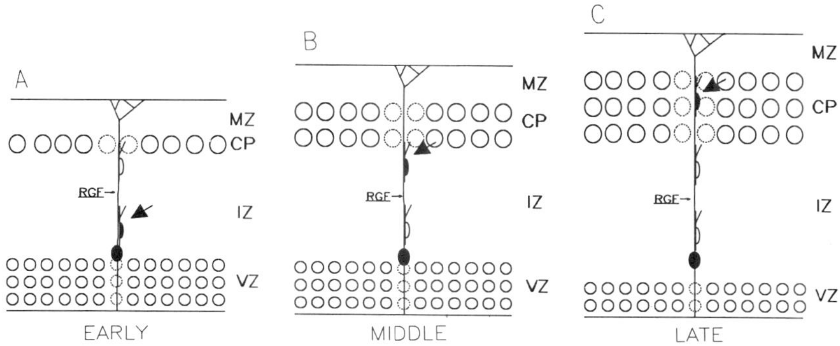

Figure 4. A schematic illustration of the "stages" of migration and of the interaction between migrating neurons and radial glial fibers. After leaving the proliferative zone, the young neuron is guided by a radially aligned glial cell as it moves toward its final position in the cortical plate. The progression of one such young neuron from the proliferative zone through the intermediate zone to the cortical plate is illustrated by a single black cell marked by an arrow in each of the three drawings A, B and C. The migratory process can be divided into three stages. First (A), as a young neuron leaves the proliferative population it becomes apposed to a radial glial fiber and acquires a polarity directed toward the pial surface. Next (B), it enters the locomotory phase and traverses the intermediate zone (IZ) maintaining its apposition to the radial glial fiber and its polarity as it moves through the zone. Later (C), when it reaches the top of the cortical plate (C), it loses its apposition to the radial glial fiber and reorganizes its polarity in order to differentiate into a mature neuron. disruption of any of the three steps of the migratory process can result in ectopic neurons. Abbreviations: VZ, ventricular zone; IZ, intermediate zone; CP, cortical plate,; MZ, marginal zone.

scope of this review; therefore, the discussion in this chapter will be confined to the limited aspect of dendritic growth.

If any of the three phases which comprise the process of neuronal migration is disrupted, an *abnormality in cell position results.* Neurons which fail to reach their appropriate position are said to be ectopic (or heterotopic) (Rakic, 1975a). Neuropathologists have described a variety of defects in cell position. In humans, the best studied examples of defects in neuronal positioning are in the cerebral cortex, where abnormalities in neuronal migration have been associated with a variety of diseases and syndromes ranging from extremely severe mental retardation and failure to thrive to "rather minor" behavioral disorders. Some of the behavioral disorders which have been associated with the disruption of the migratory process include schizophrenia (Kovelman and Scheibel 1984, 1986), dyslexia (Galaburda et al., 1983), fetal alcohol syndrome, methylmercury poisoning, hydrocephalus, methanol exposure, mental retardation, seizures, lissencephaly, and craniofacial anomalies (Miller, 1986, 1987; Choi et al., 1978; Choi and Kudo, 1981; Otake and Schull, 1984; Evrard et al., 1978; Mikhael and Mattar, 1978; Richman et al., 1975; Zimmerman et al., 1983). The presumption is that in these disorders normal functional competence is not achieved at least in part because the abnormally positioned neurons produced from the disruption of neuronal migration do not make normal connections. However, from human pathological data it is difficult to learn the developmental fate of neurons that fail to migrate to their proper positions. It is not known, for example, if these abnormally positioned neurons make connections with the rest of the brain; nor is it known whether any connections they do make are with their normal targets or with some other targets. Most importantly, it is not known how these abnormalities in connectivity (if they exist) might affect the function of the area of the brain in which these cells were normally destined to reside. Thus, the exact relationship between the severity of the functional compromise and abnormal neuronal position is not clear at this time. Testing hypotheses about this relationship is obviously not possible in humans; however, the use of single gene mutations in the mouse which affect the development of the CNS provides a unique insight into these issues (Caviness and Rakic, 1978; Nowakowski, 1985, 1988, 1991; Nowakowski and Wahlsten, 1985a, 1985b; Pearlman, 1985). Numerous mutations are being analyzed to answer a variety of developmental questions. This review will concentrate on understanding how the abnormally positioned cells which result from disruptions of neuronal migration make and receive connections with their normally positioned targets in other parts of the brain.

WHAT IS AN INBRED STRAIN?

Inbred strains of mice were first produced in the early part of the twentieth century as a way to study the genetic basis for cancer and for the variety of coat colors that exist in wild-type mice (Staats, 1966). The typical method used to create an inbred strain is illustrated in Figure 5. Essentially this involves choosing two parent mice from a wild population and then brother-sister mating their progeny for twenty consecutive generations. With each successive generation two things happen: 1) the amount of genetic diversity among the offspring is reduced, and 2) various genes which exist in heterozygous forms in the wild-type mouse are forced to homozygosity in the inbred offspring. After twenty generations of brother-sister mating, two siblings are alike at 98% of their genetic loci, and each inbred mouse has 99.9% of its genes forced to homozygosity (E. Green, 1981). During the process of inbreeding, however, the genes which are forced to homozygosity differ in each of the inbred strains that are made (Figure 5). Thus, each inbred strain has a different subset of alleles at each of the various genetic loci, but within each inbred strain the siblings are essentially genetically identical. Since the turn of the century, several hundred inbred strains have been made (M. Green, 1981), and each strain can be considered to carry a sample of the genes that are present in a normal wild population of mice. The more common inbred strains (e.g., C57BL/6J and BALB/cJ) have been inbred for well over 100 generations.

For most available mouse neurological mutants, the gene action in the

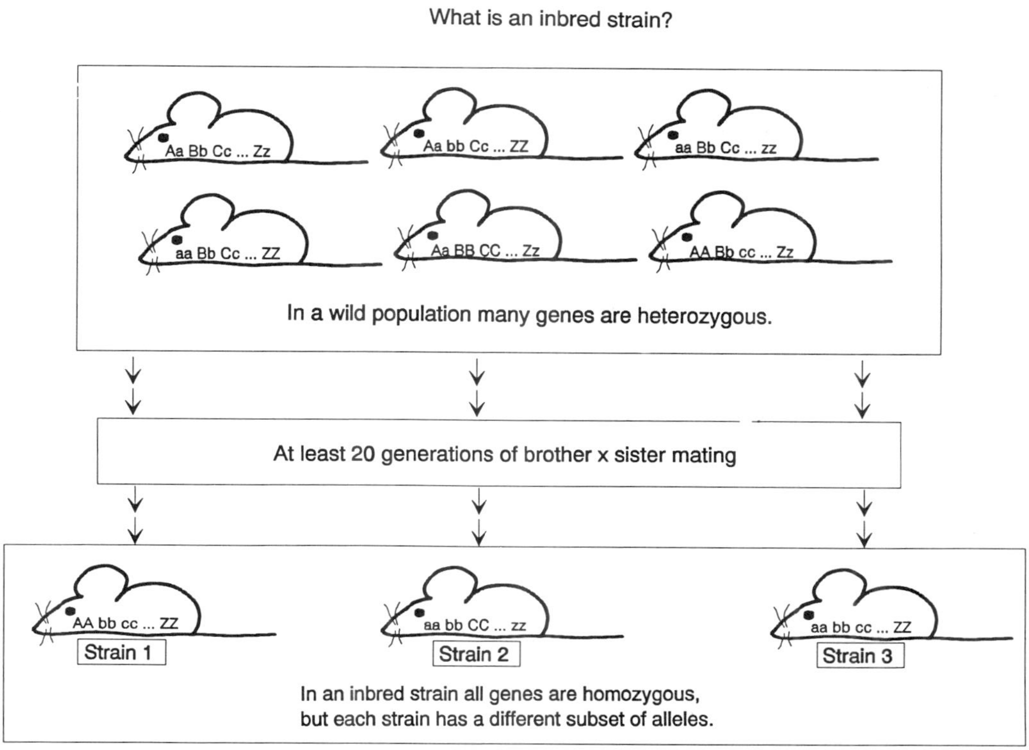

Figure 5. General strategy for producing an inbred strain of mice. For further details, see text.

developing CNS produces an adult brain which is functionally compromised. In fact, most neurological mutations in the mouse produce overt changes in the behavior of the animal, mostly involving locomotory behavior. The reason for this is quite simply that these obvious behavioral changes are most easily detected and/or screened for in large mouse colonies. For example, there are many mouse mutants known that affect the development of the cerebellar cortex (e.g., Caviness and Rakic, 1978; Herrup, 1983; Mullen and Herrup, 1979). In fact, the availability of this variety of mutations is one of the major reasons that so much is known about cerebellar development. Similarly large collections of available mouse mutants are known that affect the development of the vestibular system and other areas and which produce problems in locomotion (M. Green, 1981). Unfortunately, a comparably extensive assortment of mutations that affect the development of the cerebral cortex has not been available. Indeed, until recently only the reeler mutation (gene symbol: *rl*) was known to affect the development of the cerebral cortex (Caviness and Sidman, 1973a, 1973b; Caviness and Rakic, 1978; Pearlman,

1985). In the case of reeler, the mutation is an autosomal recessive gene that affects neuronal migration in many parts of the CNS (Caviness, 1973, 1982, 1986; Stanfield and Cowan, 1979a,b; Stanfield et al., 1979). The main reason that there are so few mutations known to affect the development of the cerebral cortex is the fact that apparently such mutations generally produce only covert behavioral changes, i.e., changes that are not easily detectable upon routine observation of the animal. Reeler is a notable exception in that *rl/rl* mice display obvious motor deficits. Recently, however, several new, genetically based disturbances of cerebral cortical development have been described (Nowakowski, 1988, 1991b). These new mutations have been discovered by comparing the anatomy of the hippocampus in inbred strains of mice. These comparisons provide a standard against which to judge what is normal and what is abnormal, and have resulted in the identification of new mutations which affect cell proliferation and cell migration.

Because the animals of an inbred strain provide an opportunity to make a large number of observations on essentially genetically identical individuals, the "normal" anatomy, development, physiology, etc. of any particular structure can be defined as that exhibited by virtually all animals of a particular inbred strain. In the case of the anatomy and development of the hippocampal formation, normal has been defined arbitrarily as the hippocampal formation of a mouse of the C57BL/6J inbred strain. There is, of course, no *a priori* reason for contending that the brains of C57BL/6J mice are "more normal" than those of any other inbred strain. However, the Jackson Laboratory (Bar Harbor, Me.) maintains many mutants on this strain, which is one of the most widely-available of the inbred strains. Also, an excellent atlas of the CNS of the C57BL/6J mouse is available (Sidman et al., 1971). C57BL/6J is, therefore, a convenient standard, and as such has become, *de facto*, the normal mouse for neurological analysis.

THE DEVELOPMENT OF THE HIPPOCAMPAL FORMATION

The major subdivisions of the hippocampal formation are the dentate gyrus, the hippocampus, and the subiculum (Lorente de No, 1934; Angevine, 1965). The main cellular layer of the dentate gyrus is the horseshoe-shaped granule cell layer. External to the granule cell layer is the molecular layer, and internal to it is the hilus (or area CA4). The hippocampus is subdivided into areas CA1, CA2 and CA3. From ventricle to pia the laminae of the hippocampus are: the alveus, the stratum oriens, the pyramidal cell layer, the stratum radiatum, and the stratum lacunosum-moleculare. In area CA3 there is an additional lamina, the stratum lucidum, which is situated between the pyramidal cell layer and the stratum radiatum and which contains the mossy fibers arising from the granule cells of the dentate gyrus. This highly laminated organization of the hippocampal formation of the normal mouse makes it an ideal location in which to assess the affects of mutant genes on the process of cell migration during the development of the CNS.

The normal development of the hippocampal formation has been studied extensively in a variety of species (Cowan et al., 1980; Rickmann et al., 1987; Nowakowski and Rakic, 1981; Nowakowski, 1988; Bayer, 1980a,b). As in all other regions of the central nervous system, the developmental process entails the three basic cellular mechanisms described above: 1) cell proliferation, 2) cell migration, and 3) cell differentiation. Except for the granule cells of the dentate gyrus, the neurons of the hippocampal formation are generated during characteristic prenatal intervals in

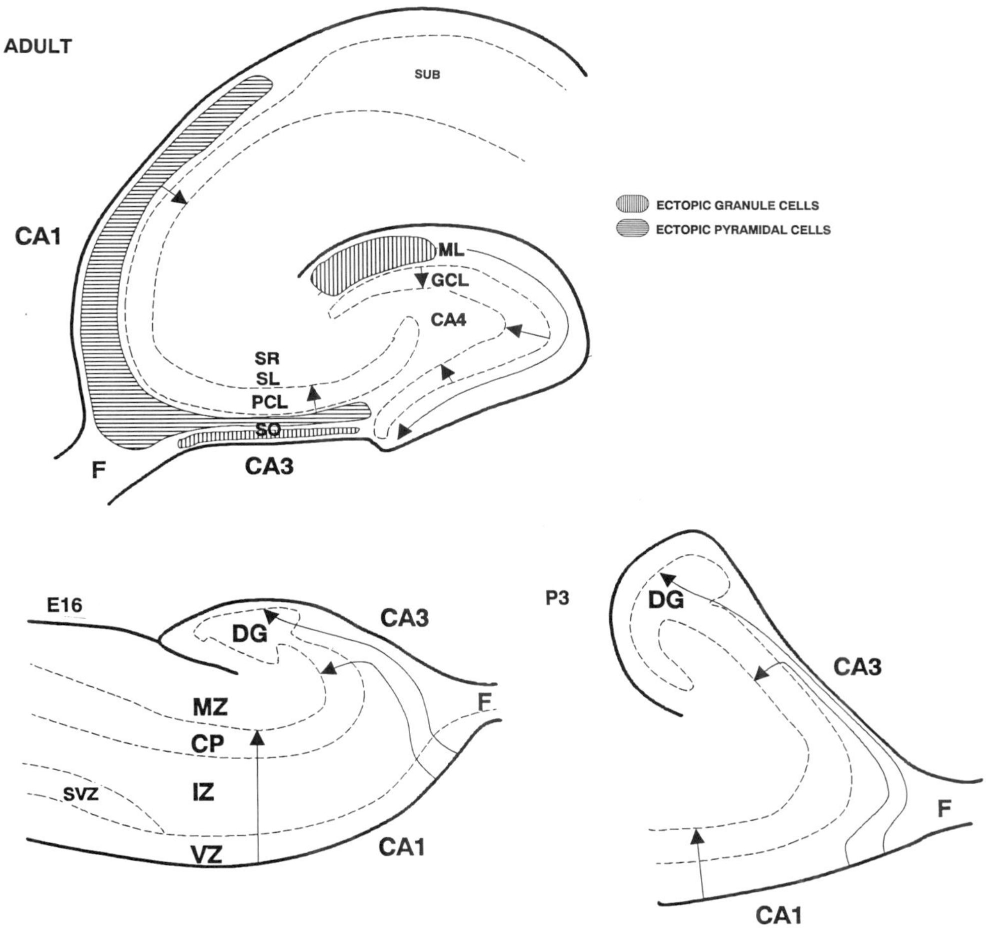

Figure 6. Schematic diagrams indicating the spatiotemporal gradients and migratory pathways of neurons comprising the mouse hippocampal formation. In the drawing at the top the arrows indicate in the adult the direction of the spatiotemporal gradient of neuron origin; the tip of the arrowhead indicates the position of the last-born neurons, while the tail of the arrow indicates the position of the first-born neurons. Shaded areas indicate the cytoarchitectonic positions in which ectopic neurons are found in a variety of mouse mutants. (For details, see text.) In the bottom two drawings, arrows illustrate the migratory pathways from the ventricular zone (VZ) to areas CA1, CA3, and the dentate gyrus (DG) followed by young neurons on E16 and P3 (Nowakowski, 1988). Abbreviations: F, fimbria; GCL, granule cell layer; ML, molecular layer; PCL, pyramidal cell layer; SL, stratum lucidum, SO, stratum oriens; SR, stratum radiatum; SUB subiculum; SVZ, subventricular zone.

the mouse (Angevine, 1965; Nowakowski, 1985; see Figure 3, top) as well as in other species (Rakic and Nowakowski, 1981; Bayer, 1980a,b; Schlessinger et al., 1975; Wyss and Sripanidkulchai, 1985). Most of the dentate gyrus granule cells are generated postnatally during the first 30 days after birth (Angevine, 1965), although there is evidence in the rat that this period may be considerably longer (Kaplan and Hinds, 1977; Bayer et al., 1982). All of the neurons of the hippocampal formation are generated in one of two proliferative zones described above. Most of the neurons, including all of the hippocampal pyramidal cells, are generated in the ventricular zone lining the lateral ventricle (Nowakowski and Rakic, 1981; Rakic and Nowakowski, 1981). In contrast, while some of the granule cells of the dentate gyrus are generated in the ventricular zone, most are generated in an intrahilar proliferative zone (Nowakowski and Rakic, 1981; Eckenhoff and Rakic, 1984). It is important to note, however, that the proliferating cells that comprise the intrahilar proliferative zone are themselves derived from the ventricular zone (Nowakowski and Rakic, 1981).

In order to reach either the intrahilar proliferative zone or their final adult positions, the neuroblasts and young neurons produced in the ventricular zone migrate along radial glial fibers across a complicated terrain (Nowakowski and Rakic, 1979; Rickmann et al., 1987). The migratory pathways followed by neurons destined to reside in the subiculum and areas CA1 and CA2 are fairly direct (Nowakowski, 1985). The migratory path followed by neurons that are destined to reside in area CA3, however, not only is tortuous but lengthens even as the young neurons move along it to their ultimate destination (Figure 6, bottom; see Nowakowski, 1985; Rickmann et al., 1987). The young neurons destined for the dentate gyrus and the neuroblasts destined for the intrahilar proliferative zone pursue a migratory path which is adjacent to the pathway followed by the CA3-bound neurons but situated closer to the pial surface of the transverse fissure. Thus, while the cells destined for area CA3 and the dentate gyrus migrate along radially-oriented glial fibers, their movement is along a path which is initially perpendicular to the ventricular surface but which later becomes largely parallel to a pial surface because of the distortions produced by the growing hippocampus and dentate gyrus (Figure 6).

HIPPOCAMPAL MUTANTS

The development of the hippocampal formation is known to be affected by seven mutations and one genetic variant (See Table 1), all of which share the phenotypic characteristic of neuronal ectopia. The presence of ectopic neurons indicates that the process of neuronal migration is disrupted either directly or indirectly by each of these mutations.

The Hippocampal Lamination Defect Mutation

Of the mutations known to affect neuronal migration, the Hippocampal lamination defect mutation (gene symbol: *Hld*) produces the most localized effect on the development of the hippocampal formation. This autosomal dominant mutation (Nowakowski, 1984) is characterized by an inversion of the laminar organization of the pyramidal cell layer of area CA3c. This inversion is the result of a disruption of migration of only those late-generated pyramidal cells destined for area CA3c (Figure 7); the late-generated pyramidal cells destined for area CA1, as well as all of the early-generated cells, are normally positioned (Barber et al., 1974; Vaughn et al., 1977). The late-generated pyramidal cells are generated on embryonic days 15 and 16 in the proliferative zone lining the lateral ventricle in both the normal (i.e. +/+ or wild-type) and *Hld/Hld* mouse (Figure 6). The young neurons destined for area CA3c leave the ventricular zone and migrate across a broad intermediate zone until they reach the border with the developing cortical plate after approximately seven days (Nowakowski, 1985). In the +/+ mouse they continue to migrate past the previously generated pyramidal cells to take up their final position at the top of the cortical plate; in the *Hld/Hld* mouse, however, they stop migrating, do not bypass the previously generated cells, and remain in a position below the early-generated pyramidal cells. As a result of these developmental events, there are ectopic pyramidal cells below the lower of the two mossy fiber bundles in area CA3c (Figure 7), and there are modifications in the dendritic morphology and connections of the ectopic neurons (Nowakowski and Davis, 1985).

The Dreher Mutant Mouse

A markedly different reorganization of hippocampal anatomy is seen in the dreher mutation (gene symbol: *dr*). This autosomal recessive gene produces considerable variation in phenotype even among genetically identical mice in both homozygotes (Wahlsten et al., 1983) and heterozygotes (Patrylo et al., 1990). In *dr/dr* mice both cell proliferation and neuronal migration of both the granule cells of the dentate gyrus and the pyramidal cells of the hippocampus are affected. In the dentate gyrus, large portions of the granule cell layer are often missing, and there are often small clusters of granule cells abnormally positioned in the molecular layer. Most frequently the infrapyramidal limb of the dentate gyrus is absent; when this happens it is apparent in Timm's-stained preparations that the infrapyramidal mossy fiber layer also is absent (Nowakowski and Wahlsten, 1985 a,b), and even the dendrites of normally-positioned granule cells are irregularly oriented (Figure 8). In area CA3 there are sometimes too few neurons and sometimes too many. When there are too many pyramidal cells, there are often pyramidal neurons and sometimes even granule cells abnormally positioned in the stratum oriens. These abnormally positioned cells seem to be distributed along their normal migratory pathways. Timm's-stained preparations indicate that the

Table 1. Eight murine migration mutants are known to affect neuronal migration in the developing hippocampal formation.

Gene Symbol	Gene Name	Chromosome	Genetic Background
$dr^{\underline{sst\text{-}J}}$	dreher	1	C3B6/J(N17)
Hld	Hippocampal lamination defect	--	BALB/cByJ
$rl^{\underline{ORL}}$	reeler	5	Noninbred
--	--	--	NZB/BlNJ
bal	balding	--	C57BL/6J
$Lps^{\underline{d}}$	Lipopolysaccharide response defect	4	C3H/HeJ
$me^{\underline{v}}$	viable motheaten	6	C57BL/6J
bg	beige	13	C57BL/6J

abnormally positioned granule cells send a small bundle of mossy fibers to terminate on the abnormally positioned pyramidal cells. (Nowakowski and Wahlsten, 1985 a,b). Curiously, they do not seem to send any input to the basal dendrites of normally positioned CA3c pyramidal neurons, even though this otherwise normal target is closer. Experiments using tritiated thymidine autoradiography to elucidate the nature of the developmental abnormality in dreher have demonstrated that 1) the abnormally positioned pyramidal cells in the stratum oriens are late-generated and 2) within the pyramidal cell layer of area CA3 the late-generated pyramidal neurons fail to bypass the early-generated ones (Nowakowski, unpublished observations).

Many of the CA3c pyramidal cells whose somata are situated in the pyramidal cell layer have dendritic trees which look entirely normal (Figure 8). Such pyramidal cells have essentially normal looking apical dendrites and robust basal dendrites with dendritic excrescences similar in quantity and size to those seen in littermate controls and other normal mice. In particular, the location of the dendritic excrescences on both the basal and apical dendrites corresponds to the position of the two mossy fiber bundles (arrowheads in Figure 8). Some of the CA3c pyramidal cells, however, do not have normal dendritic trees (Figure 8), even though their somata are located in the pyramidal cell layer. The most frequently observed abnormality is the occurrence of fine-caliber dendritic branches extending out of the apical dendrite (Figure 8) or the apical portion of the soma (Figure 8) and laterally through the pyramidal cell layer or at an upwardly directed angle towards the stratum radiatum. The ectopic pyramidal cells in the stratum oriens usually

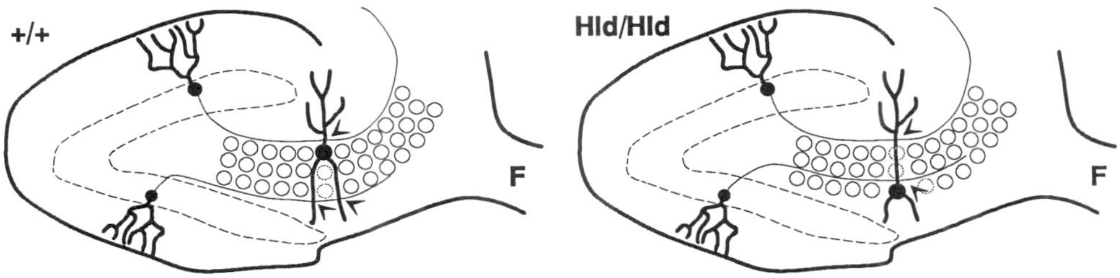

Figure 7. Schematic diagram indicating the position and mossy fiber input of late-generated pyramidal cells in area CA3c of wildtype (+/+) and Hld/Hld mutant mice. In +/+ mice (left), late-generated pyramidal cells occupy the top of the pyramidal cell layer and receive mossy fiber input at tow positions (arrowheads): on their apical dendrites, where they pass through the suprapyramidal mossy fiber layer, and on their basal dendrites, where they pass through the infrapyramidal mossy fiber layer. In Hld/Hld mice (right), late-generated pyramidal cells fail to migrate past earlier generated ones and occupy the bottom of the pyramidal cell layer in area CA3c. These ectopic pyramidal cells receive mossy fiber input at two positions on their apical dendrites (arrowheads), once where they pass through the suprapyramidal mossy fiber layer and once where they pass through the infrapyramidal mossy fiber layer (Nowakowski and Davis, 1985; Nowakowski, 1988).

have a single, thick, long apical dendrite. Overall, the pattern of their dendritic arbor is quite similar to that of normally positioned pyramidal cells (Figure 8). Some of the cells have fine-caliber secondary branches coming off of the apical dendrite within the pyramidal cell layer (Figure 8), but others send their apical dendrites through the pyramidal cell layer without emitting such branches. Most of the dendritic arbors of ectopic pyramidal cells in the stratum radiatum are characterized by an inverted shape (Figure 8). They usually have one main dendrite which extends toward the pyramidal cell layer and which bifurcates in the vicinity of the stratum lucidum (Figure 8). One of the branches usually extends through the pyramidal cell layer to the stratum oriens where it ends without ramifying (Figure 8).

The NZB/BlNJ Inbred Strain

Recently polymorphisms indicating the existence of a mutation affecting the development of the hippocampal formation been discovered in the NZB/BlNJ inbred strain (Nowakowski, 1986, 1988). In the hippocampal formation of NZB/-BlNJ mice there are abnormalities in cell position in both the dentate gyrus and the hippocampus. Clusters of abnormally positioned granule cells are found in the molecular layer of the dentate gyrus. These clusters of granule cells seem to be regularly-spaced along the surface of the suprapyramidal limb of the dentate gyrus, although they are sometimes located along the surface of the infrapyramidal limb. In area CA3 there are small clusters of pyramidal cells abnormally positioned in the stratum lucidum and stratum radiatum. In both the dentate gyrus and hippocampus the abnormalities in cell position occur most frequently in the ventral half of the hippocampal formation.

The existence of these abnormalities in cell position in the NZB/BlNJ inbred strain is interesting for two reasons. First, the abnormally positioned pyramidal and granule cells in NZB/BlNJ have migrated too far. This is in marked contrast to the cell position defects found in the hippocampal formation of the *Hld* and reeler mice, in which the abnormally positioned cells have not migrated far enough. Second, this abnormality in cell position in the hippocampal formation is similar to that of the neocortex of NZB/BlNJ mice, in which Sherman and co-workers (1985) have described islands of ectopic neurons in layer I of the neocortex in about 30% of NZB/BlNJ mice. Furthermore, it has been noted that there are similar ectopic clusters of neurons in the neocortex of human dyslexics, and it has been suggested that both the murine and human abnormalities may be related to autoimmune disorders (Sherman et al., 1985).

We have examined the dendritic trees of the ectopic neurons in the molecular layer of the dentate gyrus of NZB/BlNJ mice and have found that they are characterized by five distinct morphological abnormalities: 1) the initial orientation of the primary dendrites can be either apical or basal; 2) the basally directed dendrites do not reach the granule cell layer but usually curve towards the pial surface; 3) many of the dendrites end before reaching the pial surface; 4) the soma may have spines; and 5) the axon can exit from the cell body at any point or from a basal dendrite and extend up into the molecular layer. Each of the ectopic granule cells displays one or more of these abnormalities but not necessarily all of them,

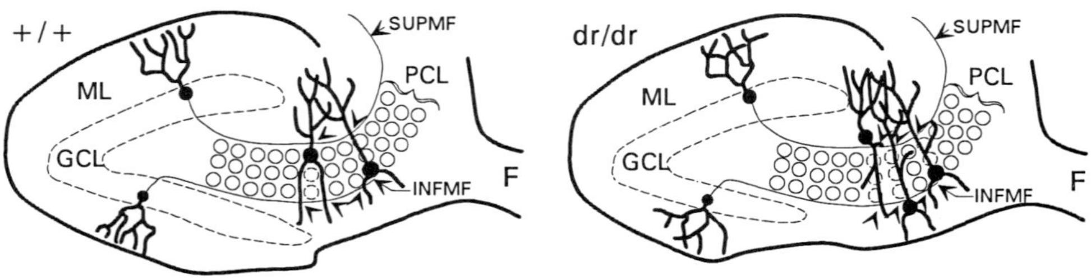

Figure 8. Schematic diagram of normally positioned and ectopic neurons in wild-type (+/+) and dreher (dr/dr) mice. In both normal and dreher mice, the ectopic pyramidal cells receive input from the mossy fibers wherever they pass through either one of the two mossy fiber bundles (arrowheads). Also, note the irregular orientation of the dendrites in the granule cells of the dentate gyrus of the dreher mouse. For details, see the text. Abbreviations: F, fimbria; GCL, granule cell layer; INFMF, infrapyramidal mossy fiber layer; PCL, pyramidal cell layer; ML, molecular layer; SUPMF, suprapyramidal mossy fiber layer.

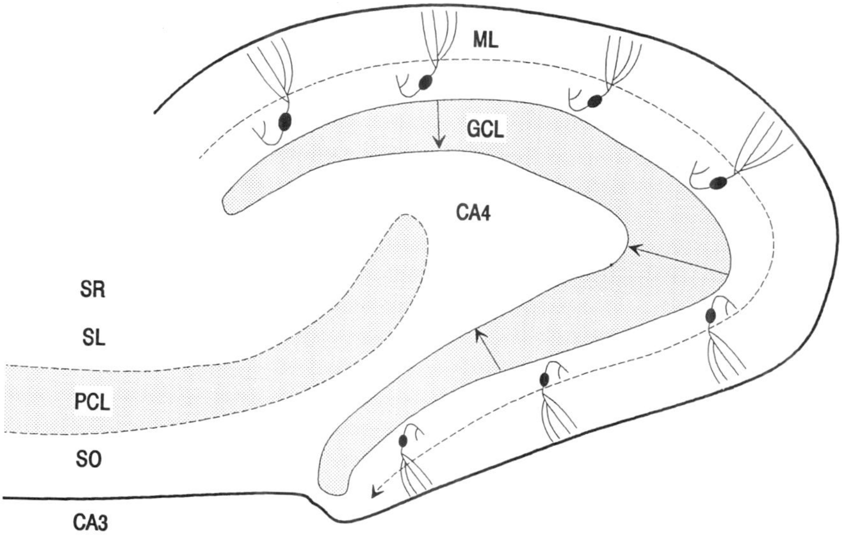

Figure 9. Schematic diagram of the orientation of the dendrites of the ectopic granule cells in the molecular layer of the dentate gyrus of NZB/BINJ mice (Nowakowski et al., submitted). Note that all of the basal dendrites of the ectopic granule cells turn towards the suprapyramidal tip of the granule cell layer.

and the degree of expression of each type of abnormality varies from granule cell to granule cell. The dendrites that originate from the apical surface arise either as a single, main dendrite or as more than one process from separate areas of the cell body. They sometimes arborize extensively, but usually they have only a few branches which do not always reach all the way to the pial surface. Most of the ectopic granule cells have a single dendrite that extends out of the basal aspect of the ectopic neuron towards the granule cell layer. In general, the basally directed dendrite leaves the cell body from the basolateral surface that is facing the *supra*pyramidal tip of the granule cell layer. As a result, the basal portion of the dendritic tree is usually directed at a slight angle towards the *supra*pyramidal tip of the dentate gyrus. The basal dendrites are never observed to enter the granule cell layer; instead they turn towards the pial surface (Figure 9) or run parallel to the granule cell layer. Furthermore, the recursion of the branches back towards the pial surface almost always occurs in the same direction; they usually make their turn towards the *supra*pyramidal tip of the dentate gyrus (Figure 9).

The features of the dendrites of the ectopic granule cells reflect their interaction(s) with the constituents of their environment. Moreover, these interactions are similar to those documented to occur for the molecular layer interneurons of the cerebellar cortex (Rakic, 1972, 1975). For example, the orientation of the apical and basal dendrites of the ectopic granule cells with respect to the *supra*pyramidal-to-*infra*pyramidal spatiotemporal gradient of cell birth indicates that during development the basally directed dendritic processes are growing into an area occupied by processes from slightly more mature granule cells. The underlying assumption of these ideas is that the ectopic granule cells do not differ from their normally positioned counterparts intrinsically; rather, any observed differences in their morphology are the result of environmental influences acting on them as a result of their ectopic position. The correlation of cell position and dendrite growth has been previously well-described for the molecular layer interneurons of the cerebellar cortex (Rakic, 1972, 1975a). In the cerebellum the shape and form of the dendritic trees of these neurons is dependent on both the position of the cell body in the molecular layer and the interactions of the growing dendrites with the parallel fibers that comprise the bulk of the molecular layer. The "rules" followed by the developing dendritic processes of the granule cells of the dentate gyrus appear to be identical to those followed by the molecular layer interneurons of the cerebellar cortex. In essence, a dendrite from either class of neuron proceeds as if it is maximizing the number of contacts it makes with its afferents. In the case of the cerebellum, the afferents to the molecular layer interneurons are the parallel fibers. In the case of the dentate gyrus, the afferents to the granule cells are the major axon systems (i.e., the commissural, associational, septal, entorhinal, etc.) of the molecular layer. The attractive feature of this idea is that it can also explain the differences between the upright, goblet-shape of the dentate granule cells and the stellate shape of the cerebellar molecular layer interneurons. The explanation lies in the fact that the orientation of the individual axons comprising the afferent input to the dentate gyrus is more-or-less a series of columnar "bouquets," while the afferent input in the cerebellum is that of parallel fibers organized tangential to the pial surface.

RELATIONSHIP OF IMMUNE DYSFUNCTION AND NEURONAL MIGRATION

Recently, we have observed that four single autosomal mutations that are known to produce immune system dysfunctions also have pleiotropic effects on neuronal migration during the development of the central nervous system (Nowakowski, 1988). Two of these mutants, motheaten ($me^{\underline{v}}/me^{\underline{v}}$) and beige (*bg/bg*) have similar disorders in the hippocampal formation and the cerebellar cortex (Figure 10A, B). In the hippocampal formation of both motheaten and beige a disruption of the migration of granule cells results in a trail of granule cells along the migratory route which extends from the ventricular zone to the dentate gyrus. Additional ectopic granule cells are located in the molecular layer of the dentate gyrus, and there are also ectopic pyramidal cells in the stratum oriens of area CA3.

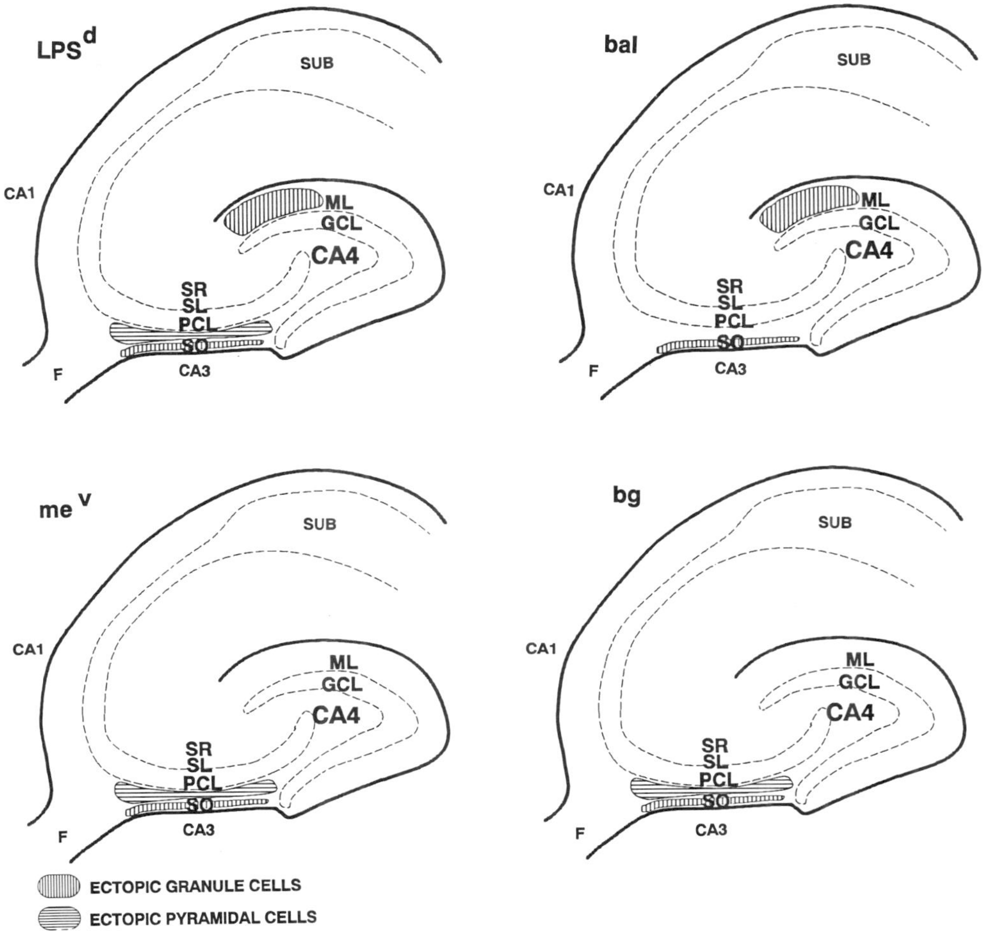

Figure 10. Schematic drawings of the hippocampal formation of four mouse mutants which exhibit both immune system dysfunctions and abnormalities in neuronal migration in the developing hippocampal formation: **LPS^d**, lipopolysaccharide response defect; **bal**, balding; **me^v**, motheaten viable; **bg**, beige. The general location of ectopic neurons in each of the four mutants is indicated by the shaded area (see key below drawing). Abbreviations: F, fimbria; GCL, granule cell layer; ML, molecular layer; PCL, pyramidal cell layer; SL, stratum lucidum; SR, stratum radiatum; SUB, subiculum (Nowakowski, 1988).

In the cerebellar cortex, islands of ectopic granule cells are located subpially, in the former position of the external granule cell layer. The other two mutants, lipopolysaccharide response defect (*LPS^d/LPS^d*) and balding (*bal/bal*), also have evidence of a disruption in the migration of granule cells in the hippocampal formation (Figure 10C, D). The distribution of granule cells along the migratory pathway to the dentate gyrus is similar to that in the motheaten and beige mutations. However, there are no ectopic granule cells in the molecular layer, and the migration of granule cells in the cerebellar cortex does not appear to be adversely affected by these mutations. Ectopic pyramidal cells in area CA3, such as those found in

Table 2. The incidence of ectopic neurons in the hippocampal region and the cerebellar cortex in the eight mutants listed in TABLE I. For details see the text.

Mutant	Granule Cells of Dentate Gyrus in		Pyramidal Cells of CA3 in		Layer I of Entorhinal Cortex	Granule Cells in ML of Cerebellar Cortex
	ML	CA3	S.R.	S.O.		
$dr^{sst\text{-}J}$	+	+	+	+	+	+
Hld				+		+
rl^{Orl}				+	+	+
NZB	+		+		+	+
bal	+	+				
Lps^{d}	+	+				
me^{v}		+		+		+
bg		+		+		+

motheaten and beige, are present in LPSd but not in balding. Thus, four genetically distinct, single, autosomal mutations (three of which (me^{v}, *bg*, *bal*) arose spontaneously in the C57BL/6J inbred strain) produce phenotypically similar disruptions in neuronal migration during the development of the central nervous system. The immune dysfunctions of these four mutants are quite dissimilar (M. Green, 1981). Interestingly, neuronal migration in the hippocampal formation and the cerebellum appears normal in nude mice (*nu/nu*) which are genetically athymic. These results indicate that there is common gene expression during B cell differentiation and neuronal migration.

GENETIC PLEIOTROPISM

Table 2 summarizes the effect of each of these mutations on the organization and development of the hippocampal region. The phenotypes resulting from these mutations range from a selective disruption of the migration of late-generated pyramidal cells to area CA3c to broadly distributed disruptions of cell position in all parts of the hippocampal formation. The dreher mutation seems to affect both cell proliferation and migration but not of all cell populations (Nowakowski and Wahlsten, 1985a,b). The reeler mutation affects the migration of all neurons but has minimal affects on cell number (Stanfield and Cowan, 1979a,b; Stanfield et al., 1979). In NZB/BlNJ mice it seems that migration of both pyramidal and granule cells is affected. The *Hld* mutation seems to affect the migration of only the late-generated pyramidal cells that are destined for area CA3c. The me^{v} and *bg* mutants affect both granule cells in the dentate gyrus and pyramidal cells in area CA3 of the hippocampus, while the *bal* and LPS^{d} mutants affect only the migration of the granule cells in the dentate gyrus. This variation in the effects of these mutations on the development of the hippocampal formation indicate that: 1) the mutant genes are probably expressed in different cell types, 2) the mutant genes are probably expressed at different times during development, and 3) a basic developmental process such as neuronal migration is influenced and perhaps controlled by a variety of cell-cell interactions which are functionally related to several different genes.

Table 2 also summarizes our observations on the distribution of the effects of each of these genes in other regions of the CNS, notably the cerebellum (Nowakowski, unpublished). For example, six of the mutations have ectopic pyramidal cells in area CA3; these same six mutations also have ectopic granule cells in the molecular layer of the cerebellar cortex. This association may reflect the existence of common gene expression during the migration of these two diverse cell types. The overlap in the phenotypes of the various mutations provides insight into the extent of common gene expression during neuronal migration.

RELEVANCE TO HUMAN DISEASE

Neuronal Migration and Neuropathology

Neuronal migration has been implicated in a number of human diseases that affect cerebral cortical development and function, e.g., dyslexia (Galaburda et al., 1983), autism (Bauman and Kemper, 1985), epilepsy (Meencke and Janz, 1984); thanatophoric dwarfism (Ho et al., 1984); schizophrenia (Kovelman and Scheibel, 1984, 1986), fetal alcohol syndrome (Miller, 1986, 1989), radiation exposure (Otake and Schull, 1984), Fukuyama-type muscular dystrophy, and others (Evrard et al., 1978; Choi and Kudo, 1981; Graff-Radford et al., 1986; Galloway and Roessmann, 1987). The relationship of the developmental defects of the mutant mice being studied to human neuropathology may be of particular relevance with respect to the dysgenesis reported in dyslexia, epilepsy, thanatophoric dwarfism, and schizophrenia. Pathological reports for patients suffering from dyslexia, epilepsy and schizophrenia all describe islands of ectopic neurons in the hippocampus, neocortex and/or cerebellar cortex (Galaburda et al., 1983; Meencke and Janz, 1984; Kovelman and Scheibel, 1984, 1986). These reports of microdysgenesis of cortical structures indicate that disruptions of neuronal migration have occurred during intrauterine life. The similarity of these human pathological descriptions to the malformations found in the mice being analyzed is striking. Also, the constellation

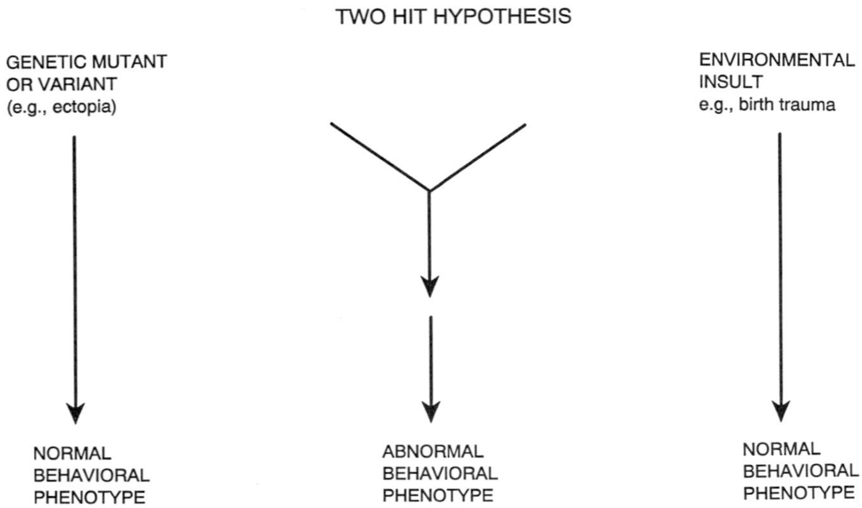

Figure 11. Schematic representation of the "Two Hit Hypothesis" described in the text. This hypothesis is suggested to provide a biological basis for the inheritance of a predisposition or susceptibility to a late-onset disease. According to this hypothesis, an abnormal behavioral phenotype may result from the additive effect of an otherwise non-deleterious genotype and an environmental event (or independent genotype) which also is relatively benign when both occur in the same organism. See text for further details. (Nowakowski, 1988.)

of CNS and peripheral abnormalities (Ho et al., 1984) and the incomplete recessiveness of thanatophoric dwarfism (McKusick, 1983) are similar to our findings for the dreher mouse (Nowakowski and Wahlsten, in preparation).

Two-hit Hypothesis

Many neurological diseases, including such diverse disorders as Alzheimer's disease, multiple sclerosis, dyslexia and schizophrenia, are widely believed to have both genetic and environmental contributions to their etiology (e.g., Murray et al., 1985; Murray and Lewis, 1987; Martin, 1987). This idea stems from the observations that these, as well as other neurological disorders, occur more frequently in the siblings of an affected individual than in the general population, but as yet an obvious mode of inheritance (such as autosomal dominant or recessive) has not been demonstrated (McKusick, 1983). In the case of schizophrenia, there is a significant familial component and high (but not 100%) concordance in many twin studies (e.g., Crow et al., 1989; Suddath et al., 1990). The suggestion is, therefore, that people afflicted with such disorders have a genetic composition that predisposes them by providing a permissive arena for the action of some second event later in life. The genetic composition and the second, environmentally related event (e.g., LaFosse and Mednick, this volume; Suddath et al., 1990) are by themselves relatively benign, such that neither alone produces any overt pathology or behavioral change (Figure 11). This idea is similar to the proposed two-hit models proposed for the genetic (somatic or germline) mutations that occur during oncogenesis (Land et al., 1983; Sinn et al., 1987). In this context, the possibility of a "family" of mouse mutations that affect the developing hippocampal region could be of great significance in understanding how such a two-hit hypothesis could contribute to the etiology of schizophrenia. The "two-hit hypothesis" provides a convenient conceptual framework for dealing with the specific concept of an interaction of genetic and environmental components of schizophrenia and with the more general concept of the inheritance of a predisposition.

Stochastically acting genes

An alternative view to the two-hit hypothesis is to consider the possible mode of inheritance of schizophrenia. Perhaps the easiest way to understand this issue is to examine one of the weak links in this field -- namely discordance in identical twins, which is frequently used as an argument that diseases, disorders, behaviors or traits of the CNS are not inherited (e.g., Corballis and Morgan, 1978; Plomin, 1990). Various environmental influences and cytoplasmic factors (Corballis and Morgan, 1978; Plomin, 1990) have been suggested as necessary to account for discordant twin data. However, there is a simple genetic mechanism that could account for discordance in the studies of identical twins (Nowakowski, 1991,c). Simply stated, this suggestion is that *there exist some alleles at some genetic loci whose action in producing a given phenotype is stochastic*. In its simplest form the stochastic action of the allele would be to produce an equal proportion of each of two possible phenotypes. A well-documented precedent in mammalian genetics for such a stochastic action by a gene can be found at the *situs inversus* locus in the mouse (Layton, 1976). There exist two alleles at this locus: *Iv*, the dominant form, and *iv*, the recessive form (Layton, 1976; Brueckner et al., 1989). Mice which are homozygous *(Iv/Iv)* or heterozygous *(Iv/iv)* for the dominant allele have typical left-sided asymmetry of the viscera. Mice which are homozygous for the recessive allele *(iv/iv)* have a 50% chance of developing a reversed asymmetry (Layton, 1976). In addition, the *iv/iv* offspring of both reversed asymmetric and typically asymmetric mice also have a 50% chance of developing reversed asymmetry (Figure 12) even after many generations of inbreeding (Layton, 1976). The simplest interpretation of these findings is that the *Iv* allele "biases" the development of the viscera to promote the establishment of their typical asymmetry, and

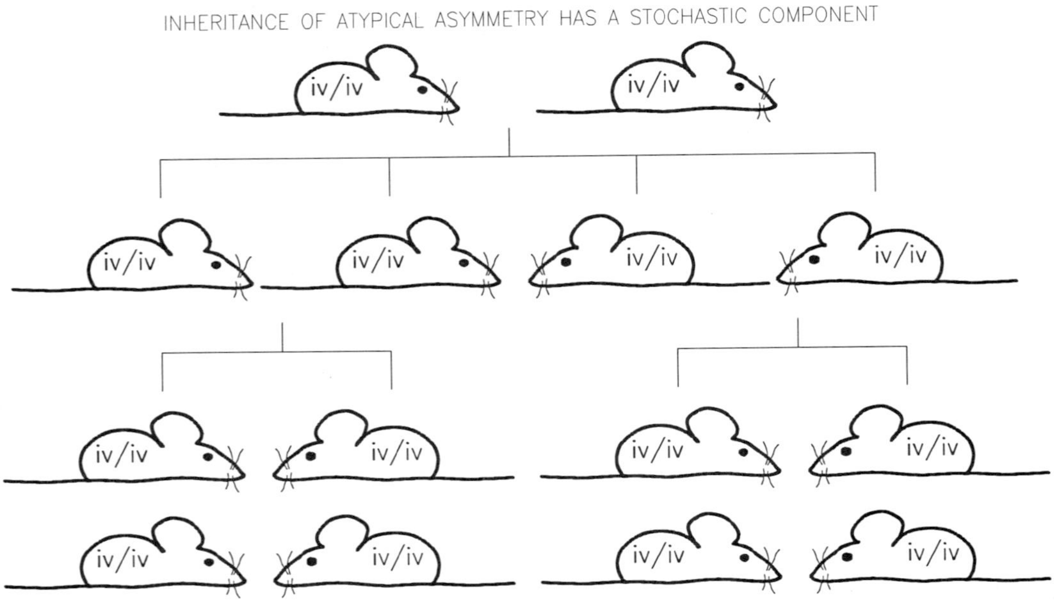

Figure 12. The determination of the direction of asymmetry in mice which are homozygous for the iv allele at the situs inversus locus is stochastic. this means that an equal proportion of iv/iv mice have each type of asymmetry regardless of the direction of asymmetry of their parents.

that the *iv* allele is a "loss of function" mutation which, therefore, removes this bias. In the absence of bias, the "sidedness" of the asymmetry is decided at random, and, hence, a 50% incidence of each type results. It is useful to note that the apparent random direction of the asymmetry in the *iv/iv* mice is not likely to be due to the influence of other genetic loci, because the experiments have been performed on inbred strains (Layton, 1976; Brueckner et al., 1989) which are, in essence, genetically homogeneous (E. Green, 1981). The *iv* locus has recently been localized to chromosome 12 (Brueckner et al., 1989).

A stochastically acting "biasing" gene (like *iv*) could account for discordance in CNS asymmetry in schizophrenia. A hypothetical, stochastically-acting allele at a gene which affects some function during CNS development and which is necessary to avoid developing schizophrenia would, by analogy with *iv*, produce a 50% rate of schizophrenia in homozygotes. Thus, in the case of identical twins homozygous for the hypothetical allele, 25% of the pairs would both be normal, 50% of the pairs would be discordant, and 25% would both develop schizophrenia. Thus, in identical twins carrying this stochastically-acting gene, one would expect to find a 1:2 ratio of pairs of identical twins concordant for schizophrenia to pairs of identical twins discordant for atypical asymmetry. This is a concordance rate of only 33%. (Note that the pairs with no schizophrenia would not be detected.) This rate is clearly much lower than the 100% concordance rate expected for genes that lack a stochastic component and in agreement with known concordance rates for schizophrenia (Crow et al., 1989; Suddath et al., 1990). It would be expected that a stochastically acting biasing gene like *iv* would act during the early development of the brain; indeed, a plausible developmental basis for the action of such a gene has recently been proposed (Nowakowski, 1991c). Caution is necessary, however, because one could imagine that a person homozygous for a hypothetical allele that allows schizophrenia to develop in a stochastic fashion might have his or her fate biased in one direction or the other by the environment, such as suggested by the two-hit hypothesis.

ACKNOWLEDGEMENTS

Supported by grants from the Scottish Rite Schizophrenia Research Program, from the U.S. National Science Foundation (BNS-8921020), and the U.S.P.H.S. (R01-NS20861).

REFERENCES

Altman, J., and Bayer, S.A. 1979. Development of the diencephalon in the rat: V. Thymidine-radiographic observations on internuclear and intranuclear gradients in the thalamus. J. Comp. Neurol. 188: 473-500.

Altman, J., and Bayer, S.A. 1981. Development of the brain stem in the rat: V. Thymidine-radiographic study of the time of origin of neurons in the midbrain tegmentum. J. Comp. Neurol. 198: 677-716.

Angevine, J.B., Jr. 1965. Time of neuron origin in the hippocampal region: An autoradiographic study in the mouse. Exp. Neurol. (Suppl.) 2: 1-71.

Angevine, J.B., Jr. 1970. Time of neuron origin in the diencephalon of the mouse: An autoradiographic study. J. Comp. Neurol. 139: 129-188.

Angevine, J.B., Jr., and Sidman, R.L. 1961. Autoradiographic study of cell migration during histogenesis of cerebral cortex in the mouse. Nature 192: 766-768.

Barber, R.P., Vaughn, J.E., Wimer, R.E., and Wimer, C.C. 1974. Genetically-associated variations in the distribution of dentate granule cell synapses upon the pyramidal cell dendrites in mouse hippocampus. J. Comp. Neurol. 156: 417-434.

Bauman, M., and Kemper, T.L. 1985. Histoanatomic observations of the brain in early infantile autism. Neurol. 35: 866-874.

Bayer, S.A. 1980a. Development of the hippocampal region in the rat. I. Neurogenesis examined with 3H-thymidine autoradiography. J. Comp. Neurol. 190: 87-114.

Bayer, S.A. 1980b. Development of the hippocampal region in the rat. II. Morphogenesis during embryonic and early postnatal life. J. Comp. Neurol. 190: 115-134.

Bayer, S.A. 1982. Changes in the total number of dentate granule cells in juvenile and adult rats: A correlated volumetric and 3H-thymidine autoradiographic study. Exp. Brain Res. 46: 315-323.

Bayer, S.A., Yackel, J.W., and Puri, P.S. 1982. Neurons in the rat dentate gyrus granular layer substantially increase during juvenile and adult life. Science 216: 890-892.

Boulder Committee 1970. Embryonic vertebrate central nervous system: Revised terminology. Anat.Rec. 166: 257-261.

Brueckner, M., D'Eustachio, P, and Horwich, A.L. 1989. Linkage mapping of a mouse gene, *iv*, that controls left-right asymmetry of the heart and viscera. Proc. Natl. Acad. Sci. USA 86: 5035-5038.

Caviness, V.S., Jr. 1973. Time of neuron origin in the hippocampus and dentate gyrus of normal and reeler mutant mice: an autoradiographic analysis. J. Comp. Neurol. 151: 113-120.

Caviness, V.S., Jr. 1982. Neocortical histogenesis in normal and reeler mice: A developmental study based on [3H]thymidine autoradiography. Dev. Brain Res. 4: 293-302.

Caviness, V.S., Jr. 1986. Genetic abnormalities of the developing nervous system. In Diseases of the Nervous System, ed. A.K. Asbury, G.M. McKhann, and W.I. McDonald, pp. 22-35.

Caviness, V.S., Jr., and Rakic, P. 1978. Mechanisms of cortical development: A view from mutations in mice. Ann.Rev.Neurosci. 1: 297-326.

Caviness, V.S., Jr., and Sidman, R.L. 1973a. Retrohippocampal, hippocampal and related structures of the forebrain in the reeler mutant mouse. J. Comp. Neurol. 147: 235-254.

Caviness, V.S., Jr., and Sidman, R.L. 1973b. Time of origin of corresponding cell classes in the cerebral cortex of normal and reeler mutant mice: An autoradiographic analysis. J. Comp. Neurol. 148: 141-152.

Choi, B.H., and Kudo, M. 1981. Abnormal migration and gliomatosis in epidermal nevus syndrome. Acta Neuropathol. 53: 319-325.

Choi, B.H., Lapham, L.W., Amin-Zaki, L., and Saleem, T. 1978. Abnormal neuronal migration, deranged cerebral cortical organization, and diffuse white matter astrocytosis of human fetal brain: A major effect of methylmercury poisoning in utero. J. Neuropathol. Exp. Neurol. 37: 719-733.

Cooper, M.L., and Rakic, P. 1981. Neurogenetic gradients in the superior and inferior colliculi of the rhesus monkey. J. Comp. Neurol. 202: 309-334.

Corballis, M.C. and Morgan, M.J. 1978. On the biological basis of human laterality: I. Evidence for a maturational left-right gradient. Behav. and Brain Sci. 2: 261-336.

Cowan, W.M., Stanfield, B.B., and Kishi, K. 1980. The development of the dentate gyrus. Curr. Top. Dev. Biol. 15: 103-157.

Crow, T.J., Ball, J., Bloom, S.R., Brown, R., Bruton, C.J., and Colter, N. 1989. Schizophrenia as an anomaly of development of cerebral asymmetry: A postmortem study and a proposal concerning the genetic basis of the disease. Arch. Gen. Psychiatry 46: 1145-1150.

Eckenhoff, M.F., and Rakic, P. 1984. Radial organization of the hippocampal dentate gyrus: A Golgi, ultrastructural and immunocytochemical analysis in the developing rhesus monkey. J. Comp. Neurol. 223: 1-21.

Evrard, P., Caviness, V.S.,Jr., Prats-Vinas, J., and Lyon, G. 1978. The mechanism of arrest of neuronal migration in the Zellweger malformation: An hypothesis based upon cytoarchitectonic analysis. Acta Neuropathol. 41: 109-117.

ffrench-Constant, C., and Raff, M.C. 1986. Proliferating bipotential glial progenitor cells in adult rat optic nerve. Nature 319: 499-502.

Flechsig, P. 1920. Anatomie des menschlichen Gehirns und Ruckenmarks auf myelogenetischer Grundlage. Leipzig: Georg Theime.

Galaburda, A.M., Sherman, G.F., and Geschwind, N. 1983. Developmental dyslexia: Third consecutive case with cortical anomalies. Soc. Neurosci. Abstr. 9: 940.

Galloway, P.G., and Roessmann, U. 1987. Diffuse dysplasia of cerebral hemispheres in a fetus. Possible viral cause?. Arch. Pathol. Lab. Med. 111: 143-145.

Graff-Radford, N.R., Bosch, E.P., Stears, J.C., and Tranel, D. 1986. Developmental Foix-Chavany-Marie syndrome in identical twins. Ann. Neurol. 20: 632-635.

Green, E. 1981. Genetics and Probability in Animal Breeding Experiments. New York: Macmillan.

Green, M.C. 1981. Genetic Variants and Strains of the Laboratory Mouse. Stuttgart: Gustav Fisher Verlag.

Goldman, S.A., and Nottebohm, F. 1983. Neuronal production, migration, and differentiation in a vocal control nucleus of the adult female canary brain. Proc. Natl. Acad. Sci. USA 80: 2390-2394.

Herrup, K. 1983. Role of staggerer gene in determining cell number in cerebellar cortex. I. Granule cell death is an indirect consequence of staggerer gene action. Brain Res. 313: 267-274.

Hickey, T.L., and Hitchcock, P.F. 1968. Neurogenesis in the cat lateral geniculate nucleus: A 3H-thymidine study. J. Comp. Neurol. 228: 186-199.

Hinds, J.W. 1968. Autoradiographic study of histogenesis in the mouse olfactory bulb: I. Time of origin of neurons and neuroglia. J. Comp. Neurol. 134: 287-304.

Ho, K.L., Chang, C.H., Yang, S.S., and Chason, J.L. 1984. Neuropathologic findings in thanatophoric dysplasia. Acta Neuropath. (Berl.) 63: 218-228.

Ifft, J.D. 1972. An autoradiographic study of the time of final division of neurons in the rat hypothalamic nuclei. J. Comp. Neurol. 144: 193-204.

Kaplan, M.S. 1977. Neurogenesis in the 3-month-old rat visual cortex. J. Comp. Neurol. 195: 323-338.

Kaplan, M.S., and Hinds, J.W. 1977. Neurogenesis in the adult rat: Electron microscopic analysis of light radioautographs. Science 197: 1092-1094.

Kovelman, J.A., and Scheibel, A.B. 1984. A neurohistological correlate of schizophrenia. Biol. Psychiatry 19: 1601-1621.

Kovelman, J.A., and Scheibel, A.B. 1986. Biological substrates of schizophrenia. Acta Neurol. Scand. 73: 1-32.

Land, H, Parada, L.F., and R.A. Weinberg 1983. Cellular oncogenes and multistep carcinogenesis. Science 222: 771-778.

Layton, W.M., Jr. 1976. Random determination of a developmental process. J. Hered. 67: 336-338.

Lorente de No, R. 1934. Studies on the structure of the cerebral cortex. II. Continuation of the study of the ammonic system. J. f. Psych. Neurol. 46: 113-117.

Martin, J.B. 1987. Molecular genetics: Applications to the clinical neurosciences. Science 238:765-777.

McKusick, V.A. 1983. Mendelian Inheritance in Man. Baltimore: Johns Hopkins University Press. Meencke, H.-J., and Janz, D. 1984. Neuropathological findings in primary generalized epilepsy: a study of eight cases. Epilepsia 25: 8-21.

Mikhael, M.A., and Mattar, A.G. 1978. Malformation of the cerebral cortex with heterotopia of the gray matter. Journal of Computer Assisted Tomography 2: 291-296.

Miller, M.W. 1985. Cogeneration of retrogradely labeled corticocortical projection and GABA-immunoreactive local circuit neurons in cerebral cortex. Dev. Brain Res. 23: 187-192.

Miller, M.W. 1986. Effects of alcohol on the generation and migration of cerebral cortical neurons. Science 233: 1308-1311.

Miller, M.W. 1987. The effect of prenatal exposure to alcohol on the distribution and the time of origin of corticospinal neurons in the rat. J. Comp. Neurol. 257: 372-382.

Miller, M.W. 1989. Effect of prenatal exposure to ethanol on the development of the cerebral cortex: II. Cell proliferation in the ventricular and subventricular zones of the rat. J. Comp. Neurol. 287: 326-338.

Mountcastle, V.B. 1978. An organizing principle for cerebral function: The unit module and distributed system. In The Mindful Brain, ed. G. Edelman and V.B. Mountcastle, pp. 7-50. Cambridge, Massachusetts: MIT Press.

Mullen, R., and Herrup, J. 1979. Chimeric analysis of mouse cerebellar mutants., In Neurogenetics: Genetic Approaches to the Study of the Nervous System, ed. X.O. Breakfield, pp. 173-196. New York: Elsevier.

Murray, R.M., and Lewis, S.W. 1987. Is schizophrenia a neurodevelopmental disorder? Brit. Med. J. 295: 681-682.

Murray, R.M., Lewis, S.W., and Reveley, A.M. 1985. Towards an aetiological classification of schizophrenia. Lancet 1(8436): 1023-1026.

Nornes, H.L., and Das, G.D. 1974. Temporal patterns of neurons in spinal cord of rat: I. An autoradiographic study -- time and sites of origin and migration and settling pattern of neuroblasts. Brain Res. 73: 121-138.

Nottebohm, F. 1985. Neuronal replacement in adulthood. Ann. NY Acad. Sci. 457: 143-161.

Nowakowski, R.S. 1984. The mode of inheritance of a defect in lamination in the hippocampus of the BALB/c mouse. J. Neurogenetics 1: 249-258.

Nowakowski, R.S. 1985. Neuronal migration in the hippocampal lamination defect (Hld) mutant mouse. In Cellular and Molecular Control of Direct Cell Interactions, ed. H.J. Marthy, pp. 133-154. New York: Plenum.

Nowakowski, R.S. 1986. Abnormalities in neuronal migration in the hippocampal formation of the NZB/BlNJ mouse. Soc. Neurosci. Abstr. 12: 317.

Nowakowski, R.S. 1987. Basic Concepts of CNS development. Child Development 58: 568-595.

Nowakowski, R.S. 1988. Development of the hippocampal formation in mutant mice. Drug Dev. Res. 15: 315-336.

Nowakowski, R.S. 1991a., Some Basic Concepts of the Development of the CNS. In Fetal Neural Development in Adult Shcizophrenia, ed. Mednick, S. A., Cannon, T.D., Barr, C.E. and Lyon, M., Cambridge University Press, in press.

Nowakowski, R.S. 1991b., Genetic Disturbances of Neuronal Migration: Some Examples from the Limbic System of Mutant Mice. In Fetal Neural Development in Adult Schizophrenia, ed. Mednick, S. A., Cannon, T.D., Barr, C.E. and Lyon, M., Cambridge University Press, in press.

Nowakowski, R.S. 1991c., Mechanisms of Asymmetrical Development in the Human CNS. In Neurodevelopment, Aging and Cognition, ed. Kostovic, I., Birkhauser, in press.

Nowakowski, R.S., and Davis, T.L. 1985. Dendritic arbors and dendritic excrescences of abnormally positioned neurons in area CA3c of mice carrying the mutation "hippocampal lamination defect". J. Comp. Neurol. 239: 267-275.

Nowakowski, R.S., and Rakic, P. 1979. The mode of migration of neurons to the hippocampus. A Golgi and electron microscopic analysis in foetal rhesus monkey. J. Neurocytol. 8: 697-718.

Nowakowski, R.S., and Rakic, P. 1981. The site of origin and route and rate of migration of neurons to the hippocampal region of the rhesus monkey. J. Comp. Neurol. 196: 129-154.

Nowakowski, R.S., and Wahlsten, D. 1985a. Anatomy and development of the hippocampus and dentate gyrus in the shaker short-tail (sst) mutant mouse. Anat. Rec. 211: 140A.

Nowakowski, R.S., and Wahlsten, D. 1985b. Asymmetric development of the hippocampal region in the shaker short-tail (sst) mutant mouse. Soc. Neurosci. Abstr. 11: 989.

Otake, M., and Schull, W.J. 1984. In utero exposure to A-bomb radiation and mental retardation; a reassessment. Brit. J. Radiol. 57: 409-414.

Patrylo, P.R., Sekiguchi, M., and Nowakowski, R.S. 1990. Heterozygote effects in *dreher* mice. J. Neurogenetics 6: 173-181.

Pearlman, A.L. 1985. The visual cortex of the normal mouse and reeler mutant. In The Cerebral Cortex, ed. E.G. Jones and A.A. Peters pp. 1-18. New York: Plenum Press.

Plomin, R. 1990. The role of inheritance in behavior. Science 248: 183-188.

Rakic, P. 1971. Neuron-glia relationship during granule cell migration in developing cerebellar cortex: A Golgi and electron microscopic study in macacus rhesus. J. Comp. Neurol. 141: 283-312.

Rakic, P. 1972. Mode of migration to the superficial layers of fetal monkey neocortex. J. Comp. Neurol. 145: 61-83.

Rakic, P. 1975a. Cell migration and neuronal ectopias in the brain. Birth Defects: Original Article Series 11(7): 95-129.

Rakic, P. 1975b. Timing of major ontogenetic events in the visual cortex of the rhesus monkey. In Brain Mechanisms in Mental Retardation, pp. 3-40. New York: Academic Press.

Rakic, P. 1977. Genesis of the dorsal lateral geniculate nucleus in the rhesus monkey: Site and time of origin, kinetics of proliferation, routes of migration and pattern of distribution of neurons. J. Comp. Neurol. 176: 23-52.

Rakic, P. 1978. Neuronal migration and contact guidance in the primate telencephalon. Postgraduate Medical Journal 54: 25-40.

Rakic, P. 1982. Early developmental events: Cell lineages, acquisition of neuronal positions, and areal and laminar development. Neurosci. Res. Prog. Bull. 20: 439-451.

Rakic, P. 1985. Limits of neurogenesis in primates. Science 227: 1054-1056.

Rakic, P. 1988. Specification of cerebral cortical areas. Science 241: 170.

Rakic, P., and Nowakowski, R.S. 1981. The time of origin of neurons in the hippocampal region of the rhesus monkey. J. Comp. Neurol. 196: 99-128.

Rakic, P., Stensaas, L.J., Sayre, E.P., and Sidman, R.L. 1974. Computer-aided three-dimensional reconstruction and quantitative analysis of cells from serial electron microscopic montages of foetal monkey brain. Nature 250: 31-34.

Richardson, E.P., Jr. 1982. Myelination in the human central nervous system. In Histology and Histopathology of the Nervous System, vol. I, ed. W. Haymaker and R.D. Adams pp. 146-173. Springfield: Thomas.

Richman, D.P., Stewart, R.M., Hutchinson, J.W., and Caviness, V.S., Jr. 1975. Mechanical model of brain convolutional development. Science 189: 18-21.

Rickmann, M., Amaral, D.G., and Cowan, W.M. 1987. Organization of radial glial cells during the development of the rat dentate gyrus. J. Comp. Neurol. 264: 449-479.

Schmidt, J.T. 1985a. Selective stabilization of retinotectal synapses by an activity-dependent mechanism. Fed. Proc. 44: 2767-27772.

Schlessinger, A.R., Cowan, W.M., and Gottlieb, D.I. 1975. An autoradiographic study of the time of origin and the pattern of granule cell migration in the dentate gyrus of the rat. J. Comp. Neurol. 159, 149-176.

Sherman, G.F., Galaburda, A.M., and Geschwind, N. 1985. Cortical anomalies in brains of New Zealand mice: a neuropathologic model of dyslexia. Proc. Natl. Acad. Sci. USA 82: 8072-8074.

Sidman, R.L. 1961. Histogenesis of mouse retina studied with thymidine-H3. In Structure of the Eye, ed. G. Smelser pp. 487-506. New York: Academic Press.

Sidman, R.L., Angevine, J.B., and Taber-Pierce, E. 1971. Atlas of the Mouse Brain and Spinal Cord. Cambridge, Massachusetts: Harvard University Press.

Sidman, R.L., and Rakic, P. 1973. Neuronal migration with special reference to developing human brain: A review. Brain Res. 62: 1-35.

Sinn, E., Muller, W., Pattengale, P., Tepler, I., Wallace, R., and Leder, P. 1987. Coexpression of MMTV/v-Ha-ras and MMTV/c-myc genes in transgenic mice: synergistic action of oncogenes in vivo. Cell 49: 465-475.

Smart, I.H.M., and McSherry, G.M. 1982. Growth patterns in the lateral wall of the mouse telencephalon: II. Histological changes during and subsequent to the period of isocortical neuron production. J. Anat. 134: 415-442.

Staats, J. 1966. The laboratory mouse. In Biology of the Laboratory Mouse, ed E. Green, pp. 1-9. New York: Dover.

Stanfield, B.B., Caviness, V.S., Jr., and Cowan, W.M. 1979. The organization of certain afferents to the hippocampus and dentate gyrus in normal and reeler mice. J. Comp. Neurol. 185: 461-484.

Stanfield, B.B., and Cowan, W.M. 1979a. The development of the hippocampus and dentate gyrus in normal and reeler mice. J. Comp. Neurol. 185: 423-459.

Stanfield, B.B., and Cowan, W.M. 1979b. The morphology of the hippocampus and dentate gyrus in normal and reeler mice. J. Comp. Neurol. 185: 393-422.

Suddath, R.L., Christison, G.W., Torrey, E.F., Casanova, M.F., and Weinberger, D.R. 1990. Anatomical abnormalities in the brains of monozygotic twins discordant for schizophrenia. New Eng. J. Med. 322: 791-794.

Taber-Pierce, E. 1972. Time of origin of neurons in the brain stem of the mouse. Prog. in Brain Res. 40: 53-66.

Temple, S., and Raff, M.C. 1986. Clonal analysis of oligodendrocyte development in culture: Evidence for a developmental clock that counts cell divisions. Cell 44: 773-779.

Vaughn, J.E., Matthews, D.A., Barber, R.P., Wimer, C.C., and Wimer, R.E. 1977. Genetically-associated variations in the development of hippocampal pyramidal neurons may produce differences in mossy fiber connectivity. J. Comp. Neurol. 173: 41-52.

Wahlsten, D., Lyons, J.P., and Zagaja, W. 1983. Shaker short-tail, a spontaneous neurological mutant in the mouse. J. Hered. 74: 421-425.

Walsh, C., Polley, E.H., Hickey, T.L., and Guillery, R.W. 1983. Generation of cat retinal ganglion cells in relation to central pathways. Nature 302: 611-614.

Wyss, J.M., and Sripanidkulchai, B. 1985. The development of Ammon's horn and the fascia dentata in the cat: A [3H]thymidine analysis. Dev. Brain Res. 18: 185-198.

Zimmerman, R.A., Bilaniuk, L.T., and Grossman, R.I. 1983. Computed tomography in migratory disorders of human brain development. Neuroradiology 25: 257-263.

IS THE DIFFERENTIAL LOCALIZATION OF SPECIFIC PLASMA PROTEINS IN THE DEVELOPING NEO- AND ARCHICORTEX A REFLECTION OF DIFFERENCES IN TRANS-BARRIER TRANSPORT? POSSIBLE IMPLICATIONS FOR THE NEUROPATHOLOGY OF SCHIZOPHRENIA

Mette Stagaard Janas, Torben Moos, and Kjeld Møllgård

Medical Anatomy A and Center for Neuroscience
The Panum Institute, University of Copenhagen
Copenhagen, Denmark

INTRODUCTION

The mature central nervous system (CNS) is well protected against both mechanical injuries and alterations in the environment outside of the brain barriers. The mechanical protection is provided by a bony vault, various membranes, and by the cerebrospinal fluid (CSF) which serves to support and cushion the CNS against trauma. The buoyancy of CSF is indicated by the fact that a brain weighing 1500 g in the air weighs only 50 g when immersed in CSF. Just as the skull and the "hydraulic suspension" of the brain provide a mechanical protection, the tight junctions between endothelial cells in CNS capillaries, epithelial cells in choroid plexuses and arachnoidal cells in meninges, provide the underlying diffusion restraint of the brain barriers upon which all other mechanisms act (see Dziegielewska & Saunders, this volume).

The immediate impression of the immature CNS is that the fetal and neonatal brain may be less well protected and therefore more readily subjected to adverse external influences. The types of damage caused by pre- and perinatal complications seem to reflect a vulnerability of the developing brain, which may be due to mechanical influences or to alterations in the internal environment of the fetus. Both types of damage have been indicated to be involved in the etiology of schizophrenia (Mednick, 1970; Cannon and Mednick, 1989; Lyon et al., 1989). The hippocampal formation has been pointed to as one of the areas with neuro-pathological changes in brains of schizophrenics (Falkai and Bogerts, 1986; Roberts and Bruton, 1990). Therefore, we have selected the developing *archicortex* as a candidate area for studying the neuropathology of schizophrenia, and the developing *parietal neocortex* as an area of no involvement, a control region.

The human plasma protein *α_2HS glycoprotein* seems to play an important role in human embryonic and fetal brain development (Dziegielewska et al., 1987). It has been suggested that this glycoprotein binds heavy metals, specifically zinc (Shaw, 1979) and that its importance is based on its transport function of heavy metals (Colclasure et al., 1988) and on its presumptive trophic action during early brain development (Møllgård et al., 1990). Although characterized by a rather low concentration in both plasma and CSF during development (Dziegielewska et al., 1987), α_2HS glycoprotein seems to be an obvious candidate for further studies of differential plasma protein localization in the developing human archi- and neocortex.

PENETRATION OF MACROMOLECULES ACROSS THE BLOOD-BRAIN BARRIER IN MATURE MAMMALS

The existence of a mechanism to exclude substances from the brain has been known since the beginning of this century, although several decades passed before the morphological basis of the barrier system (the tight junction) was identified (Reese and Karnovsky, 1967; Brightman and Reese, 1969). Behnsen's original work from 1927 represents an early detailed analysis performed to investigate the "permeability" of both the developing and adult mouse brain. Detailed figures depict the staining of the adult mouse brain following subcutaneous injections of the dye trypan blue, which is now known to be stoichiometrically bound to albumin.

In the figures published by Behnsen (1927), staining of three different types of cells can be recognized consistently: 1) The cells of the circumventricular organs: choroid plexus, subfornical organ, organum vasculosum laminae terminalis, median eminence and neurohypophysis, pineal gland, and area postrema are all markedly stained due to a localized lack of an endothelial blood-brain barrier as was later shown by Brightman and co-workers (1975); they also showed that the brain barrier resides at the epithelial cell level as a blood-CSF barrier, which prevents further penetration of macromolecules. 2) Neurons of hypothalamic nuclei such as the paraventricular, supraoptic, and arcuate nuclei which project to circumventricular organs are stained as are 3) the cranial nerve and spinal cord motor neurons with projections beyond the blood-brain barrier. The staining of hypothalamic nuclei and motor neurons is thought to be caused by retrograde axonal transport in axons projecting beyond the blood-brain barrier either to the circumventricular organs or to the periphery (Sparrow, 1981; Moos et al., 1990).

It is impressive as will be discussed below, that many of Behnsen's speculations about his findings are so close to the knowledge of today, in spite of the fact that at the time of discovery there was no information about the morphological basis of the brain barriers, or of the circumvention of the barriers by retrograde axonal transport. Likewise, nothing was known about the plasma proteins and their capability to bind endogenous and exogenous substances or of their transport functions.

PLASMA PROTEINS IN THE IMMATURE MAMMALIAN BRAIN

In recent years data have accumulated indicating that even in early stages of development, the brain barrier system is very complex (Møllgård and Saunders, 1986; Møllgård et al., 1987; Dziegielewska and Saunders, 1988) and that it prevents passive diffusion of plasma proteins and other macromolecules across the blood-brain barrier (c.f. Møllgård and Saunders, 1986) and the CSF-brain barrier (Fossan et al., 1985). The brain development and brain barrier maturation occur over a prolonged period of time, the length of which varies with the species examined, but the underlying principles for the blood-brain and blood-CSF barriers "the tight junction" and in the case of the CSF-brain barrier "the strap junction" (Møllgård et al., 1987) are present already from the beginning.

In the immature brain of neonatal mouse, Behnsen (1927) described a more intense staining of the same areas than were stained in the adult brain, and an additional prominent staining in regions, where the blood-brain barrier at least in the mature brain is known to be intact. The neurons of these regions do not project beyond the barriers, so that retrograde axonal transport could not account for the presence of the dye-albumin complex. Granule cells of the dentate gyrus and pyramidal cells of the hippocampus are regional cell types which are intensely labelled in the developing mouse brain; in contrast e.g. the neocortex never exhibited any staining. The difference in staining between the developing archi- and neocortex is not readily explained even by today's knowledge. As Behnsen also summarized: "Diese Durchlässigheits-unterschiede scheinen uns insofern nicht ohne Bedeutung, als man annehmen muss, dass wie für die Farbstoffe, so auch für andere Stoffe (Nährstoffe, Gifte) ein erleichterte Zutritt zu den entsprechenden Teilen der nervösen Substanz besteht." ("This difference in permeability does not seem unimportant, because one must assume that a facilitated entry into the brain regions in question, that exists for the dyes also exists for other molecules such as nutrients and poisonous substances.")

In the developing sheep, the initial appearance of the cortical plate in the neocortex is at around *35 days* of gestation (gestational period is *147 days*), whereas its appearance in the archicortex is slightly later, around *day 40.* An immunocytochemical comparison of the distribution of the 4 quantitatively most important proteins both in plasma and CSF: *fetuin* (the homologue of α_2HS glyco-protein in the human, see below), *albumin, α fetoprotein and transferrin* (Dziegielewska et al., 1980) revealed marked differences in early developing sheep neo- and archicortex (Reynolds and Møllgård, 1985).

At the stage of neocortical plate appearance, *fetuin*-positive cells are much more numerous in the marginal zone of the archicortex than in the corresponding area of the neocortex. In spite of a high CSF concentration of *albumin* and *α feto-protein* in fetal sheep brain, these proteins have a very restricted distribution in the developing neocortex, whereas most of the cells in the developing archicortex are positive for those proteins; a proportion of these cells are larger and have particularly darkly stained perikarya. This is in contrast to the reactivity seen for *transferrin* in the developing neocortex where perikarya are markedly non-reactive, whereas the incoming fibers above and below the neocortical plate are strongly positive (Møllgård et al., 1984). A different pattern of reactivity for transferrin is seen in the developing archicortex at day 35 where many large cells are stained, whereas staining of the fiber systems is sparse. Data on the plasma protein distribution in the sheep archicortex after day 40 are not available.

PLASMA PROTEINS IN THE IMMATURE HUMAN BRAIN

During prenatal development of the human brain, several plasma proteins e.g. *albumin, α fetoprotein,* α_2*HS glycoprotein,* α_2 *macroglobulin, prealbumin,* and *transferrin* are localized in well-defined cell populations. This intracerebral presence is not necessarily indicative of an immature blood-brain barrier, but may rather be a reflection of an intracerebral synthesis (Møllgård et al., 1988b). The hippocampal formation is known to contain large amounts of zinc, which must be delivered from the periphery by one of four plasma proteins with known zinc-binding properties: α_2HS glycoprotein, albumin, α_2 macroglobulin, and transferrin (Shaw, 1979). For some of these proteins there are known or proposed receptors on the endothelial cells (e.g. Jeffries et al., 1984) which may be involved in the specific transport across the blood-brain barrier (transcytosis), permitting ligands with or without the binding protein to gain access to specific, localized areas of the brain (cf Møllgård et al., 1990). Numerous properties have been ascribed to *fetuin and* α_2*HS glycoprotein,* but in spite of the similarity of their primary structure (Kellerman et al., 1989; Dziegielewska et al., 1990), there is so far very little correspondence in the properties claimed for them (for summary, see Dziegielewska et al., 1987). Among the proposed functions are for fetuin: anti-proteolytic properties (e.g. Galembeck and Cann, 1974) and binding thyroxin (Fisher and Lam, 1974) and lipid (Kumbla et al., 1989), and for α_2HS glycoprotein: transport functions, DNA-binding (Lewis and André, 1978) and zinc-binding (Shaw, 1979), and potentials for acting as a growth factor (Dziegielewska et al., 1987; Møllgård et al., 1990).

The distribution of a given plasma protein changes continuously during development; thus it is present in various regions and nuclei following a specific

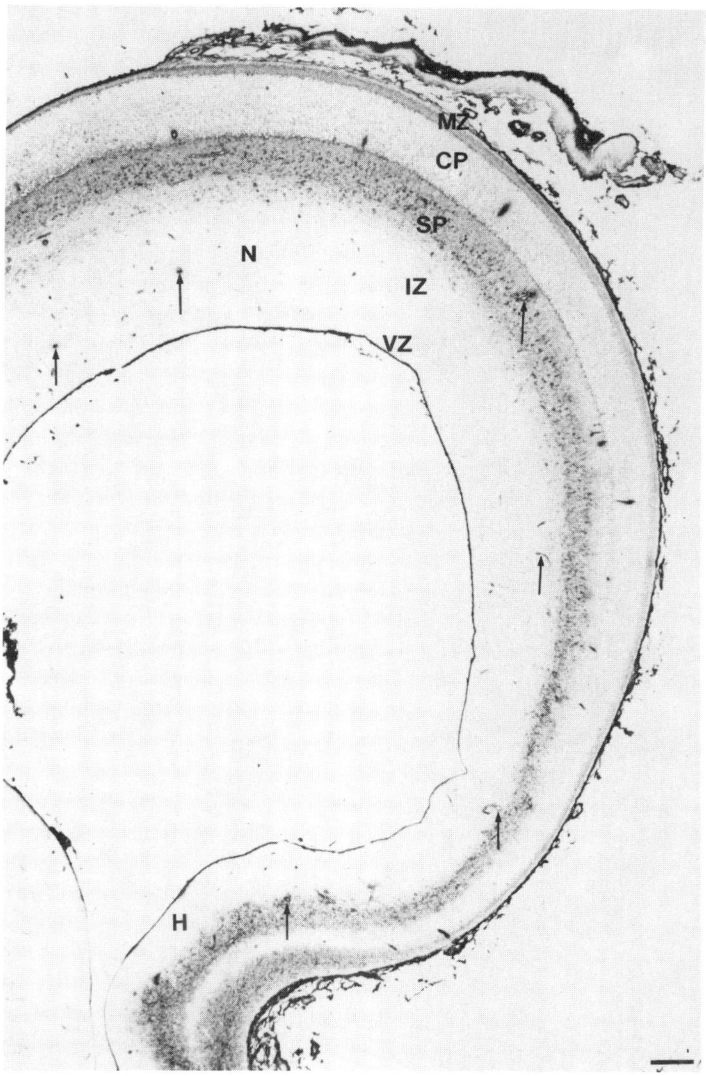

Figure 1. An 11 week old human fetus, immunostained for α_2HS glycoprotein showing the characteristic staining pattern with a strongly reacting developing subplate zone (SP), separated from a positive marginal zone (MZ) by the cortical plate (CP), which exhibits only a weak reactivity in the neuropil. The ventricular zone (VZ) is unstained. Slender arrows indicate stained vessels throughout the cerebral wall. Larger magnifications of the midlateral neocortex (N) and hippocampus (H) are shown in Figs. 2A & B). Bar = 40μm.

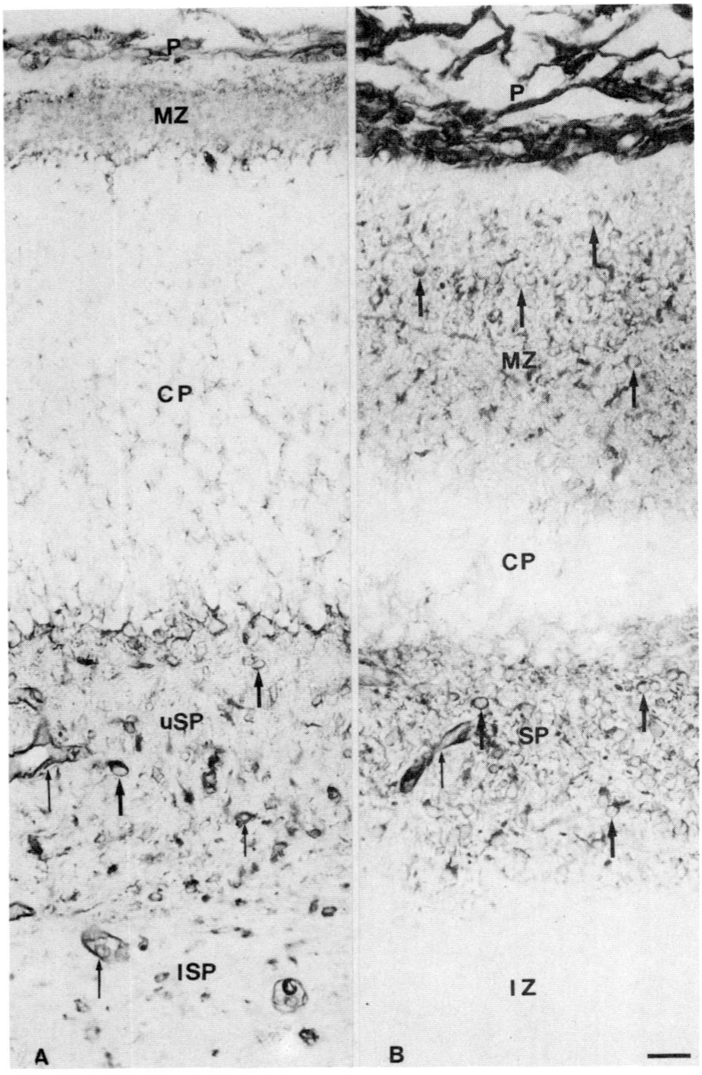

Figure 2. The midlateral neocortex (A) and the hippocampus (B) from an 11 week old human fetus, immunostained for α_2HS glycoprotein. The marginal zone (MZ in A) of the neocortex is characterized by a punctuate staining of cross-sectioned fibers, whereas the corresponding region in the hippocampus (MZ in B) exhibits numerous perikarya (arrows) which are α_2HS glycoprotein positive. The immunoreactivity of the cortical plates (CP) and the intermediate zone of the hippocampus (IZ) is sparse. Numerous neuronal perikarya (arrows in B) are stained in the subplate (SP) of the hippocampus, but only a few perikarya are present in the upper (uSP) part of the neocortical subplate (arrows in A). The vasculature of the pia (P) and the SP is strongly immunoreactive (slender arrows). Bar = 20 μm.

temporal pattern, and often shows a differential localization in the various cell types at different stages of development (Møllgård et al., 1979; 1988b). At the stage of neocortical plate appearance (7 weeks), α_2HS glycoprotein positive cells are much more numerous in the *marginal zone* of the archicortex than in the neocortical marginal zone, where in contrast incoming fiber systems are strongly stained. Later at 11 - 15 weeks, during the formation of the subplate zone (Fig. 1), immunoreactive cells disappear entirely from the marginal zone of the neocortex, whereas a further increase in number of α_2HS glycoprotein-positive perikarya is seen within the hippocampal marginal zone (compare Figs. 2A & B). At the same stage, immunostained neurons have appeared within the *subplate zone* of both neo- and archicortex, although much more pronounced in the latter (Figs. 2A & B). At the subplate stage (16 - 22 weeks) (Møllgård et al., 1990) the expanded neocortical subplate exhibits appreciable numbers of immunoreactive neurons throughout its extent. In the hippocampal formation, stained perikarya remain concentrated only in the hilus of the dentate gyrus, which thus in terms of immunoreactivity corresponds to the neocortical subplate.

There are some indications that the hippocampal endothelium of young rats may be involved in transcytosis (Møllgård et al., 1988a), although comparative ultrastructural studies of endothelial cells of the cerebral microvasculature of the developing neo- and archicortex are not available. The endothelial cells of the hippocampal formation exhibit numerous coated and uncoated vesicular profiles, endosomes and multivesicular bodies (Møllgård et al., 1988a), which may be involved in the uptake of some nutrients and trace substances; this could explain regional differences in plasma protein content in the brain. The endothelium of the neocortex on the other hand, is characterized by a scarcity of vesicles, which is presumed to explain the lack of transcellular transport of macromolecules across the mature blood-brain barrier (Reese and Karnovsky, 1967; Brightman and Reese, 1969).

PLASMA PROTEINS IN DISEASED IMMATURE AND MATURE HUMAN BRAIN

Scrutinizing the field for clinical parallels in which plasma proteins are involved in the pathogenesis of disease, we have focussed attention on two different brain disorders.

<u>An acquired condition</u>: kernicterus where an excess of the toxic sub-stance bilirubin probably bound to albumin penetrates into the brain. This causes severe perinatal neurological symptoms and persistent psychomotor impairment (Larroche, 1984; van de Bor et al., 1989).

<u>A genetic disease</u>: hereditary hepato-lenticular degeneration in which the

primary defect seems to be a failure of the specific copper-binding protein ceruloplasmin to bind copper. The clinical onset of this disease usually occurs during the second or third decade, and the course of disease is protracted (Adams, 1967).

The jaundice seen postnatally in mature or preterm infants may -- if untreated -- progress to kernicterus at unexpectedly low levels of plasma bilirubin (Turkel et al., 1982). As unconjugated bilirubin may not be lipid-soluble (Brodersen, 1979) and as penetration of bilirubin into the brain does not seem to be due to barrier immaturity (cf Møllgård and Saunders, 1986), a localized break down (cf Nitsch and Hubauer, 1986) or by-passing of the blood-brain barrier may allow bilirubin to gain access to the brain (Chiueh et al., 1978). Levine et al. (1982) have proposed that the underlying problem in kernicterus, especially in the preterm infant, may be an alteration or damage of the blood-brain barrier which allows the albumin-bilirubin complex, rather than bilirubin *per se* to penetrate into the endothelium of the brain. Albumin may then in turn shuttle the ligand bilirubin into the brain. Animal experiments have indicated this may indeed occur (Chiueh et al., 1978; Levine et al., 1982). Interestingly, hippocampus is one of the sites commonly affected, whereas the neocortex is only very rarely affected (cf Smith, 1974; Larroche, 1984).

In many respects, an adult counterpart to neonatal kernicterus is *hepatolenticular degeneration*, also known as Wilson's disease, which develops during the second to third decade of life. This hereditary disease is characterized by a progressive accumulation of copper, which at a certain level becomes toxic leading to hepatic cirrhosis and degeneration of lenticular and caudate nuclei and more rarely of other brain nuclei. An approximate tenfold increase in the amounts of copper has been observed in brain tissue, but the distribution of CNS lesions caused by the excess copper in hepatolenticular degeneration does not coincide with the normal intracerebral distribution of copper. Thus, the locus ceruleus, which has the highest copper concentration of all brain regions, is not lesioned in Wilson's disease. The metabolic abnormality in Wilson's disease seems to be a failure of the plasma protein ceruloplasmin to bind copper, and the current hypothesis is that the copper gains access to the brain via uptake of an albumin-copper complex (cf Duchen and Jacobs, 1984). In that way copper uptake escapes normal homeostatic regulation; the result is an accumulation of the trace heavy metal, with ensuing localized brain lesions.

CONCLUSION

We have pointed to a differential staining of some plasma proteins and discussed the distribution in selected brain regions during normal development and in two conditions in the developing and mature brain. Brain regions with high plasma protein content are also characterized either by a high heavy metal content as the hippocampus (zinc), the locus ceruleus and the diseased corpus striatum (copper) and e.g. also globus pallidus, subthalamic and dentate nuclei (iron), or by retrograde axonal transport e.g. in hypothalamic nuclei and motor neurons in brain stem and spinal cord. This is in contrast to the very rare involvement of the neocortex, which is characterized by an overall low content of heavy metals and no projections beyond the barriers. Disturbances of transports systems of heavy metals including abnormalities of transport proteins and their receptors, located either extra- or intracerebrally, seem to cause deficiency of its ligand within the developing or maturing brain. This may result in altered cell proliferation and differentiation (cf. Warkany and Petering, 1972; Espinosa at al., 1989) or cause cell damage or death (Duchen and Jacobs, 1984; Stibler and Jacken, 1990). It is conceivable that a diminished metal ion supply may trigger or stimulate other transporting systems (Stagaard et al., 1990). A resulting increased activity of receptor-mediated uptake of albumin-ligand complexes might lead to concomitant uptake of the ligand in regions and in amounts which are abnormal. Whether this difference between the developing and mature archi- and neocortex is caused by regional differences in the requirement of the plasma proteins, heavy metal ions, hormones, vitamins, fatty acids, or toxic substances or of a still unidentified ligand of a given plasma protein remains to be elucidated. Since the developing human brain is also synthesizing plasma proteins (Møllgård et al., 1988b), which may handle the intracerebral transport of potentially toxic ligands of plasma proteins, we find it attractive to investigate the distribution of α_2HS glycoprotein and other plasma proteins in the developing human hippocampal formation and its microvasculature and to compare the distributions with the ones found in the parietal neocortex. Further studies will compare the findings in normal fetal material with those in fetuses which are potentially at high risk for having inherited a predisposition for schizophrenia.

ACKNOWLEDGEMENTS

We wish to thank Dr. K. M. Dziegielewska for helpful discussions and criticism, and K. Ottesen for excellent photographic work. The study was supported by the NOVO Foundation and NIMH grant # 44188.

REFERENCES

Adams, R. D. (1967) Hereditary hepatocerebral degeneration of Wilson-Westphal-Strümpell with reference to acquired hepatocerebral degeneration. In: *Future of neurology*. Ed.: Bammer, H. G. Stuttgart, Georg Thieme Verlag, pp 45-69.

Behnsen, G. (1927) Über die Farbstoffspeicherung im Zentralnervensystem der Weissen Maus in Verschiedenen Alterszuständen. *Z Zellforsch Anat,* 4: 515-572.

Brightman, M. W., Prescott, L., and Reese, T. S. (1975) Intercellular junctions of special ependyma. In: *Brain-Endocrine Interaction, II.* Karger, Basel. Eds.: Knigge, K. M. et al. pp. 146-156.

Brightman, M. W., and Reese, T. S. (1969) Junctions between intimately apposed cell membranes in the vertebrate brain. *J Cell Biol,* 40: 648-677.

Brodersen, R. (1979) Bilirubin, solubility and interaction with albumin and phospholipid. *J Biol Chem,* 254: 2364-2369.

Cannon, T. D., Mednick, S. A., and Parnas, J. (1989) Genetic and perinatal determinants of structural brain deficits in schizophrenia. *Arch Gen Psych, 46:883-889.*

Chiueh, C. C., Sun, C. L., Kopin, I. J., Fredericks, W. R., and Rapoport, S. I. (1978) Entry of ^{3}H-norepinephrine, ^{125}I-albumin and Evans Blue from blood into the brain following unilateral osmotic opening of the blood-brain barrier. *Brain Res,* 145: 291-301.

Colclasure, G. C., Lloyd, W. S., Lamkin, M., Gonnerman, W., Troxler, R. F., Offer, G. D., Bürgi, W., Schmid, K., and Nimberg, R. B. (1988) Human serum α_2HS glycoprotein modulates *in vitro* bone resorption. *J Clin Endocrinol Metabol.* 66: 187-191.

Duchen, L. W., and Jacobs, J. M. (1984) Nutritional deficiencies and metabolic disorders. In: *Greenfield's Neuropathology.* (4th ed). Eds.: J. H. Adams, J. A. N. Corsellis and L. W. Duchen. London: Edward Arnold, pp 573-626.

Dziegielewska, K. M., and Saunders, N. R. (1988) The development of the blood-brain barrier: proteins in fetal and neonatal CSF, their nature and origins. In: *Handbook of Human Growth and Biological Development.* Eds.: E. Meisami and P. J. Timiras, Boca Raton: CRC Press. pp 169-191.

Dziegielewska, K. M., and Saunders, N. R. (1990) The internal environment of the developing brain. In: *Developmental Neuropathology of Schizophrenia.* Ed.: S. A. Mednick. this vol.

Dziegielewska, K. M., Evans, C. A. N., Fossan, G., Lorscheider, F. L., Malinowska, D. H., Møllgård, K., Reynolds, M. L., Saunders, N. R., and Wilkinson, S. (1980) Plasma proteins in fetal sheep brain: blood-brain barrier and intracerebral distribution. *J Physiol,* 300: 441-455.

Dziegielewska, K. M., Møllgård, K., Reynolds, M. L., and Saunders, N. R. (1987) A fetuin-related glycoprotein (α_2HS) in human embryonic and fetal development. *Cell Tiss Res,* 248: 33-41.

Dziegielewska, K. M., Brown, W. M., Casey, S.-J., Christie, D. L., Foreman, R. C., Hill, R. M., and Saunders, N. R. (1990) The complete cDNA and amino acid sequence of bovine fetuin. Its homology with α_2HS glycoprotein and relation to other members of the cystatin superfamily. *J Biol Chem,* 265: 4354-4357.

Espinosa de los Monteros, A., Pena, L. A., and Vellis, J. de (1989) Mini review: Does transferrin have a special role in the nervous system? *J Neurosci Res,* 24: 125-136.

Falkai, P., and Bogerts, B. (1986) Cell loss in the hippocampus of schizophrenics. *Eur Arch Psych Neurol Sci,* 236: 154-161.

Fisher, D. A., and Lam, R. W. (1974) Thyroid hormone binding by bovine and bovine fetuin. *Endocrinology,* 94: 49-54.

Fossan, G., Cavanagh, M. E., Evans, C. A. N., Malinowska, D. H., Møllgård, K., Reynolds, M. L., and Saunders, N. R. (1985) CSF-brain permeability in the immature sheep fetus: A CSF-brain barrier. *Dev Brain Res,* 18: 113-124.

Galembeck, F., and Cann, J. R. (1974) Fetuin as a trypsin inhibitor. *Arch Biochem Biophys,* 164: 326-331.

Jeffries, W. S., Brandon, M. R., Hunt, S. V., Williams, A. F., Gatter, K. C., and Mason, D. Y. (1984) Transferrin receptor on endothelium of brain capillaries. *Nature,* 312: 162-163.

Kellerman, J., Haupt, H., Auerswald, E.-A., and Müller-Ester, W. (1989) The arrangement of disulfide loops in human α_2HS glycoprotein. Similarity to the disulfide bridge structures of cystatins and kininogens. *J Biol Chem,* 64: 14121-14128.

Kumbla, L., Cayatte, A. J., and Subblah, M. T. R. (1989) Association of a lipoprotein-like particle with bovine fetuin. *FASEB J,* 3: 2075-2080.

Larroche, J.-C. (1984) Perinatal brain damage. In: *Greenfield's Neuropathology.* (4th ed). Eds.: J. H. Adams, J. A. N. Corsellis and L. W. Duchen. London: Edward Arnold, pp 451-490.

Levine, R. L., Fredericks, W. R., and Rapoport, S. I. (1982) Entry of bilirubin into the brain due to opening of the blood-brain barrier. *Pediatrics,* 69: 255-259.

Lewis, J. G., and André, C. M. (1978) A serum DNA-binding protein absent in malignant disease. *FEBS Letters,* 92: 211-213.

Lyon, M., Barr, E. C., Cannon, T. D., Mednick, S. A., and Shore, D. (1989) Fetal neural development and schizophrenia. *Schizophrenia Bulletin,* 15: 149-161.

Mednick, S. A. (1970) Breakdown in individuals at high risk for schizophrenia: Possible predisposition perinatal factors. *Mental Hygiene,* 54: 50-63.

Moos, T., Stagaard, M., and Møllgård, K. (1990) In adult rat CNS, granular and non-granular immunoreaction product of plasma proteins is correlated to their uptake or synthesis. *Histochem,* submitted.

Møllgård, K., and Saunders, N. R. (1986) Annotation: The development of the human blood-brain and blood-CSF barriers. *Neuropathol Appl Neurobiol,* 12: 337-358.

Møllgård, K., Jacobsen, M., Jacobsen, G. K., Clausen, P. P., and Saunders N. R. (1979) Immunohistochemical evidence for an intracellular localization of plasma proteins in human fetal choroid plexus and brain. *Neurosci Letters, 14:* 85-90.

Møllgård K., Reynolds, M. L., Jacobsen, M., Dziegielewska, K. M., and Saunders, N. R. (1984) Differential immunocytochemical staining for fetuin and transferrin in the developing cortical plate. *J Neurocytol,* 13: 497-502.

Møllgård, K., Balslev, Y., Lauritzen, B., and Saunders, N. R. (1987) Cell junctions and membrane specializations in the ventricular zone (germinal matrix) of the developing sheep brain: a CSF-brain barrier. *J Neurocytol,* 16: 433-444.

Møllgård, K., Balslev, Y., and Saunders N. R. (1988a) Structural aspects of the blood-brain and blood-CSF barriers with respect to endogenous proteins. In: *Peptide and amino acid transport mechanisms in the central nervous system.* Eds.: L. Rakic, H. Davson, D. J. Begley and B. V. Zlokovic. London and Belgrade: Macmillian Press and Serbian Academy of Science and Arts, pp 93-101.

Møllgård, K., Dziegielewska, K. M., Saunders, N. R., Zakut, H., and Soreq, H. (1988b) Synthesis and localization of plasma proteins in the developing human brain: Integrity of the fetal blood-brain barrier to endogenous proteins of hepatic origin. *Dev Biol,* 128: 207-221.

Møllgård, K., Stagaard, M., Dziegielewska, K. M., Saunders, N. R., and Kostovic, I. (1990) Transient expression of α_2HS glycoprotein immunoreactivity in the marginal and subplate zones of the developing human neo- and archicortex. *Eur J Neurosci,* in press.

Nitsch C., and Hubauer, H. (1986) Distant blood-brain barrier opening in subfields of the rat hippocampus after intrastriatal injections of kainic acid but not ibotenic acid. *Neurosci Letters,* 64: 53-58.

Reese, T. S., and Karnovsky, M. J. (1967) Fine structural localization of a blood-brain barrier to exogenous peroxidase. *J Cell Biol,* 34: 207-217.

Reynolds, M. L., and Møllgård, K. (1985) The early distribution of plasma proteins in the neocortex and early allocortex of the developing sheep brain. *Anat Embryol,* 171: 41-60.

Roberts, G. W., and Bruton, C. J. (1990) Annotation: Notes from the graveyard: Neuropathology and schizophrenia. *Neuropathol Appl Neurobiol,* 16: 3-16.

Shaw, J. C. L. (1979) Trace elements in the foetus and young infant. I. Zinc. *Am J Diseases in Children,* 133: 1260-1268.

Smith, J. F. (1974) *Pediatric Neuropathology.* McGraw-Hill, New York. pp: 90-91.

Sparrow, J. R. (1981) Immunocytochemical localization of plasma proteins in neuronal perikarya. *Brain Res,* 212: 570-572.

Stagaard, M., Moos, T., and Møllgård, K. (1990) Is the genetic vulnerability of schizophrenia linked to abnormal development of the ventricular system and the brain barrier systems in the human fetal brain? In: *Fetal Neural Development and Schizophrenia.* Ed.: S. A. Mednick. Cambridge University Press, in press.

Stibler, H., and Jacken, J. (1990) Carbohydrate deficient serum transferrin in a new systemic hereditary syndrome. *Arch Disease in Childhood,* 65: 107-111.

Turkel, S. B., Miller, C. A., Gutenberg, M. E., Moynes, D. R., and Hodgman, J. E. (1982) A clinical pathological reappraisal of kernicterus. *Pediatrics,* 69: 267-272.

van de Bor, M., van Zeben-van der Aa, T. M., Verloove-Vanhorick, S. P., Brand, R., and Buys, J. H. (1989) Hyperbilirubinemia in preterm infants and neurodevelopmental outcome at 2 years of age: Results of a national collaborative survey. *Pediatrics,* 83: 915-920.

Warkany, J., and Petering, H. G. (1972) Congenital malformations of the central nervous system in rats produced by maternal zinc. *Teratology,* 5: 319-334.

DOPAMINERGIC INNERVATION OF THE CEREBRAL CORTEX: DEVELOPMENTAL AND ORGANIZATIONAL DIFFERENCES IN PRIMATES AS COMPARED TO RODENTS

Brigitte Berger
Hopital Salpêtrière
Paris, France

INTRODUCTION

In their recent review on the neuropathology of schizophrenia, Roberts and Crow (1987) concluded that schizophrenic brains may have a structural defect that could have resulted from an embryonic insult or a developmental anomaly preferentially affecting the temporal lobe. They further raised the provocative question of whether one cell type and consequently one transmitter would be consistently affected. This question could apply especially to dopamine (DA) and to the dopaminergic system. Its involvement in the pathophysiology of schizophrenia has been considered for more than 25 years and pharmacological evidence supports the key role of DA in psychosis. Different hypotheses have been proposed (Crow, T, 1987; Reynolds, G, 1989), considering either an increase or a decrease of DA activity but direct evidence for a disturbance of DA function is still lacking (Carlsson, A, 1988). Insufficient attention might well have been paid to the DA system of the cerebral cortex. Indeed, most of the biological data concerning the DA system in schizophrenia have been obtained either by analyzing subcortical brain areas, mainly the basal ganglia and sometimes the limbic system or bodily fluids such as CSF or urinary excretion whereas the DA innervation of the cerebral cortex has not been investigated in great detail (Crow, 1987; Bridge, T., Kleinman, J., Karoum, F, & Wyatt, J, 1986; Doran, A, Boronov, J, Weinberger, D, Wokowitz, O, Breier, A, & Pickar, D, 1987; Hetey, L, Berg, R, & Schlesinger, T 1987; Karoum, F, Karson, C, Bigelow, L, Lawson, W, & Wyatt, R, 1987; Oke, A, Adams, R, Winblad, B, & von Knorring, L, 1988). In fact, current understanding of the functional organization of the cortical DA system in primates has been largely based on direct inferences from data obtained in rodent where the cortical DA innervation is relatively restricted (Bjorklund, A, & Lindvall, O, 1984). However, a growing collection of data obtained these last three years by our group (Berger, B, Trottier, S, Gaspar, P, Verney, C, & Alvarez, C, 1986; Berger, B, Trottier, S, Verney, C, Gaspar, P, & Alvarez, C, 1988; Gaspar, P, Berger, B, Febvret, A, Vigny, A, & Henry, J, 1989) and others (Lewis, D, Campbell, M, Foote, S, Goldstein, M, & Morrison, J, 1987; Lewis, D, Foote, S, Goldstein, M, & Morrison, J, 1988; Campbell, M, Lewis, D, Foote, S., & Morrison, J, 1987) points to a major expansion of the cortical DA innervation in both human and nonhuman primates as compared to rodents. The region- and lamina-specific redistribution of the DA input which accompanies the growth and differentiation of the primate neocortex suggests an involvement of this amine in the functions of additional cortical targets. Moreover, the developmental rate of these DA projections as well as the characteristics of the DA mesocortical subpopulations also differ in primate (Berger, B, Gaspar, P, & Verney, C, 1990). This suggests that the DA fields of the cerebral cortex should be taken into consideration in addition to the subcortical regions, in the search for abnormalities of the DA system in psychosis and this target should not be necessarily limited to the prefrontal cortex, contrary to the indications issued from data collected in rodent brain.

REGIONAL AND LAMINAR DISTRIBUTION OF DA TERMINAL FIELDS IN THE CEREBRAL CORTEX OF PRIMATES

Different techniques have been used by different groups to visualize the DA circuitry. They explored distinct properties of the aminergic system: synthesis of the neurotransmitter, storage, or high affinity transport across the axonal membrane. 1) Tyrosine hydroxylase (TH) immunocytochemistry labels the first biosynthetic enzyme for catecholamines which is present in all catecholaminergic neurons whether DA or noradrenaline-containing, whereas dopamine-betahydroxylase (DBH), the final biosynthetic enzyme for NA, is not contained in DA neurons. Thus, double labeling immunocytochemical studies for TH and DBH should be necessary to identify the DA innervation (Gaspar, et al., 1989). In fact, TH immunocytochemistry seems to demonstrate preferentially DA terminals in monkey cerebral cortex at least with some antibodies (Noack, H, & Lewis, D, 1989). 2) DA immunocytochemistry reveals the intraneuronal endogenous content of DA (Van Eden, C, Hoorneman, E, Buijs, R, Matthissen, M, Geffard, M, & Yulings, H, 1987; Goldman-Rakic, P, Leranth, C, & Williams, S, 1989) and 3) specific in vitro loading with exogenous tritiated DA shows the full extent of the dopaminergic processes (Berger et al., 1986; Berger et al., 1988). These techniques gave largely similar results although there was some variation in the laminar distribution or in the specificity which depended on the species investigated (for instance human versus monkey). We preferred the in vitro radioautographic method that we worked out with L. Descarries and his group (Descarries, L, Lemay, B, Doucet, G, & Berger, B, 1987): it is highly specific, gives a better account of the DA terminals as compared to the axonal trajectories and allows a quantified study of their density and distribution.

The DA innervation of the monkey cerebral cortex is widespread, extending from the frontal to the occipital pole and characterized by a regionally specific pattern of laminar distribution (Fig.1). DA projections are diffuse to all cortical layers in the agranular cortices (motor and anterior cingulate cortices for instance, with a clustering in layer IIIa in the supplementary and premotor cortices), but display a characteristic bilaminar pattern (highest amount of terminals in layers I and V-VI) in the granular somatosensory and association cortices. Consequently, the DA innervation is most dense in the motor and anterior cingulate cortex and displays a decreasing density gradient rostralwards and caudalwards; moreover, layer IV which receives the specific thalamocortical projections is almost deprived of DA innervation (Berger et al., 1986; Berger, 1988; Lewis et al., 1987). In addition, a predominance for association over primary sensory regions is apparent in the somatosensory, auditory and visual cortex (Berger et al., 1988; Lewis et al., 1987; Campbell et al., 1987). Quantitative data confirmed this pattern of distribution and revealed another typical feature of the laminar distribution of cortical DA terminals in primate: the highest density in layer I throughout the cortical mantle, in all types of cortex (Berger et al., 1988).

The radioautographic method that requires an in vitro loading of tritiated dopamine did not give satisfactory results on postmortem human material. We thus used the aforementioned double labeling immunocytochemical technique. Careful topographic comparison of the synthetic enzymes of catecholamines, tyrosine hydroxylase and dopamine-beta-hydroxylase (used as marker of the noradrenergic system) revealed, as in monkey, the extent of DA innervation to all cortical areas, with a clear predominance in the primary and secondary motor areas, the anterior cingulate cortex and the insula; moreover, as in monkey, the laminar pattern of distribution clearly differed in the agranular and the granular cortices (Gaspar et al., 1989).

COMPARISON BETWEEN THE DA TERMINAL FIELDS IN RAT AND MONKEY

A main difference between rodent and primate consists in the restricted DA terminal fields in rat cerebral cortex (Fig.1). Extensive cortical zones, in fact most of the primary sensorimotor and association areas, receive minor or no DA projections in rat (Bjorklund et al., 1984; Berger et al., 1990; Berger, B, Verney, c, Alvarez, C, Vigny, A, & Helle, K, 1985) whereas they are innervated in primates (Berger et al., 1988; Lewis et al., 1987); they include the motor, premotor and supplementary motor areas, and the parietal, temporal and posterior cingulate

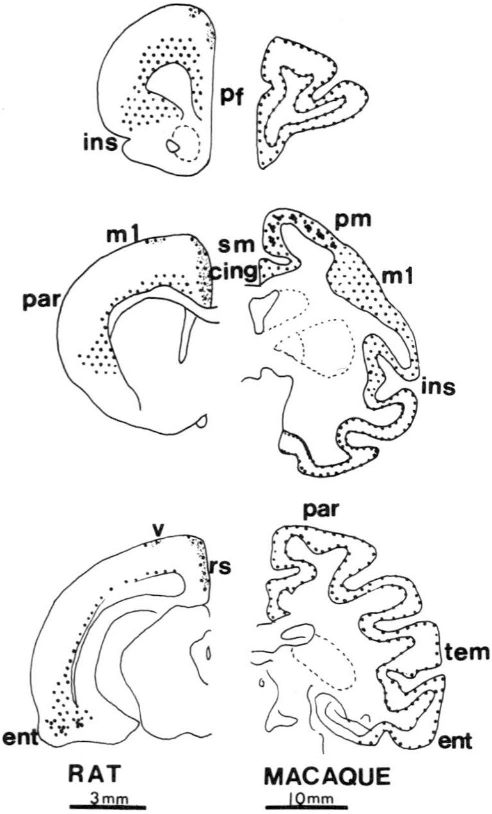

Fig.1. Schematic coronal sections of rat and macaque brain illustrated at different scale. Dots indicate the regional and laminar distribution of DA afferents in the cerebral cortex without reference to the density differences. Many arguments (see text) support the hypothesis of two classes of cortical DA afferents in rat, ending in the deeper layers (large dots) or the superficial layers (small and large dots) respectively. In monkey, the expanded DA projections display a general bilaminar pattern except in the agranular cortices (cing, sm, pm, m1, ins) which are diffusely innervated; clusters of DA terminals are figured in layer III. Whether these DA projections in primate are provided by a single or by several different classes of DA neurons as in rodent has not yet been investigated.

Abbreviations: Cing, cingulate cortex; ent, entorhinal cx; ins, insula; m1, primary -motor cx; par, parietal cx; pf, prefrontal cx; pm, premotor cx; rs, retrosplenial cx; sm, supplementary motor cx; tem, temporal cx; v, visual cortex.

cortices. A few cortical areas are equally innervated in rodent and primate, either densely as in the prefrontal or the limbic cortex (anterior cingulate, insular, piriform, perirhinal and entorhinal cortices), or poorly as in the visual areas (Berger et al., 1988; Lewis et al., 1987; Papadopoulos, G, Parnavelas, J, and Buijs, R, 1989; Phillipson, O, Kilpatrick, I, & Jones, M, 1986). The laminar distribution of DA terminals also differs in the two species (Fig.1). In primate, the molecular layer is a widespread laminar target; layer I is the most densely innervated lamina throughout the cortical mantle and virtually the only target in the primary visual cortex, whereas in rodent, only the anterior cingulate cortex and, to a lesser extent, the entorhinal cortex receive a dense contingent of DA terminals in the superficial layers I-III (Descarries et al., 1987).

HETEROGENEITY OF MESOCORTICAL DA SYSTEMS

The heterogeneity of the mesocortical DA systems is now well established in rat. The two classes of DA afferents that could be distinguished in rat cerebral cortex on the basis of their rate of development and of the regional and laminar topography of projections (Berger, B, Verney, C, Febvret, A, Vigny, A, & Helle, K, 1985), also differ by other chemoanatomical and functional characteristics: they have a different mediolateral origin in the ventral mesencephalon, DA group A10 for the first, DA group A9 for the second, display differences in collateralization and have distinct metabolic characteristics (Rev. in Berger et al., 1990). Finally, we have recently provided evidence that DA axons projecting to the superficial layers of the cingulate, motor, retrosplenial and visual cortices are not colocalized with neurotensin (NT)(Febvret, A, Berger, B, Gaspar, P, & Verney, C, in press) in contrast with the DA projections to the prefrontal cortex (Studler, J, Kitabgi, P, Tramu, G, Herve, D, Glowinski, J & Tassin, J, 1988) and to the other deep cortical targets (Studler et al., 1988). Whether they are colocalized with cholecystokinin as the latter are (Seroogy, K, Ceccatelli, S, Schalling, M, Hokfelt, T, Frey, P, Walsh, J, Dockray, G, Brown, J, Buchan, A, & Goldstein, M, 1988), remains to be investigated. The entorhinal cortex which receives DA projections from other DA cells of the A10 and A8 groups (Bjorklund et al., 1984) also displays different patterns of colocalized or not-colocalized DA and NT innervation (Febvret et al., in press).

In primate brain, the expansion of the DA projections to the whole cortical mantle is even more impressive when compared to the DA neuronal population. The 400 fold increase of the cortical surface in man (Hofman, M, 1988) contrasts with an only 20 fold increase of the mesencephalic DA neuronal population (Halliday, G, & Tork, I, 1986). This suggests a high level of collateralization and/or a very expanded projection territory for each DA neuron. It would thus be of interest to determine whether a particular neuronal subset participates preferentially in the more extensive cortical DA projections in primate, especially those to the superficial layers which are the most developed as compared to rodent. This is a task for future research, as very little information is available concerning the topographical organization of the DA mesocortical projections in primates (Lewis, D, Morrison, J, & Goldstein, M, 1989; Porrino, L, & Goldman-Rakic, P, 1982). However, the different vulnerability of the different mesencephalic DA cell groups to the neurotoxin MPTP or to degeneration in Parkinson's disease (Hirsch, E, Graybiel, A, & Agid, Y, 1988) provides some indirect evidence of a physiological heterogeneity among these cells.

OTHER POTENTIALLY IMPORTANT PHYLOGENETIC CHANGES IN THE DA CIRCUITRY IN PRIMATE CEREBRAL CORTEX

Lack of Colocalization with Neurotensin (NT) in Cortical DA Terminals

In adult human brain, we have recently shown that the overall regional and laminar distribution of NT afferents differs from that of DA terminals; moreover, double labeling procedures disclosed no fibres containing both NT and DA, even in zones where the two innervations were abundant (Gaspar, P, Berger, B, & Febvret, A, 1990). Preliminary observations in the mesencephalon (Deutch, A, Goldstein, :M, Baldino, F, & Roth, R, 1988) and cerebral cortex (personal unpublished results) in monkeys, provided similar results. Striking differences in the co-expression of DA and cholecystokinin (CCK) in mesencephalic neurons were also observed between rodent and primate (Palacio, M, Savasta, M, & Mengod, G, 1989). These results, which still need confirmation, question previous hypotheses regarding the role of an imbalance of peptide and dopamine co-transmission in the pathophysiology of psychoses (Gariano, R, & Groves, P, 1989). However, the lack of co-existence with NT and CCK in particular mesencephalic DA neurons might not be a permanent phenotype: the possibility of a transient co-expression, either in pathological states such as schizophrenia (Schalling, M, Friberg, K, Bird, E, Goldstein, M, Schiffmann, S, Mailleux, P, Vanderhaeghen, J, & Hokfelt, T, 1989) or during ontogeny, similar to the transient multi-localization of TH with peptides observed in the rodent amygdala, for example (Verney, C, Gaspar, P, Febvret, A, & Berger, B, 1988), has to be explored further.

From an evolutionary perspective, it could be hypothetized that the DA neurons that develop preferentially in primates, are the ones that are not colocalized with NT and that project to the superficial layers of the cerebral cortex in rodent.

Differences Between Rodent and Primates in the Expression of DARPP-32, a Protein Enriched in Dopaminoceptive Neurons

DARPP-32 is a cAMP- and DA-regulated phosphoprotein, associated with dopaminoceptive neurons bearing dopamine D-1 receptors in basal ganglia (Hemmings, H, Walaas, S, Ouimet, C, & Greengard, P, 1987). In rodent cerebral cortex, neurons that stain most strongly for DARPP-32 were observed in layer VI where high densities of D-1 receptor sites have also been reported (Ouimet, C, Miller, P, Hemmings, H, Waslaas, S, & Greengard, P, 1984). We have shown that in contrast with the observations made in rodent, the distribution of DARPP32-like immunoreactivity (LIR) in monkey cerebral cortex is characterized by its laminar extension to neurons of layer V and by its progressive regional restriction during postnatal maturation (Berger, B, Febvret, A, Greengard, P, & Goldman-Rakic, P, 1990). In fetuses, DARPP-32-LIR was expressed in the subplate of the cortical anlage at an early stage of prenatal development, similarly to DA afferents. In young monkeys (newborn and 6 week-old), a large number of DARPP32-positive neurons with the morphological characteristics of pyramidal cells were observed throughout the cerebral cortex in layer V-VI and to a lesser extent in layer II and uppermost III. In the parietal, insular, temporal and occipital cortices, DARPP-32 positive neurons were arranged in a monolayer in layer Va. These neurons were most numerous in the ventral temporal cortex. The labeled pyramidal neurons formed characteristic dendritic bundles branching several times in layer I. In the association and somatosensory areas, the basal dendrites of the DARPP-32-positive neurons in layers V-VI and the prominent tufting of their apical dendrites in layer I contributed to an essential bilaminar pattern similar to the bilaminar pattern of distribution of the DA afferents. Particularly noteworthy was the coincidence between the superficial dendritic tufts of the Darpp-32-LIR neurons in layer I and the dense DA projections to this layer. DARPP-32 labeling along with the DA innervation also matched remarkably well the distribution of D-1 receptors in somatosensory and association areas (Lidow, M, Goldman-Rakic, P, Gallager, D, Geschwind, D, & Rakic, P, 1989; Richfield, E, Young, A, & Penney, J, 1989). These data support the hypothesis that DARPP-32 is enriched in dopaminoceptive cells bearing D-1 receptors in primate cerebral cortex and may be used in first approximation as a marker of those neurons (Berger et al., 1990). Moreover, the predominance of DARPP-32-like immunoreactivity in pyramidal cells is in agreement with the ultrastructural observations which indicate a preferential input of DA terminals on pyramidal neurons (Goldman-Rakic et al., 1989; Verney, C, Alvarez, C, Geffard, M, & Berger, B, 1990).

DARPP-32 labeled neurons, which were widely distributed in the young monkey cerebral cortex became much restricted in the adult. DARPP-32 labeling almost disappeared from the motor, visual and prefrontal cortices and only weakly labeled neurons were present in the parietal cortex. However, the usual pattern with long ascending dendrites to layer I was observed in the ventral temporal gyrus and in the association areas of the paralimbic belt: caudal orbito-frontal cortex, insula, temporal pole, entorhinal and anterior cingulate cortex. These developmental changes of DARPP-32-LIR in the cerebral cortex contrasted with the lack of similar modifications in the subcortical areas (striatum for instance) and are apparently characteristic of primate as they have not been observed in the rat.

DEVELOPMENTAL DIFFERENCES OF CORTICAL DA INNERVATION BETWEEN RODENT AND PRIMATE

A complex developmental schema characterizes the cortical DA innervation in rat brain since the two main contingents that contribute to this innervation develop at different time, one prenatally and the other postnatally. The first contingent reaches the frontal pole in the last third of embryonic life, by E16 (Verney, C, Berger, B, Adrien, J, Vigny, A, & Gay, M, 1982; Kalsbeek, A, Voorn, P, Buijs, R, Pool, C, & Yulings, H, 1988) and extends to the entorhinal and visual cortices at birth. It displays a striking rostro-caudal gradient of decreasing density from the prefrontal cortex to the visual cortex and distributes predominantly to the deeper cortical layers V-VI. The second class of DA afferents reaches its cortical targets (superficial cingulate, motor and visual cortices) only after birth, during the first and second postnatal weeks and does not assume the adult distribution pattern until the fourth week (Berger et al., 1985).

Only a few data are available on the development of the cortical DA innervation during primate fetal life. In a study on the ontogenesis of cortical monoaminergic innervation in rhesus monkeys which is now in progress in our laboratory (in collaboration with P.S.Goldman-Rakic, New Haven), we observed already on embryonic day 7O, TH-positive fibers in the cortical anlage (Berger, B, Verney, C, & Goldman-Rakic, P, in press). Since the gestation lasts 165 days in macaques, this means that DA afferents have reached the cerebral cortex by the first half of gestation, in contrast to the situation in rodent. This precocious development of the DA projections (and of the other monoaminergic projections as well) is in agreement with the early generation of the monoaminergic neurons in the brainstem and parallels the early generation of the cortical neurons. From the beginning on, the ingrowth of the DA fibers displayed a bilaminar pattern, predominating in the marginal zone (prospective molecular layer) and the subplate and the highest density of DA afferents was observed in the insula and in the entorhinal cortex. At birth, the topographical and laminar distribution of DA afferents was like that in adult.

In the frontal lobe of 5 and 6 month-old human fetuses, we also observed a DA innervation in the whole depth of the future cingulate and motor cortices whereas a more bilaminar pattern predominated in more rostral areas (Berger et al., in press). This region-specific distribution of the dopaminergic innervation was similar to that observed in the adult human cortex. Thus in primate, the arrival of the first dopaminergic afferents clearly takes place before the end of the first half of fetal life and proceeds rapidly until birth in contrast with the obervations made in rodent.

FUNCTIONAL IMPLICATIONS

DA Innervation of Motor Areas in Primate

The dense DA input to the motor areas as well as to the interconnected anterior cingulate cortex in primates, indicates that the target of DA influence on motor mechanisms is probably not limited to the striatum as had previously been suggested. Neurons sensitive to iontophoretically applied DA have indeed been detected in the primate motor cortex (Sawaguchi, T, Mtsumura, M, & Kubota, K, 1986). The DA system could thus exert an effect on motor control directly at the cortical level, in addition to that produced through the basal ganglia via long cortico-subcortical loops (Alexander, G, Delong, M, & Stick, P, 1986). In this perspective it is noteworthy that the clusters of DA afferents in layer IIIa of the motor cortices are reminiscent of the columnar organization which characterizes the cortico-cortical afferents (Goldman, P, & Nauta, W, 1977) while a patchy concentration of efferent somata is observed in layers III and II (Jones, & Wise, S, 1977; Leichnetz, G, 1986). DA afferents might thus modulate the ipsilateral cortico-cortical neurons lying mainly in layer IIIa. From a physiopathological point of view, a dysfunction or a lesion of the DA input to the motor areas, especially to the premotor and supplementary motor cortex which play a role in the planning, initiation and sensory guidance of movement (Wiesendanger, M, 1986; Wise, S, 1985) could be involved in the different kinds of motor disorders observed in psychoses and Parkinson's disease.

Neuronal Targets of DA Innervation in Primate

The high density of DARPP-32-labelled pyramidal cells observed not only in layer VI but also in layer V of all cortical areas suggests that DA might primarily modulate not only the cortico-thalamic projections as in rodent but the vast array of cortico-subcortical output pyramidal neurons located in the deep cortical layers as well as a small proportion of these neurons that participate in corticocortical projections. The functional importance of this modulation is suggested by the lack of equivalence in rodent (Ouimet et al., 1984) of the prominent and widespread distribution of DARPP-32-LIR pyramidal cells in layer V observed in primate cortex (Berger et al., 1990). The bilaminar pattern of DA and DARPP-32 positivity in the somatosensory and association cortices indicates that DA terminals could thus modulate the neurotransmission of the same pyramidal neurons both in layer I and in layers V-VI. Interestingly, D-2 receptors, mapped using the selective D-2 antagonist raclopride, also accumulate in layer V (Goldman-Rakic, P, Lidow, M, & Gallager, D, 1990) and might be synergistically involved with D-1 receptors (Walters, J, Bergstrom, D, Carlson, J, Chase, T, & Brfaun, A, 1987) in the modulatory effect of DA on these output pyramidal neurons.

As mentioned before, different classes of DA neurons in the mesencephalon might provide the innervation of the superficial and deep cortical layers in primate, layer I receiving projections from the substantia nigra and layers V-VI from the ventral tegmental area and midline nuclei as in rodent. In that case, a given pyramidal neuron would be submitted to different modulatory influences on its apical and basal dendrites (Berger et al., in press).

Major Importance of the DA Input to Layer I in Primate

In rats, only the anterior cingulate cortex receives a rich contingent of DA terminals in the molecular layer (Descarries et al., 1987) whereas in primate, layer I is the most densely innervated cortical lamina (Berger et al., 1988). This raises the question of a secondary phylogenetic development of the superficial DA innervation first restricted to a few areas in rodent, then extending to the molecular layer of the whole cortex in higher mammals. This increase of the DA projections to layer I, contrasting with the regression of the NA input to this layer (Lewis, D, & Morrison, J, 1989), suggests a growing importance of the inhibitory role of DA on the transfer of information in the molecular layer.

An ultrastructural finding, in both rodent (Verney et al., 1990) and primate (Goldman-Rakic et al., 1989), which appears to be functionally important, is the involvement of DA terminals in triadic complexes. They include, in addition to the symmetrical DA synapse, another bouton forming an asymmetrical synapse (presumed to be excitatory) on the same pyramidal dendritic spine or shaft. This configuration allows a direct pre- or postsynaptic interaction of DA with other neurotransmitters. This may apply particularly to afferents that share the same laminar distribution as DA projections and presumably form asymmetrical synapses; in monkey, this is the case of the extended amygdalo-cortical projections (Amaral, D, & Price, J, 1984), the "nonspecific" thalamocortical afferents issued from the paracentral and midline thalamic nuclei (Friedman, D, Li, L, & Ungerleider, L, 1989) and the cortico-cortical connections of the feedback type (Selemon, L, & Goldman-Rakic, 1988). The latter comprise projections from layer III of higher order integrative cortical zones back to layer I of primary or secondary cortical fields. Interestingly, these three afferent systems increase in primates in proportion to the development of association cortices and of the DA innervation.

The DA control of this type of connection could be implicated in the abnormal sensory gating process which has been described in schizophrenia (Freedman, R, Adler, L, Gerhardt, G, Waldo, M, Baker, N, rose, G, Drebing, C, Nagamato, H, Bickford-Wimer, P, & Franks, R, 1987). This hypothesis is supported by recent data showing that dopaminergic stimulation disrupts sensorimotor gating in the rat (Peng, R, Mansbach, R, Braff, D, & Geyer, M, 1990).

Physiological Role of DARPP-32

In several subcortical areas, DARPP-32 was localized to dopaminoceptive neurons possessing dopamine receptors of the D-1 subclass and appears to serve as an intracellular third messenger mediating the action of dopamine at these receptors (Hemmings et al., 1987). Interest in this protein has been stimulated by the discovery that it acts as a potent inhibitor of protein phosphatase-I and is thus presumably involved in the regulation of the state of phosphorylation of other phosphoproteins in dopaminoceptive neurons. This could be one component of the DA regulated physiological processes in neurons bearing D-1 receptors. Several schemas have been proposed, illustrating a possible role for the phosphorylated DARPP-32 in amplifying the effects of cAMP on other substrates of cAMP-dependent protein kinase or in mediating the interaction of DA with other first messengers such as for instance glutamate (Hemmings et al, 1987). The activation of NMDA receptors situated on the medium size spiny neurons of rodent neostriatum indeed prevents the phosphorylation of DARPP-32 and therefore its activity (Halpain, S, Girault, J, Zorn, S, & Greengard, P, 1989). Glutamate containing neurons represent about 50% of all neurons in the somatic sensory cortex of monkeys (Conti, F, Rustioni, A, Petrusz, P, & Towle, A, 1987) and these neurons are mostly pyramidal cells. What proportion of DARPP-32-LIR pyramidal cells are also glutamatergic remains to be determined. Abnormalities of DARPP-32 might exist for instance in those cases of schizophrenia with a presumably altered glutamatergic transmission (Kerwin, R, Patel, S, Meldrum, B, Czudek, C, & Reyholds, G, 1988; Deutsch, S, Mastropaolo, J, Schwartz, L, Rosse, R, & Morihisa, J, 1989).

The developmental changes from fetal life to adulthood in the expression of DARPP-32 point to a possible role for this molecule and/or D-1 receptors during pre- and postnatal development of the primate cerebral cortex. Acting as an intracellular third messenger for DA, DARPP-32 could also be involved in those pathological processes in which a role of DA has been proved or suspected. The levels of DARPP-32 are not altered in Parkinson's disease nor in progressive supranuclear palsy (Girault, J, Raisman, R, Agid, Y, & Greengard, P, 1989) but this question obviously deserves further investigation in psychoses. Indeed, in spite of the fact that DARPP-32 seems preferentially associated with D-1 receptors and that D-2 rather than D-1 receptors have been implicated in the pathophysiology of schizophrenia, they are linked by complex pharmacological and functional interactions (Clarke, D, & White F, 1987). D1 dopamine receptor activation is required for postsynaptic expression of D2 agonist effects (Walters et al, 1987) and stimulation of D-1 receptors has been shown to exert a permissive role in the expression of D-2 mediated behavioral responses (Longoni, R, Spina, L, & Di Chara, G, 1987; White, F, Bednarz, L, Wachtel, S, Hjorth, S, & Brooderson, R, 1988; Jackson, D, Ross, S, & Larsson, L, 1989). The functional relationship of these two DA receptors with the receptor D-3 that was recently cloned in rodent (Sokoloff, P, Giros, B, Martres, M,Bouthenet, M, & Schwartz, J, 1990) will certainly be a matter of intensive research in the near future.

In conclusion, the major expansion of DA projections to the cerebral cortex in monkey and human brain suggests that cortical DA might be involved in more complex modulatory functions in primate than in rodent and consequently deserves further investigation in psychoses. This holds true particularly for the medial temporal lobe where developmental abnormalities have been repeatedly reported (Bogerts, B, Ashtari, M, Degreef, G, Alvir, J, Bilder, R, and Lieberman, J, 1990) and which is endowed with a dense DARPP-32-LIR population even in the adult primate.

REFERENCES

Alexander, G.E., Delong, M.R. and Stick, P.L. (1986) Parallel organization of functionally segregated circuits linking basal ganglia and cortex. Ann. Rev. Neurosci., 9: 357.

Amaral, D.G. and Price, J.L. (1984) Amygdalo-cortical projections in the monkey (Macaca fascicularis). J.Comp.Neurol. 230:465.

Berger, B., Febvret, A., Greengard, P. and Goldman-Rakic, P.S. (1990) DARPP32, a phosphoprotein enriched in dopaminoceptive neurons bearing dopamine D1 receptors: distribution in the cerebral cortex of the newborn and adult rhesus monkey. J.Comp.Neurol. 299:1.

Berger, B., Verney, C. and Goldman-Rakic, P.S. (1991) Prenatal monoaminergic innervation of the cerebral cortex: differences between rodents and primates. In Neurodevelopment, Aging and Cognition, Kostovic, I., Knezevic, S. and Spilich, G., ed., Birkhauser, Boston.

Berger, B., Trottier, S., Gaspar, P., Verney, C. and Alvarez, C. (1986) Major dopamine innervation of the cortical motor areas in the Cynomolgus monkey. A radioautographic study with comparative assessment of serotonergic afferents. Neurosci.Lett. 72:121.

Berger, B., Gaspar, P. and Verney, C. (1990) Dopaminergic innervation of the cerebral cortex: unexpected differences between rodent and primate. T.I.N.S. in press.

Berger, B., Trottier, S., Verney, C., Gaspar, P. and Alvarez, C. (1988) Regional and laminar distribution of the dopamine and serotonin innervation in the macaque cerebral cortex: a radioautographic study. J.Comp.Neurol. 273:99.

Berger, B., Verney, C., Alvarez, C., Vigny, A. and Helle, K.B. (1985) New dopaminergic terminal fields in the motor, visual (area 18b) and retrosplenial cortex in the young and adult rat. Immunocytochemical and catecholamine histochemical analyses. Neuroscience 15:983.

Berger, B., Verney, C., Febvret, A., Vigny, A., and Helle, K.B. (1985) Postnatal ontogenesis of the dopaminergic innervation in the rat anterior cingulate cortex (area 24). Immunohistochemical and catecholamine fluorescence histochemical analysis. Brain Research, 21:31.

Björklund, A. and Lindvall, O. (1984) Dopamine containing systems in the CNS. in A. Björklund and T. Hökfelt (eds): Handbook of Chemical Neuroanatomy, Vol.2, Classical transmitters in the CNS, part 1. Elsevier, p.55.

Bogerts, B., Ashtari, M., Degreef, G., Alvir, J.M.J., Bilder, R.M., Lieberman, J.A. (1990) Reduced temporal limbic structure volumes on magnetic resonance images in first episode schizophrenia. Psychiat. Res. 35:1.

Bridge, T.P., Kleinman,J.E., Karoum, F. and Wyatt, J.R. (1986) Postmortem central catecholamines and antemortem cognitive impairment in elderly schizophrenics and controls. Neuropsychobiol. 14:57.

Campbell, M.J., Lewis, D.A., Foote, S.L. and Morrison, J.H. (1987) Distribution of choline acetyltransferase, serotonin, dopamine-beta-hydroxylase, tyrosine hydroxylase immunoreactive fibers in monkey primary auditory cortex. J.-Comp.Neurol. 261:209.

Carlsson, A. (1988) The current status of the dopamine hypothesis of schizophrenia. Neuropsychopharmacol. 1:179.

Clarke, D. and White, F.J. (1987) Review: D1 dopamine receptor. The search for a function: a critical evaluation of the D1/D2 dopamine receptor classification and its functional implications. Synapse 1:347.

Conti, F., Rustioni, A., Petrusz, P. and Towle, A.C. (1987) Glutamate positive neurons in the somatic sensory cortex of rats and monkeys. J.Neurosci. 7: 1987.

Crow, T.J. (1987) The dopamine hypothesis survives but there must be a way ahead. Brit.J.Psychiat. 151:460.

Descarries, L., Lemay, B., Doucet, G. and Berger, B. (1987) Regional and laminar density of the dopamine innervation in adult rat cerebral cortex. Neuroscience 21:807.

Deutch, A.Y., Goldstein, M., Baldino, F. and Roth, R.H. (1988) Telencephalic projections of the A8 dopamine cell group. In "The Mesocorticolimbic dopamine system." Ann. N.Y. Acad. of Sci. 537:27.

Deutsch, S.I., Mastropaolo, J.B., Schwartz, L., Rosse, R.B. and Morihisa, J.M. (1989) A glutamatergic hypothesis of schizophrenia: Rationale for pharmacotherapy with glycine. Clin.Neuropharmacol. 12:1.

Drebing, C., Nagamato, H., Bickford-Wimer, P. and Franks, R. (1987) Neurobiological studies of sensory gating in schizophrenia. Schizophrenia 13:669.

Doran, A.R., Boronov, J., Weinberger, D.R., Wolkowitz, O.M., Breier, A. and Pickar D. (1987) Structural brain pathology in schizophrenia revisited. Neuropsychopharmacol. 1:25.

Febvret, A., Berger, B., Gaspar, P. and Verney, C. (1991) Further indication that distinct dopaminergic subsets project to the rat cerbral cortex: lack of colocalization with neurotensin in the superficial dopaminergic fields of the anterior cingulate, motor retrosplenial and visual cortices. Brain Res., in press.

Freedman, R., Adler, L.E., Gerhardt, G.A., Waldo, M., Baker, N., Rose, G.M., Friedman, D.P., Li, L. and Ungerleider, L.G. (1989) Origins of thalamic projections to layer I of the cerebral cortex of the monkey. Soc. Neurosci. Abstr. 15:311.

Gariano, R.F. and Groves, P.M., (1989) A mechanism for the involvement of colocalized neuropeptides in the actions of antipsychotic drugs, Biol. Psychiat., 26:303.

Gaspar, P., Berger, B., Febvret, A., Vigny, A. and Henry J.P. (1989) Catecholaminergic innervation of the human cerebral cortex as revealed by comparative immunohistochemistry of tyrosine hydroxylase and dopamine-beta-hydroxylase. J. Comp. Neurol. 279:249.

Gaspar, P., Berger, B. and Febvret A. (1990) Neurotensin innervation of the human cerebral cortex: lack of colocalization with catecholamines, Brain Research, in press.

Girault, J.A., Raisman, R., Agid, Y. and Greengard, P. (1989) Striatal phosphoproteins in Parkinson disease and progressive supranuclear palsy. Proc. Nat. Acad. Sci. 86:2493.

Goldman, P.S. and Nauta, W.J.H. (1977) Columnar distribution of cortico-cortical fibers in the frontal association, limbic and motor cortex of the developing rhesus monkey. Brain Res. 122:393.

Goldman-Rakic, P.S., Leranth, C., and Williams, S.M. (1989) Dopamine synaptic complex on pyramidal neurons in primate cerebral cortex. Proc. Nat. Acad. Sci. 86:9015 .

Goldman-Rakic, P.S., Lidow, M.S., and Gallager, D.W. (1990) Overlap of dopaminergic, adrenergic and serotonergic receptors and complementarity of their subtypes in primate prefrontal cortex. J. Neurosci. 10:2125.

Halliday, G.M. and Törk, I. (1986) Comparative anatomy of the ventromedial mesencephalic tegmentum in the rat, cat, monkey and human. J. Comp. Neurol. 252:423.

Halpain, S., Girault, J.A., Zorn, S. and Greengard, P. (1989) NMDA receptor activation regulates the phosphory-lation state of DARPP-32. Soc. Neurosci. Abs. 15:533.

Hemmings, H.C. Jr, Walaas, S.I., Ouimet, C.C. and Greengard, P. (1987) Dopaminergic regulation of protein phosphorylation in the striatum: DARPP-32. T.I.N.S. 10:377.

Hetey, L., Berg, R. and Schlesinger, T. (1987) Characterization of synaptosomal dopamine uptake in postmortem brain regions of schizophrenics. Neurochem. Pathol. 7:221.

Hirsch, E., Graybiel, A.M. and Agid, Y. (1988) Melanized dopaminergic neurons are differentially susceptible to degeneration in Parkinson's disease. Nature 334:345.

Hofman, M.A. (1988) Size and shape of the cerebral cortex in mammals. II. The cortical volume. Brain. Behav. Evol. 32:17.

Jackson, D.M., Ross, S.B. and Larsson, L.G. (1989) Dopamine D-2 receptor agonist induced behavioural depression: critical dependence upon postsynaptic dopamine D-1 function. A behavioural and biochemical study. N.S. Arch. Pharmacol. 340:355.

Jones, E.G. and Wise, S.P. (1977) Size, laminar and columnar distribution of efferent cells in the sensory-motor cortex of monkeys. J. Comp. Neurol. 175:391.

Kalsbeek, A., Voorn, P., Buijs, R.M., Pool, C.W. and Uylings, H.B.M. (1988) Development of the dopaminergic innervation in the prefrontal cortex of the rat. J. Comp. Neurol. 269:58.

Karoum, F., Karson, C.N., Bigelow, L.B., Lawson, W.B. and Wyatt, R.J. (1987) Preliminary evidence of reduced combined output of dopamine and its metabolites in chronic schizophrenia. Arch. Gen. Psychiat. 44:604.

Kerwin, R.W., Patel, S., Meldrum, B.S., Czudek, C. and Reynolds, G.P. (1988) Asymmetrical loss of glutamate receptor subtype in left hippocampus in schizophrenia. The Lancet 583.

Leichnetz, G.R. (1986) Afferent and efferent connections of the dorsolateral precentral gyrus (area 4, hand/arm region) in the macaque monkey, with comparison to area 8. J. Comp. Neurol. 254:460.

Lewis, D.A. and Morrison, J.H. (1989) Noradrenergic innervation of monkey prefrontal cortex: a dopamine-beta-hydroxylase immunohistochemical study. J. Comp. Neurol. 282:317.

Lewis, D.A., Morrison, J.H. and Goldstein, M. (1989) Brainstem dopaminergic neurons project to monkey parietal cortex. Neurosc. Letters 86:11.

Lewis, D.A., Campbell, M.J., Foote, S.L., Goldstein, M. and Morrison, J.H.(1987) The distribution of tyrosine hydroxylase immunoreactive fibers in primate neocortex is widespread but regionally specific. J. Neurosci.7:279.

Lewis, D.A., Foote, S.L., Goldstein, M. and Morrison, J.H. (1988) The dopaminergic innervation of monkey prefrontal cortex: a tyrosine hydroxylase immunohistochemical study. Brain Res. 449:225.

Lidow, M.S., Goldman-Rakic, P.S., Gallager, D.W., Geschwind, D.H. and Rakic, P. (1989) Distribution of major neurotransmitter receptors in the motor and somatosensory cortex of the rhesus monkey. Neuroscience 32:609.

Longoni, R., Spina, L. and Di Chiara, G. (1987) Permissive role of D-1 receptor stimulation for the expression of D-2 mediated behavioral responses: a quantitative phenomenological study in rats. Life Sci. 41:2135.

Noack, H.J. and Lewis, D.A. (1989) Antibodies directed against tyrosine hydroxylase differentially recognize noradrenergic axons in monkey neocortex. Brain Res. 500:313.

Oke, A.F., Adams, R.N., Winblad, B. and von Knorring, L. (1988) Elevated dopamine/norepinephrine ratios in thalami of schizophrenic brains. Biol. Psychiat. 24:79.

Ouimet, C.C., Miller, P.E., Hemmings, H.C. Jr, Walaas, S.I. and Greengard, P. (1984) DARPP-32, a dopamine- and adenosine 3':5'-monophosphate- regulated phosphoprotein enriched in dopamine-innervated brain regions III. Immunocytochemical localization. J. Neurosci. 4:111.

Palacios, M., Savasta, M., and Mengod, G. (1989) Does cholecystokinin colocalize with dopamine in the human substantia nigra? Brain Research 488: 369.

Papadopoulos, G.C., Parnavelas, J.G., and Buijs, R.M. (1989) Light and electron microscopic immunocytochemical analysis of the dopamine innervation of the rat visual cortex. J. Neurocytol. 18:303.

Peng, R.Y., Mansbach, R.S., Braff, D.L. and Geyer, M.A. (1990) A D2 dopamine receptor agonist disrupts sensorimotor gating in rats. Implications for dopaminergic abnormalities in schizophrenia. Neuropsychopharmacol. 3:211.

Phillipson, O.T., Kilpatrick, I.C. and Jones, M.W. (1986) Dopaminergic innervation of the primary visual cortex in the rat and some correlations with human cortex. Brain Res. Bull. 18:621.

Porrino, L.J. and Goldman-Rakic, P.S. (1982) Brainstem innervation of prefrontal and anterior cingulate cortex in the rhesus monkey revealed by retrograde transport of HRP. J. Comp. Neurol. 205:63.

Reynolds, G.P. (1989) Beyond the dopamine hypothesis. The neurochemical pathology of schizophrenia. Brit. J. Psychiatry. 155:305.

Richfield, E.K., A.B.Young and J.B.Penney (1989) Comparative distributions of dopamine D-1 and D-2 receptors in the cerebral cortex of rats, cats and monkeys. J. Comp. Neurol. 286:409.

Roberts, G.W. and Crow, T.J.(1987) The neuropathology of schizophrenia, a progress report. Brit. Med. Bull. 43:599.

Sawaguchi, T., Matsumura, M. and Kubota, K. (1986) Catecholamine sensitivities of motor cortical neurons of the monkey. Neurosci. Letters, 66:135.

Schalling, M., Friberg, K., Bird, E., Goldstein, M., Schiffmann, S., Mailleux, P., Vanderhaeghen, J.J. and Hökfelt, T. (1989) Presence of cholecystokinin mRNA in dopamine cells in the ventral mesencephalon of a human with schizophrenia, Acta Physiol. Scand. 137:467.

Selemon, L.D. and Goldman-Rakic, P.S. (1988) Common cortical and subcortical targets of the dorsolateral prefrontal and posterior parietal cortices in the rhesus monkey: evidence for a distributed neural network subserving spatially guided behaviour. J. Neurosci. 8:4049.

Seroogy, K.B, Ceccatelli, S., Schalling, M., Hökfelt, T., Frey, P., Walsh, J., Dockray, G., Brown, J., Buchan, A. and Goldstein, M. (1988) A subpopulation of dopaminergic neurons in rat ventral mesencephalon contains both NT and CCK, Brain Research, 455:88.

Sokoloff, P., Giros, B., Martres, M-P., Bouthenet, M-L. and Schwartz, J-C. (1990) Molecular cloning and characterization of a novel dopamine receptor (D3) as a target for neuroleptics. Nature 347:146.

Studler, J.M., Kitabgi, P., Tramu, G., Herve, D., Glowinski, J., and Tassin, J.P. (1988) Extensive coloca-lization of neurotensin with dopamine in rat mesocortico-frontal dopaminergic neurons, Neuropeptides, 11:95.

Van Eden, C.G., Hoorneman, E.M.D., Buijs, R.M., Matthissen, M.A.H., Geffard, M. and Uylings, H.B.M. (1987) Immunocytochemical localization of dopamine in the prefrontal cortex of the rat at the light and electron microscopical level. Neuroscience 22:849.

Verney, C., Gaspar, P., Febvret, A., Berger, B. (1988) Transient tyrosine hydroxylase-like immunoreactive neurons contain somatostatin and substance P in the developing amygdala and bed nucleus of the stria terminalis of the rat. Develop. Brain Res. 42:45.

Verney, C., Alvarez,C., Geffard, M. and Berger, B. (1990) Ultrastructural double labeling study of dopamine terminals and GABA-containing neurons in rat anteromedial cerebral cortex. The Europ. J. Neurosci. (in press)

Verney, C., Berger, B., Adrien, J., Vigny, A. and Gay, M. (1982) Development of the dopaminergic innervation of the rat cerebral cortex. A light microscopic immunocytochemical study using antityrosine hydroxylase antibodies. Dev. Brain Res. 5:41.

Walters, J.R., Bergstrom, D.A., Carlson, J.H., Chase, T.N. and Braun, A.R. (1987) D1 dopamine receptor activaion required for postsynaptic expression of D2 agonist effects. Science 236:719.

Wiesendanger, M. (1986) Recent developments in studies of the supplementary motor area of primates. Rev. Physiol. Biochem. Pharmacol. 103:1.

Wise, S.P. (1985) The primate premotor cortex: past, present and preparatory. Ann. Rev. Neurosci. 8:1.

White, F.J., Bednarz, L.M., Wachtel, S.R., Hjorth, S. and Brooderson, R.J. (1988) Is stimulation of both D1 and D2 dopamine receptors necessary for the expression of dopamine-mediated behaviors? Pharmacol. Biochem. Behav. 30:189.

CLINICAL AND NEURODEVELOPMENTAL ASPECTS OF BRAIN PATHOLOGY IN SCHIZOPHRENIA

Bernhard Bogerts and Peter Falkai

Department of Psychiatry
University of Düsseldorf
Düsseldorf, Germany

INTRODUCTION

After the failure of classical neuropathological schizophrenia research to convincingly demonstrate anatomical anomalies in the brains of schizophrenics, a new era of pathomorphological interest in schizophrenia started some 10 years ago. It received strong impetus from modern neuroimaging techniques such as computed tomography (CT), magnetic resonance imaging (MRI), positron emission tomography (PET), single photon emission computed tomography (SPECT), and regional cerebral blood flow (rCBF) studies as well as from new morphometric post mortem methods.

Recent interest in the structural and functional neuroanatomy of schizophrenia has focused on several brain regions: (1) the limbic system with its important telencephalic components comprising the medial temporal lobe structures and the cingulate gyrus, (2) the prefrontal cortex, which roughly consists of frontal cortical areas anterior to the level of the genu of the corpus callosum, (3) the basal ganglia, most importantly the globus pallidus, (4) the corpus callosum, (5) the thalamus with its limbic components, that is the mediodorsal and the anterior thalamic nucleus, and (6) the cerebral ventricles. An increasing number of neuroimaging and postmortem studies show that the type of the psychopathology of the disease may depend, at least in part, on the affected brain region. Moreover, different types of etiologies may account for the structural changes.

The purpose of this article is to review (A) the more recent literature on the clinical-anatomical relationships in schizophrenic diseases, and (B) the neuromorphological studies which address the question of the etiology of the structural brain changes.

Developmental Neuropathology of Schizophrenia
Edited by S.A. Mednick *et al.*, Plenum Press, New York, 1991

PSYCHOPATHOLOGICAL-ANATOMICAL CORRELATIONS

Temporolimbic Structures: Interest in the medial temporal and related limbic structures was raised by post mortem brain studies demonstrating neuroanatomical anomalies in the hippocampus, amygdala, entorhinal cortex, parahippocampal and cingulate gyri in a substantial proportion of schizophrenics (Bogerts, 1984, 1985; Kovelman and Scheibel 1984; Brown, Colter, Corsellis, Crow, Frith, Jagoe, Johnstone, & Marsh, 1986; Falkai and Bogerts, 1986; Jakob and Beckmann, 1986; Benes, 1987; Falkai, Bogerts, & Rozumek, 1988a; Jeste and Lohr, 1989; Altshuler, Casanova, Goldberg, & Kleinman, 1990). Several MRI scan studies of temporal lobe structures (DeLisi, Dauphinais, & Gershon, 1988, Suddath, Casanova, Goldber, Daniel, Kelsoe, & Weinberger, 1989, Rossi, Stratta, D'Albenzio, Tartaro, Schiazza, di Michele, Bolino, & Casacchia, 1990; Johnstone, Owens, Crow, Frith, Alexandropolis, Bydder, & Colter, 1989; Bogerts, Ashtari, Degreef, Alvir, Bilder, & Lieberman, 1990a) are consistent with these post mortem findings. Three studies investigating the medial temporal lobe reported negative results (Christison, Casanova, Weinberger, Rawlings, & Kleinman, 1989; Heckers, Heinsen, Heinsen & Béckmann, 1990a, 1990b). The latter study was based on very old cases, a fact which might explains the negative result.

Additional support for the assumption that temporolimbic pathology can cause schizophrenia-like symptoms comes from autopsy reports of organic brain diseases mimicking schizophrenia. Viral infections with high affinity to the medial temporal lobe (e.g., herpes simplex encephalitis, rabies) often produce in the initial stages of the disease severe emotional symptoms of fear, aggression, anxiety, irritability, periods of apathy or restlessness, over-attention to external stimuli, distractibility, inappropriate sexual behavior and even paranoid symptoms and hallucinations (Greenwood, Bhalla, Gordon, & Roberts, 1983). The same symptoms can be caused by medial temporal lobe tumors, infarctions, traumas (Mulder and Daly, 1952; Davison and Bagley, 1969; Malamud, 1967; Hillbom, 1951) and temporal lobe epilepsy, especially if the lesion is on the left side (Flor-Henry, 1969). At least in the initial stages, such organic brain diseases are frequently misdiagnosed as schizophrenia.

In view of the recent progress in the neuroanatomy and neurophysiology of the limbic system, some authors have linked theoretically temporo-limbic pathology, especially dysfunction of the hippocampal formation and entorhinal cortex, to the so-called positive symptoms of schizophrenia such as delusions, hallucinations and paranoid symptoms (Bogerts, 1989, 1991; Luchins, 1990). Direct evidence linking limbic pathology to typical schizophrenic symptoms was provided by some CT scan, MRI and SPECT investigations. As of now, we know of six studies which analyzed in living patients, morphometrically or functionally, several brain regions including the temporolimbic areas relating the anatomical changes to the psychopathology:

(1) Besson, Corrigan, & Cherryman (1987) examined ventricular size and

regional spin lattice relaxation time (T1) changes in MRI scans of 23 chronic schizophrenics (15 controls). Patients with high positive symptom scores had significantly increased T1 in the left medial temporal structures, while schizophrenics with high negative symptoms (social withdrawal, apathy, anhedonia, lack of drive and initiative) had significant higher signal intensity in the left frontal region.

(2) In a CT scan study of nine schizophrenics (nine controls) McCarley, Faux, Shenton, LeMay, Cane, Ballinger, & Duffy (1989) reported that positive symptoms correlate with left Silvian fissure enlargement, while negative symptoms correlate with right Silvian fissure size. Since Silvian fissure enlargement mainly indicates temporal brain tissue reduction, this finding points towards left temporal lobe dysfunction in positive schizophrenia, whereas right temporal pathology is associated with negative symptoms.

(3) The most detailed in vivo study of clinical-anatomical correlations in schizophrenia has recently been performed by Degreef, Ashtari, Bogerts, Bilder, Jody, Alvir, & Lieberman (1991). Using a high resolution MRI system, different components of the ventricular system of 40 first episode schizophrenics (25 controls) were related to negative and positive symptoms. To determine that the structural changes were not secondary to the treatment or the chronicity of the disease itself MR scans were obtained at the beginning of the disease and before the patients had received substantial neuroleptic medication. Psychopathology in patients was measured prior to treatment by the SANS scale for negative symptoms and the SADS-PD scale for positive symptoms. The most consistent and highly significant correlations between psychotic symptoms and ventricular enlargement were seen in the anterior and posterior temporal horn. The positive symptoms correlated significantly only with left posterior temporal horn enlargement. The negative symptoms correlated with right and left, anterior and posterior temporal horn enlargement. This study revealed that there is a much higher association of a broad range of typical positive and negative schizophrenic symptoms with temporo--limbic than with frontal, parieto-occipital, diencephalic or cerebellar components of the ventricular system.

The posterior temporal horn is surrounded by hippocampus and white matter containing afferent and efferent fibers to the parahippocampal gyrus. The anterior temporal horn is surrounded by amygdala and anterior hippocampus and fibers from and to the anterior temporal lobe structures. Since ventricular enlargement in many brain diseases is related to dysfunction of the surrounding brain structures, the data of this study suggest left hippocampal and parahippocampal dysfunction involvement in the pathogenesis of positive symptoms, whereas more general right and left medial temporal lobe dysfunction contributes to the development of negative symptoms.

(4) In a SPECT study, Anderson, Gordon, Rennie, & Meares (1990) examined six patients with and four patients without a history of hallucinations. A statistical evaluation of selected areas of interest (frontal, temporal, basal ganglia) to cerebellum ratios revealed no hypofrontality in any subject. Five subjects

demonstrated left temporal hypoperfusion, all of these patients currently experienced auditory hallucinations. None of the non-hallucinators had temporal hypoperfusion.

(5) To investigate to which extent different brain regions as visualized by computed tomography can be related to positive and negative schizophrenic symptoms, we measured the CSF spaces of various brain parts of 79 female schizophrenics which had during the whole course of the disease predominant positive (n=48), mixed (n=22) or negative (n=9) symptoms (Bogerts, Falkai, Degreef, & Lieberman, 1991). In each patient, the size of all clearly visible cortical sulci and fissures, the VBR, the maximal area of the temporal horn, and the maximal diameter of the third ventricle was measured planimetrically. There were no significant differences in VBR and third ventricle between the patients with positive and those with negative symptoms. Patients with negative symptoms tended to have larger frontal and parieto-occipital cortical sulci and had significantly larger interhemispheric fissures than the patients with positive symptoms. Compared to the negative schizophrenics, patients with positive symptoms showed a trend towards larger Silvian fissures and, more interestingly, they had a highly significantly larger left temporal horn (by 73%) but no significant enlargement of the right temporal horn. Although obtained by the relatively poor resolution of CT scan technology, the results demonstrate an association between temporal lobe pathology and positive schizophrenic symptoms. In particular, left temporolimbic pathology as indicated by left temporal horn enlargement, was most impressively associated with positive symptoms.

(6) In a recent MRI scan study of 15 young schizophrenics (15 controls) Barta, Pearlson, Powers, Richards, & Tune (1990) found a bilateral reduction of the whole temporal lobe, the amygdala and superior temporal gyrus. Shrinkage of the left superior temporal gyrus was strongly and selectively correlated with the severity of auditory hallucinations.

Summarizing these in vivo studies of neuroanatomical-psychopathological correlates, the most consistent finding to date is an association between left temporolimbic pathology and positive symptoms, whereas negative symptoms are probably associated with more diffuse structural brain changes.

Prefrontal Cortex: Prefrontal cortical dysfunction in schizophrenia has mainly been indicated by various functional brain studies such as regional cerebral blood flow studies (rCBF), positron emission tomography (PET), and single photon emission computerized tomography (SPECT) (Ingvar and Franzen, 1974, Buchsbaum, Ingvar, & Kessler, 1982; Buchsbaum, DeLisi, & Holcomb, 1984; Weinberger, Berman, & Zec, 1986; Geraud, Arne-Bes, Guell, & Bes, 1987). Several groups, however, have not observed this "hypofrontality", particularly not in acute onset medication free patients in which usually positive symptoms predominate (Mathew, Barr, Weinman, & Barr, 1982; Mathew, Wilson, Tant, Robinson, & Prakash, 1988; Sheppard, Gruzelier, Manchanda, & Hirsch, 1983; Kling, Metter, & Riege, 1986;

Gur, Resnick, & Alavi, 1987a; Gur, Resnick, & Gur, 1987b; Early, Reimann, & Raichle, 1987).

It is questionable whether the functional abnormalities observed in the frontal cortex of schizophrenics by rCBF, PET, and SPECT are associated with gross structural abnormalities. In the two first planimetric MR scan studies of the frontal brain of schizophrenics, reduced midsagittal (Andreasen et al., 1986) or horizontal (DeMyer, Gilmor, Hendrie, DeMyer, Augustyn, & Jackson, 1988) frontal lobe areas were described, but the differences to the controls disappeared after adjustment for educational level. In four subsequent investigations of frontal lobe volumes (Kelsoe et al., 1988; Suddath,Casanova, Goldber, Daniel, Kelsoe, & Weinberger, 1989; Suddath, Christison, Torrey, Casanova, & Weinberger, 1990) or frontal midsagittal areas (Andreasen, Swayze, Falum, Yates, Arndt, & McChesney, 1990b) no differences to controls were detected. There is, however, one histological study of three frontal cortical areas of schizophrenics (Benes, Davidson, & Bird, 1986) reporting reduced neuronal densities and subtle cytoarchitectural changes, and, in our above mentioned CT scan study, the frontal portions of the interhemispheric fissure were in negative schizophrenics significantly larger than in the positive symptom group.

There is evidence from some of the perfusion studies (Ingvar and Franzen, 1974; Warkentin, Nilsson, & Risberg, 1990), but also from animal experiments and organic brain diseases (for review see Kirkpatrick and Buchanan, 1990; Bogerts et al., 1991), that prefrontal cortical hypofunction is related to the so called negative schizophrenic symptoms (such as social withdrawal, apathy, anhedonia, lack of drive and initiative). Vice versa, hyperperfusion of frontal cortical areas was found during acute exacerbation of positive symptoms (Szechtman, Nahmias, & Garnett, 1988; Warkentin et al., 1990).

Reduced activity of the frontal lobes could well explain some psychopathological aspects of negative schizophrenia. Frontal lobe syndromes caused by brain tumors, injuries, lobotomy or Pick's disease are characterized by apathy, loss of drive, inappropriate affect, social withdrawal or disinhibition, poor judgement and psychomotor retardation. Many of these symptoms are commonly seen in patients with negative schizophrenia. Alternatively, it is conceivable that hypofrontality could be caused by other factors such as chronic neuroleptic treatment.

Globus Pallidus: Structural and functional disturbances of the globus pallidus have been reported by some post mortem and PET studies (Hopf, 1952; Stevens, 1982, 1986; Bogerts, 1984, 1985; Early et al., 1987; Luchins et al., 1989). Preliminary data from qualitative (Hopf, 1952; Stevens, 1982) and quantitative post mortem studies (Bogerts, Falkai, & Tutsch, 1986; Stevens 1986) and from brain perfusion studies (Early et al., 1987; Luchins, Metz, Marks, & Cooper, 1989) indicate that pallidal dysfunction occurs mainly in catatonic schizophrenics.

Catatonia is characterized by abnormal movements combined with positive as well as with negative symptoms. The external and internal pallidum, which are regarded to be parts of the extrapyramidal and limbic system (Mesulam, 1986), are involved in the neuronal modulation of movement coordination and emotional reactions. It is, therefore, conceivable that dysfunction of this brain part plays a role in the pathogenesis of catatonic symptoms.

Corpus Callosum: Structural anomalies of the midline area of the corpus callosum were demonstrated by several MRI scan and post mortem investigations (Nasrallah, Andreasen, Coffman, Olson, Dunn, Ehrhardt, & Chapman, 1986; Raine, Harrison, Reynolds, Sheard, Cooper, & Medley, 1990; Mathew, Partain, Prakash, Kulkarni, Logan, & Wilson, 1985, Uematsu and Kaiya, 1988; Rossi, Stratta, Gallucci, Passarellio, & Cassachia, 1989; Rosenthal and Bigelow, 1972, Bogerts, Lesch, Lange, Zech, & Tutsch, 1983). The findings, however, are inconsistent; there are reports of increased (Rosenthal and Bigelow, 1972) as well as of decreased (Bogerts et al., 1983; Rossi et al., 1989) midline areas. More consistent are reports of shape abnormalities (Nasrallah et al., 1986; Raine et al., 1990), in that the sex difference in anterior and posterior callosal thickness in normal controls seems to be reversed in schizophrenics, with the corpus callosum being thicker in female schizophrenics and thinner in male schizophrenics. We found one investigation correlating the size of the corpus callosum to schizophrenic symptoms: investigating midsagittal MRI scans of 31 schizophrenics (31 controls), Günther, (1990) reported significantly larger corpus callosum areas in patients with predominant positive symptoms as compared to patients with predominant negative symptoms.

Thalamus: Cell loss and reduced tissue volume of medial thalamic structures have already been described several decades ago (Fünfgeld, 1925; Bäumer, 1954; Treff and Hempel, 1958). Although two studies investigating of the same brain material (Dom, de Saedeler, Bogerts, & Hopf, 1981; Lesch and Bogerts, 1984) failed to fully replicate these findings, one recent investigation (Pakkenberg, 1990) using different brain collections again found volume and cell number reductions similar to those reported in the original studies.

If thalamic dysfunction caused schizophrenia-like symptoms, as assumed by some authors (Leonhard 1952; Huber 1957; Gross and Huber, 1972), such symptomatology might be expected in patients with known organic diseases of the thalamus. In the quite extensive literature on organic lesions of the thalamus and the diencephalon, clinical symptoms such as apathy, drowsiness, mental lethargy, stuporous conditions, disturbances of memory, and sensory phenomena such as hypesthesia, hyperpathia, and painful perceptions are described as being most characteristic (for review see Lesch and Bogerts, 1984). Positive psychotic symptoms usually do not occur. Thus, clinical symptoms associated with dysfunction of the thalamus resemble the negative symptoms of schizophrenia. This assumption is supported by the observation that in CT scans of schizophrenics third ventricular enlargement (possibly indicating atrophy of the surrounding thalamus) occurs in patients with chronic negative symptoms (Gross, Huber, & Schuttler, 1982).

Cerebral Ventricles, CT Scan Studies: In addition to the above mentioned studies, a large number of CT scan studies addressed the question of relations between brain morphology and clinical pictures of schizophrenia. Many but not all CT scan studies found that enlargement of lateral and third ventricles, widening of cortical sulci and fissures, is associated with various clinical symptoms such as poor premorbid adjustment, negative or positive symptoms, poor response to neuroleptic treatment, cognitive impairment and unfavorable outcome. (Shelton and Weinberger, 1986; Marks and Luchins, 1990).

Although the statistical power of most of these studies is sufficient since large sample sizes were used, the value of the clinical-anatomical correlations of computed tomography studies is limited. Nearly all CT studies assessed quantitatively the lateral ventricles on one standardized horizontal level (VBR, ventricles to brain ratio, i.e., the area of the lateral ventricles at their maximal extent expressed as a percent of the whole brain area at this level) or qualitatively or semiquantitatively the cerebral cortex as a whole. With CT, assessments of gross anatomical structures only are possible. Increased VBR or "cortical atrophy" means that there is a lack of tissue somewhere in the hemispheres without localizing it in a specific brain region. Since visualization of smaller brain structures by computerized tomography is limited because of its poor resolution and poor white/gray matter contrasts, separate evaluation of right and left cortical, basal ganglia or limbic areas, which are now considered to play an important role in the pathophysiology of positive and negative schizophrenic symptoms, generally have not been performed by computed tomography.

Clinical-Anatomical Correlations in Postmortem Studies

Investigations of clinical-anatomical relationships using postmortem brain material are much more problematic than the in vivo studies, since postmortem brains are usually from patients which were chronically hospitalized and had during the long course of their disease alternating periods of various schizophrenic symptoms. Most neuropathological investigations were performed in relatively old brain collections (Vogt-collection, Düsseldorf; Yakovlev-collection, Washington; Runwell collection, UK) and, therefore, retrospective assessment of patients' psychopathology by modern rating scales was difficult. However, several of the post mortem studies reported some preliminary correlations between brain morphology and clinical symptoms. In the Vogt-collection, patients which were characterized in the extensive and well preserved clinical records as having predominant paranoid and hallucinatory symptoms had the focus of pathology in the medial temporal lobe, whereas patients with predominant catatonic symptoms had more basal ganglia pathology (Stevens, 1986; Bogerts et al., 1986). Cytoarchitectural changes in the limbic allocortex have been reported to occur more frequently in hebephrenic than in paranoid patients (Jakob and Beckmann, 1986). In a qualitative study of gliosis and cell loss, Stevens (1982) found a relationship between periventricular, limbic, or hypothalamic pathology and assaultive behavior, flat affect, catatonia, and seclusiveness; disturbances of speech were associated with pathologic changes in the globus pallium; stereotypy was associated with hypothalamic and hippocampal anomalies. Because identical sections from each of these regions were not available in every case, statistical tests of these suggestive correlations could not be performed.

Investigating morphometrically postmortem brains of schizophrenics, Pakkenberg (1987) found that patients with prevailing negative symptoms had significantly larger ventricles than patients with predominant positive symptoms.

In a comprehensive semiquantitative neuropathological study, Bruton, Crow, Frith, Johnstone, Owens, & Roberts (1990) found a significant association between both brain weight and brain length with premorbid function in that the poorer the function the lighter and shorter the brain.

<u>General Comment on the Studies in Clinical-Anatomical Correlations in Schizophrenia</u>

The pathomorphological changes in schizophrenia are subtle and not comparable in magnitude to the brain tissue loss seen in the well known degenerative brain disorders. The changes cannot be seen in all schizophrenic patients. There is a considerable overlap between patients and healthy controls and, morphometrically, only a minority (some 20-30%) have values below the range of matched healthy control cases. As shown below, an additional difference (Mc Kenna and Tandon 1990) in the brains of schizophrenics with neurodegenerative disorders is that, at least in most patients, the structural changes are not progressive and probably were acquired very early in life (Weinberger, 1987; Bogerts 1989, 1990).

Another problem in relating the pathomorphological findings of the post mortem, CT, and MRI scan studies with the clinical subtypes of schizophrenia is that different types of symptoms (e.g. positive and negative symptoms, catatonic behavior and hallucinations) can occur simultaneously or in alternating periods in the same patient. The reported neuroanatomical changes, however, are believed to be stable over time and are not as mutable as the psychopathology. One answer to this problem is that the neuroanatomical findings can be considered as only one component of many pathophysiological and psychosocial factors which contribute to the clinical picture of schizophrenia. There are convincing arguments linking positive and negative psychotic symptoms to biochemical factors, such as an imbalance of cerebral dopaminergic (Meltzer and Stahl, 1976; McKenna,1987), cholinergic (Tandon and Greden, 1990), mechanisms. Moreover, the role of psychosocial factors, e.g., stress, in precipitating acute psychotic symptoms (Zubin and Spring, 1977; Curran and Cirelli, 1988) and the consequences of long term hospitalization and social depravation for the development of syndromes similar to negative schizophrenia are well known.

We believe that the various types of structural abnormalities in the brains of schizophrenics are vulnerability or trait markers, which predispose the brain to decompensate under the influence of additional neurochemical or psychosocial stressors, thus developing the typical clinical pictures of schizophrenia.

STUDIES ON THE ETIOLOGY OF THE STRUCTURAL CHANGES

The question on the etiology of the structural brain changes in schizophrenia was approached by several research strategies. Among these approaches, the search for a virus, genetic and family studies, as well as investigations of perinatal and pregnancy complications play a major role (Revely, 1987; Delisi, 1987; Gill, Taylor, & Murray, 1989). Five strategies based on morphological methods are currently applied: (1) Correlations of the structural changes with the disease duration, (2) Follow-up MRI and CT scan studies, (3) MRI and CT brain morphometry at the beginning of the disease, (4) post mortem investigations of the cortical architecture, and (5) investigations in glial cells.

CT and MRI Scan Studies

Although there are a few exceptions (Woods and Wolf, 1983; Kemali, Maj, and Galderisi, 1985; Woods, Yurgelun-Todd, Benes, Frankenburg, Pope, & McSparren, 1990), most of the CT scan studies found no correlation between ventricular or cortical sulcal enlargement and the disease duration (for review see Cannon et al. this volume) and no significant difference in ventricular size in follow-up studies (Nasrallah et al.,1986; Kemali et al., 1985; Illowski, Juliano, & Bigelow, 1988; Andreasen, Swayze, Flaum, Yates, Arndt, & McChesney, 1990b). However, there might be a small subgroup of chronic deteriorating patients which has a stepwise progressive ventricular enlargement (Woods et al., 1990). Nevertheless, the majority of CT scan studies support the view that brain pathology at least in the majority of schizophrenics is not progressive and probably predates the onset of the typical clinical symptoms. This is an important difference to the well known degenerative brain diseases such as Alzheimer's, Pick's, Parkinson's and Huntington's disease.

Ventricular enlargement and reduced temporolimbic structure volumes also have been observed in CT and MRI scans at the beginning of the disease before the patients had substantial amounts of neuroleptic drugs (Schulz, Koller, Kishore, Hamer, Gehl, & Friedel, 1983; Bogerts, 1990; Degreef et al., 1991).

Post Mortem Studies

In a recent article (Bogerts et al., 1991), we comprehensively reviewed the neuropathological studies which addressed the question of the etiology of the disease. In the present chapter, a summary of the publications reviewed in the previous article is shown in tables 1-3. The tables are completed by some most recent publications which were not included in the previous review (Crow, Ball, Bloom, Brown, Bruton, Colter, Frith, Johnstone, Owens, & Roberts, 1989; Bogerts, Falkai, Haupts, Greve, Ernst, Tapernon-Franz, & Heinzmann, et al., 1990b, Altshuler et al., 1990; Pakkenberg, 1990;. Bruton et al., 1990; Jeste and Lohr, 1989; Heckers et al., 1990a; 1990b).

We found 14 post mortem studies, the findings of which are consistent with a disorder of brain development (Table 1), six studies consistent with a disorder of an inflammatory or degenerative brain disease (Table 2), and 12 studies with no comment on the etiology of the disease (Table 3).

The reports consistent with a disorder of brain development describe:
- reduced temporolimbic (Bogerts et al., 1985; Falkai and Bogerts, 1986; Falkai et al., 1988a) as well as thalamic (Pakkenberg, 1990) structure volumes and nerve cell numbers without accompanying gliosis;
- cytoarchitectural anomalies in the hippocampal formation (McLardy, 1974; Scheibel and Kovelman, 1981; Kovelman and Scheibel, 1984; Altshuler, 1987), frontal cortex (Benes et al., 1986), cingulate gyrus (Benes, 1987), and entorhinal cortex (Jakob and Beckman, 1986; Falkai, Bogerts, & Rozumek, 1988; Falkai and Bogerts, 1989, Falkai and Bogerts, 1991);
- left lateralized temporal horn enlargement (Crow et al., 1989).

An important neurohistological indicator of a progressive degenerative or inflammatory brain disease is gliosis which means increased densities or absolute numbers of reactive glial cells, especially astrocytes. This has been described as occurring in mesiotemporal and periventricular structures (Nieto and Escobar, 1972; Stevens, 1982), in the corpus callosum (Nasrallah, McCalley-Whitters, & Rauscher, 1983a) and diffusely distributed in brains of schizophrenics [Bruton et al., 1990 (Table 2)].

If the reported structural anomalies reflect developmental disturbances, perinatal complications or inherited variations, one would not expect gliosis, since only pathological events occurring after the second trimester of pregnancy, e.g. viral infections, hypoxia or atrophic processes are associated with increased glial cell densities (Oyanagi, Yoshida, & Icuta, 1986; Larroche, 1984). The features of reactive gliosis change with age. Practically no residual gliosis is seen, even upon massive tissue destructions, during the first half of gestation. The capacity of astrocytes to react with proliferation and hypertrophy does not develop before the last trimester of gestation (Friede 1989).

Table 1. Findings consistent with a disorder of brain development

authors	number of patients (and controls)	method	findings
Mc Lardy (1974)	30 (7)	qualitative	reduced thickness of the granule cell layer in hippocampal formation without degeneration of appearance
Scheibel and Kovelman (1981)	10 (8)	qualitative	disorientation of hippocampal pyramidal cells
Bogerts et al. (1984,1985)	13 (10)	morphometric	reduced volumes of hippocampus, parahippocampal gyrus and amygdala (Vogt collection)
Kovelman and Scheibel (1984)	10 (8)	morphometric	disarray of hippocampal pyramidal cells
Benes et al. (1986,1987)	10 (10)	morphometric	reduced neuronal density without gliosis, cytoarchitectural disturbances in the prefrontal cortex, anterior cingulate and primary motor cortex
Falkai and Bogerts (1986)	13 (11)	morphometric	reduction of hippocampal pyramidal cells without gliosis
Jakob and Beckmann (1986)	64 (10)	qualitative	cytoarchitectonic abnormalities in the rostral entorhinal region, abnormal pattern of temporal sulci
Altshuler et al. (1987)	7 (6)	morphometric	correlation between hippocampal pyramidal cell and severity of clinical symptoms
Falkai et al. (1988a)	13 (11)	morphometric	lower volume and cell densities in the entorhinal cortex without gliosis
Falkai and Bogerts (1989)	11 (7)	morphometric	abnormal location of entorhinal pre-alpha cell clusters
Crow et al. (1989)	56 (56)	morphometric	selective left temporal horn enlargement found
Bogerts et al. (1990b)	18 (21)	morphometric	reduced hippocampal volume (new Düsseldorf collection)
Altshuler et al. (1990)	12 (27)	morphometric	reduced cross sectional area of parahippocampal gyrus but not hippocampus; shape abnormalities in medial temporal structures
Pakkenberg et al. (1990)	12 (12)	morphometric	reduction of total neuron and glial cell number in mediodorsal thalamic nucleus and nucleus accumbens

Table 2. Findings consistent with an inflammatory or degenerative brain disease

authors	number of patients (and controls)	method	findings
Nieto and Escobar (1972)	10(4)	qualitative	periventricular gliosis
Fisman (1975)	10(10)	qualitative	glial knots and pervascular infiltrations in the brainstem
Averback (1981)	13(35)	qualitative	cellular degeneration in the nucleus of the ansa lenticularis
Stevens (1982)	25(48)	qualitative	hypothalamic gliosis in the midbrain tegmentum, bed nucleus of the stria terminalis, basal nucleus, medial thalamus, amygdala and hippocampus.
Nasrallah et al. (1983a)	18(11)	qualitative	gliosis in the corpus callosum of late onset schizophrenics compared to early onset schizophrenia (anteriorly and posteriorly)
Bruton et al. (1990)	56(56)	qualitative	reduction of brain weight and brain length, increase of ventricular size, periventricular fibrous gliosis in half of the schizophrenic cases

All studies listed in Table 2 describing gliosis in brains of schizophrenics were performed by qualitative investigations. The major problem with these qualitative studies of gliosis is that they do not allow a quantitative-statistical comparison of glial cell densities. In six controlled quantitative studies (Falkai and Bogerts, 1986; Falkai et al., 1988a; Benes et al., 1987; Roberts, Colter, Lofthouse, Bogerts, Zech, & Crow, 1986; Roberts, Colter, Lofthouse, & Johnstone,, 1987; Casanova, Stevens, & Bigelow, 1988; Stevens and Casanova, 1988) no evidence of gliosis in the medial temporal lobe, cingulate gyrus or hypothalamic periventricular regions could be found. It has been argued that in some of these studies the applied densitometric methods for assessing GFAP (glial fibrillary acidic protein) levels were not sensitive enough to detect moderate degrees of gliosis (Casanova et al., 1987; Stevens and Casanova 1988). Moreover, all of these studies investigated relative small samples by which a moderate gliosis, if any, in subgroup of patients would not have been detected by the applied statistical tests.

We therefore performed, in our new Düsseldorf brain collection, a study on astrocyte densities in a larger sample size of schizophrenics and healthy controls. Astrocytes were stained with GFAP (Glial fibrillary astrocytic protein) in post-mortem brains of 20 chronic schizophrenic patients and 20 matched control cases.

Table 3. Studies with no comments on the etiology

authors	number of patients (and controls)	method	findings
Rosenthal and Bigelow (1972)	10(10)	morphometric	increase in corpus callosum width
Dom et al. (1981)	5(5)	morphometric	reduced microneuron density in the pulvinar of catatonic patients
Bogerts et al. (1983)	15(12)	morphometric	reduced volume of the lateral substantia nigra
Lesch and Bogerts (1984)	15(12)	morphometric	reduction of thickness of periventricular grey matter
Brown et al. (1986)	41(29)	morphometric	reduced thickness of parahippocampal cortex, temporal horn enlargement
Colter et al. (1987)	17(11)	morphometric	reduced parahippocampal white matter
Pakkenberg (1987)	29(30)	morphometric	volume reduction of both hemispheres, the cortex and subcortical white matter and brain weight, increased ventricular volume
Lohr and Jeste (1988)	15(15)	morphometric	reduced neuropil in the locus coeruleus
Jeste and Lohr (1989)	13(26)	morphometric	reduction of hippocampal volume and pyramidal cell numbers
Christison et al. (1989)	14(29)	morphometric	no disarray of hippocampal pyramidal cells
Heckers et al. (1990a)	20(20)	morphometric	unchanged volume of parahippocampal gyrus
Heckers et al. (1990b)	20(20)	morphometric	unchanged volume of hippocampus and amygdala

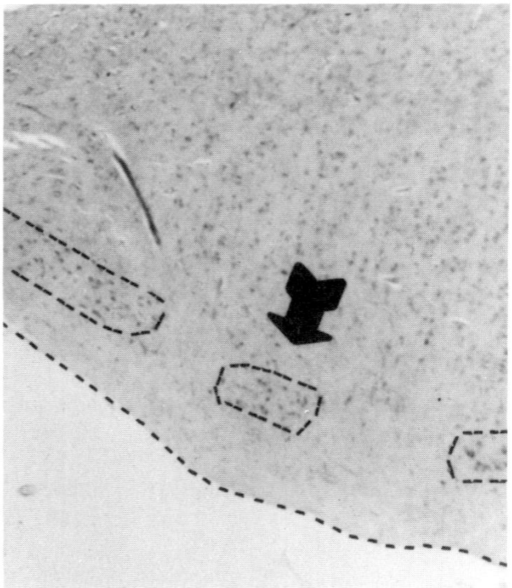

Figure 1A. Microphotography demonstrating the normal cytoarchitecture of the entorhinal cortex of a control subject (combined Nissl-Myelin-staining, x 40). The arrow indicates a pre-alpha-cell cluster with regular size and position.

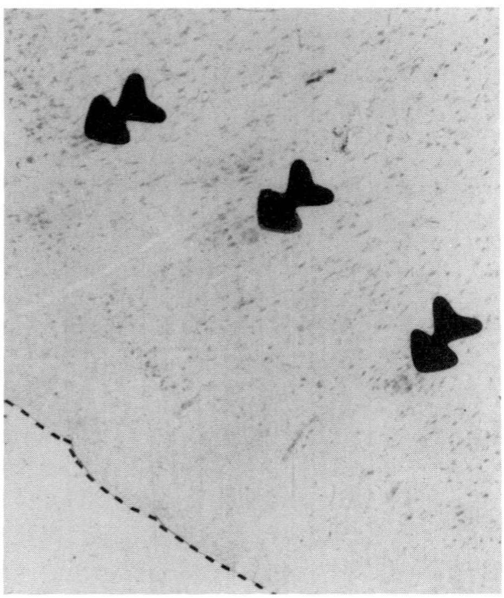

Figure 1B. Entorhinal cortex of a schizophrenic patient, matched for age and sex, with severe cytoarchitectural disturbances. Arrows indicate abnormally positioned pre-alpha-cell clusters.

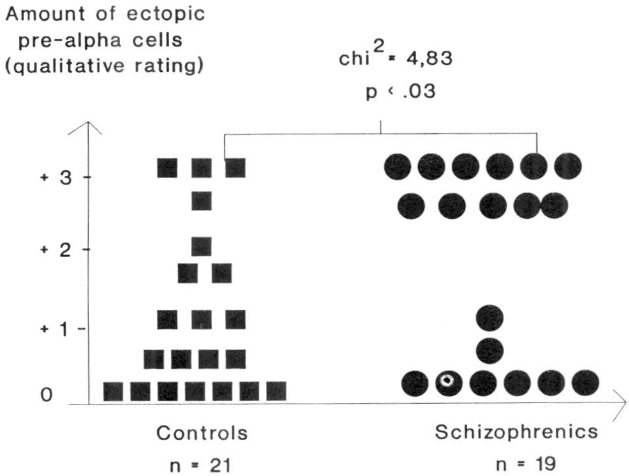

Figure 2. Distribution of heterotopic pre-alpha-cells in controls and schizophrenic patients.

From each brain, 20 micrometer coronal whole brain paraffin section were studied at three levels: (1) anterior commissure, (2) mammillary bodies and (3) posterior commissure. Using a light microscope at a magnification of 200x, GFAP-positive astrocytes were counted in the amygdaloid nucleus, mammillary bodies, medial thalamic nuclei, hypothalamic periventricular grey matter, hippocampus (CA4), and periaqueductal grey. The schizophrenic group revealed a moderate but significant increase in GFAP cell densities in the periventricular grey matter (+47%, $p<.02$), and the periaqueductal area (+39%, $p<.026$), and the right (+33%, $p<.05$) and left (+42%, $p<.01$) medial thalamic nucleus; whereas no significant gliosis could be observed in both amygdalae and hippocampi. As longstanding somatic diseases as well as vascular or senile changes were exclusion criteria, the increase in periventricular astrocyte densities was attributed to the disease itself or to its treatment. The extent of gliosis (mean increase in glial cell densities by 30-50%) was by far not as high as that observed in well known degenerative brain diseases. In the caudate of Huntington's disease, for example, a 10-fold increase in astrocyte densities can be seen (Stevens, 1988).

In order to determine whether in the same brain collection signs of a disturbed brain development could be detected, we assessed qualitatively the arrangment of pre-alpha cell clusters in the entorhinal cortex (Falkai and Bogerts, 1991). An abnormal position of these cell groups was described in two other brain collections (Jakob and Beckmann, 1986; Falkai and Bogerts, 1989) and interpreted as indicating a disturbance of cortical neuronal migration during the second trimester of pregnancy.

Table 4. Disorders of neuronal migration of the cortex causing severe mental handicap

name	cause	brain changes	physical anomalies	brain function
classical lissencephaly	unknown or autosom.-dom. perfusion failure	no or only a few abnormally broad gyri cortex abnormally thick, four layers subcortical heteroptopias	craniofacial	severe mental retardation
Miller-Dieker Syndrom	del (17) (p13.3)	see above	craniofacial and somatic	severe mental retardation
Walker-Warbur Malformation	meningo-encephalitis or autosom.-dom.	agyria, polymicrogyria, massive leptomeningeal glimesodermal proliferation obstructing the subarachnoid space, pyramidal tract anomalies, subcortical heterotopias	eye anomalies	severe mental retardation
Zellweger Syndrom	autosom.-rez. (peroxisomal deficiency)	abnormal gyral pattern bilaterally symmetrical in the centro-Sylvian region, thin five cortical layers, heterotopic cells distributed over the entire cortex	dysmorphic facies, changes in the ren and liver	rapid progressive course, death at 12-13 weeks

Table 5. Disorders of cortical neuronal migration causing circumscribed mental handicap

name	cause	brain changes	physical anomalies	brain function
Developmental Dyslexia focal dysplasias and ectopias in	unknown	symmetry of the planum temporale, anomalies, certain inferior frontal and left superior temporal regions	none	dyslexia, linguistic cognitive talents
Turners Syndrom	genetic (XO)	cortical dysplasia, white matter heterotopias, cerebellar malformations	none	mild mental retardation
Fragile-X-Syndrom	genetic	macrocephaly, white matter heterotopias	long face, large promi- ears, macro-orchidism, connective tissue, abnormalities	mental retardation
Temporal lobe epilepsy (in part)	unknown	10-15% of patients show an excess of large aberrant cells through all layers of the temporal cortex, occupying sharply delineated segments of the cortex	none	fits, psychotic episodes
Schizophrenia (in part)	unknown	50-60% of patients demonstrate an excess of heterotopic pre-alpha-cell clusters in a very circumscribed area of the entorhinal cortex	excess of minor physical anomalies	psychosis

Table 6. Examples for a congenital ventricular enlargement

name	cause	brain changes	physical abnormalities
Dandy-Walker-Syndrom	developmental anomaly before 3rd fetal month	exit in the foramina in the fourth ventricle are malformed or sealed complete or partial agenesis of the vermis, cystic dilatation of the fourth ventricle, enlarged posterior fossa with upward displacement of lateral sinuses, tentorium and torcular	enlarged head circumference bulging of the occiput
Arnold-Chiari-Malformation (type II)	developmental anomaly at the 10th fetal week	lengthening and downwards displacement of the vermis and tonsils of the cerebellum through the foramen magnum in the spinal canal	abnormally small occiptal bone

Brains of 19 schizophrenic patients were investigated. Only patients with well preserved and extensive clinical records were selected; all patients, including four patients with a late onset of the disease (> 40 years), fulfilled ICD-9 and DSM IIIr criteria for schizophrenia and were treated with neuroleptic drugs for most of their illness. Clinical symptoms, disease duration and cause of death of the patients were published recently (Bogerts, et al., 1990b). Brains from 21 age and sex matched subjects without history of neuropsychiatric disorders were taken as controls. The brains were cut into 20 microns thick whole brain coronal serial sections and then Nissl (cresylechtviolet)- and myelin (Heidenhain-Wölcke or luxol fast blue)-stained.

Abnormally positioned pre-alpha cell clusters were observed only in very small circumscribed area of the periamygdala region of the entorhinal cortex. The position of the cell clusters was rated semiquantitatively using the following grades: grade 0 meant no abnormal cell clusters; grade 1 meant one abnormal cluster; grade 2 meant two abnormal clusters; and grade 3 meant three or more abnormal cell clusters. Figure 1A shows the cytoarchitecture of a control subject with no heterotopic cell clusters (grade 0), Figure 1B gives an example of three or more ectopic cell clusters (grade 3) in a schizophrenic patient.

The results are shown in Figure 2. Sixteen of the 21 control subjects had no or one ectopic cluster, whereas eight of 19 schizophrenic patients had no or one ectopic cluster. On the other hand only five control subjects but 11 schizophrenics had a rating of grades 2 or 3. The difference between controls and schizophrenics was significant ($p < .05$, chi-square test). These aberrant heterotopic cells could only be found in the medial portion of the entorhinal cortex at the level of the anterior part of the amygdala. Abnormal pre-alpha cell clusters were seen in patients with and without a family history of the disease. Looking at the distribution of heterotopic pre-alpha cell clusters in the right and left hemisphere, it was found that seven schizophrenic patients and four control subjects had no hemispheric preference. However three schizophrenics had three or more clusters in the left entorhinal region, but only one patient revealed more than three clusters in the right hemisphere. One control subject had a predominance for the left hemisphere and none for the right.

Our most recent findings of a moderate periventricular gliosis and a mildly disturbed cytoarchitecture in a small region of the entorhinal cortex in the same brain collection is not entirely surprising. With regard to the many different clinical pictures of schizophrenia, different types of brain pathology and different types of etiologies can be expected. There might be a subgroup of patients which suffered from a mild brain damage during the last weeks of pregnancy, perinatally or later in life. A moderate degree of gliosis is consistent with this assumption. There might also be another group of patients which suffers from an early mild disorder of brain development; these are the patients which have the described cortical cytoarchitectural anomalies.

Besides schizophrenia, there are several other diseases of brain development which are associated with a disorder of cortical cell migration and/or ventricular enlargement. These diseases are summarized in tables 4 - 6. The difference in schizophrenia is that the morphological changes are more obvious and that the patients usually have severe and moderate mental handicaps (Dobyns, 1987; Stewart, Richman, & Caviness, 1975; Friede, 1989 a and b; Galaburda, Sherman, Rosen, Aboitiz, & Geschwind, 1985; Reske-Nielsen, Christensen, & Nielsen, 1982; Chudley & Hagerman, 1987; Bruton, 1988; Falkai and Bogerts, 1991; Larroche, 1984 a and b).

We assume that the frequency and relative selectivity of the structural anomalies in limbic regions of schizophrenics is the most plausible explanation for the fact that schizophrenics, but not the other disorders of brain development, are predisposed to suffer from the typical psychotic symptoms.

ACKNOWLEDGEMENT

This project is supported by the Deutsche Forschungsgemeinschaft (Bo 799/1-3) and the Alfried-Krupp-von Bohlen und Halbach Stiftung.

REFERENCES

Altshuler L, Conrad A, Kovelman JA, Scheibel A (1987) Hippocampal Pyramidal Cell Orientation in Schizophrenia. Arch Gen Psychiatry 44: 1094-1098.

Altshuler LL, Casanova MF, Goldberg TE, Kleinman JE (1990)The hippocampus and parahippocampus in schizophrenic, suicide and controls brains. Arch Gen Psychiatry 47: 1029-1034.

Anderson J, Gordon E, Rennie C, Meares RA (1990) The quantification of variability in ERPs and its application to schizophrenia. Abstract No. 6, Second International Symposium of Imaging of the Brain in Psychiatry and Related Fields. June 13 - 16, 1990 SPECT.

Andreasen NC, Nasrallah HA, Dunn V, Olson SC, Grove WM, Ehrhardt JC, Coffman JA, Crosset LHW (1986) Structural abnormalities in the frontal system in schizophrenia. A magnetic resonance imaging study. Arch Gen Psychiat 43:136-143.

Andreasen NC, Ehrhardt JC, Swayze VW, Alliger RJ, Yuh WTC, Cohen G, Ziebell S (1990 a) Magnetic resonance imaging of the brain in schizophrenia. Arch Gen Psychiatry 47: 35 - 44.

Andreasen NC, Swayze VW, Flaum M, Yates WR, Arndt S, McChesney C (1990 b) Ventricular enlargement in schizophrenia evaluated with computed tomographic scanning. Arch Gen Psychiatry 47:1008-1015.

Averback P (1981) Structural lesions of the brain in young schizophrenics. Le journal canadien des sciences neurologiques 8(1): 73 - 78.

Barta PE, Pearlson GD, Powers RE, Richards SS, Tune LE (1990)Reduced volume of superior temporal gyrus in schizophrenia; relationship to auditory hallucinations. American Journal of Psychiatry (in press).

Bäumer H (1954) Veränderungen des Thalamus bei Schizophrenie. J Hirnforsch 1:157 - 172.

Benes FM (1987) An analysis of the arrangement of neurons in the cingulate cortex of schizophrenic patients. Arch Gen Psychiat 44: 608-616.

Benes FM, Davidson B, Bird ED (1986) Quantitative cytoarchitectural studies of the cerebral cortex of schizophrenics. Arch Gen Psychiat 43: 31-35.

Besson JAO, Corrigan FM, Cherryman GR, et (1987) Nuclear magnetic brain imaging in chronic schizophrenia. Br J Psychiat 150: 161-163.

Bigelow LB, Nasrallah HA, Rauscher FP (1983) Corpus callosum thickness in chronic schizophrenia. Br J Psychiat 142: 282-287.

Bogerts B, Lesch A, Lange H, Zech M, Tutsch J (1983) Hypotrophy of the corpus callosum in schizophrenia. Neuroscience Letters, suppl. 14: 413.

Bogerts B (1984) Zur Neuropathologie der Schizophrenien. Fortschr Neurol Psychiat 52: 428-437.

Bogerts B (1985) Schizophrenien als Erkrankungen des limbischen Systems. In: Huber G (Hrsg): Basisstadien endogener Psychosen und das BorderlineProblem. Schattauer, Stuttgart, pp 163-179.

Bogerts B, Falkai P, Tutsch J (1986) Cell numbers in the pallium and hippocampus of schizophrenics. In: Shagass C et al (Hrsg) Biological Psychiatry. Elsevier, Amsterdam, pp 1178-1180.

Bogerts B (1989) Limbic and paralimbic pathology in schizophrenia: Interaction with age and stress related factors. In Schulz SC, Tamminga CA (eds) Schizophrenia: scientific progress. Oxford University Press pp 216 - 227.

Bogerts B (1990) The neuropathology of schizophrenia: Pathophysiological and neurodevelopmental implications. In Mednick SA, Cannon TD, Barr CE (eds) Fetal Neural Development and Adult Schizophrenia. Cambridge University Press, in press.

Bogerts B, Ashtari M, Degreef G, Alvir JMaJ, Bilder RM, Lieberman JA (1990a) Reduced temporal limbic structure volumes on magnetic resonance images in first episode schizophrenia. Psychiatry Res: Neuroimag 35: 1-13.

Bogerts B, Falkai P, Haupts M, Greve B, Ernst St, Tapernon-Franz U, Heinzmann U (1990b) Post-mortem volume measurements of limbic system and basal ganglia structures in chronic schizophrenia. Schizophrenia Research 3:295301.

Bogerts B, Falkai P, Degreef G, Lieberman J (1991) Neuropathological and brain imaging studies in positive and negative schizophrenia. in: Maneros A, Andreasen NC, Tsuang MT (eds.) Negative versus positive schizophrenia. Springer, Berlin (in press).

Brown R, Colter N, Corsellis JAN, Crow TJ, Frith CD, Jagoe R, Johnstone EC, Marsh L (1986) Postmortem evidence of structural brain changes in schizophrenia. Differences in brain weight, temporal horn area and parahippocampal gyrus compared with affective disorder. Arch Gen Psychiatry 43: 36-42.

Bruton C (1988) The Neuropathology of temporal lobe epilepsy. Maudsley Monographs No. 31, Oxford University Press.

Bruton CJ, Crow TJ, Frith CD, Johnstone EC, Owens DGC, Roberts GW (1990) Schizophrenia and the brain: a prospective clinico-neuropathological study. Psychological Medicine 20, 285-304.

Buchsbaum MS, DeLisi LE, Holcomb HH, et al (1984) Anteroposterior gradients in cerebral glucose use in schizophrenia and affective disorders. Arch Gen Psychiat 41: 1159-1166.

Buchsbaum MS, Ingvar DH, Kessler R, et al (1982) Cerebral glucography with positron tomography: use in normal subjects and in patients with schizophrenia. Arch Gen Psychiat 39: 251-259.

Casanova MF, Stevens JR, Bigelow L (1987) Gliosis in schizophrenia. Biol Psychiatry 22:1172-1175.

Casanova MF, Kleinman JE, Weinberger DR (1988) Neuropathological studies on the limbic system of schizophrenics. ACNP abstract No.1988.

Cannon-Spoor HE, Potkin HE, Wyatt RJ (1987) Measurement of premorbid adjustment in chronic schizophrenia. Schizophrenia Bull. 8: 470 - 484.

Christison GW, Casanova MF, Weinberger DR, Rawlings R, Kleinman JE (1989) A quantitative investigation of hippocampal pyramidal cell size, shape and variability of orientation in schizophrenia. Arch Gen Psychiatry 46: 1027 - 1032.

Chudley AE, Hagerman RJ (1987) Fragile X-Syndrom. The J of Pediatrics 110 (6): 821 - 831.

Colter N, Battal S, Crow TJ, Johnstone EC, Brown R, Bruton C (1987) White matter reduction in the parahippocampal gyrus of patients with schizophrenia. Arch Gen Psychiatry 44: 1023.

Crow TJ, Ball J, Bloom StR, Brown R, Bruton CJ, Colter N, Frith ChD, Johnstone EC, Owens DGC, Roberts GW (1989) Schizophrenia as an anomaly of development of cerebral asymmetry.

Curran JP, Cireilli VA (1988) The role psychosocial factors in the etiology, course and outcome of schizophrenia. In: Tsuang MT, Simpson JC (Hrsg) Handbook of Schizophrenia, vol 3. Amsterdam: Elsevier, pp. 275-297.

Davison K, Bagley CR (1969) Schizophrenia-like psychosis associated with organic disorders of the central nervous system. A review of the literature. In: Hertington RN (ed): Current problems in neuropsychiatry. Br J Psychiatry Special Publication No. 4: 113-187.

Degreef G, Ashtari M, Bogerts B, Bilder RM, Jody DN, Alvir JMaJ, Lieberman JA (1991) Temporal horn volumes measured from magnetic resonance images are correlated with symptoms of schizophrenia. Arch Gen Psychiatry (in press).

DeLisi LE, Dauphinais ID, Gershon E (1988) Perinatal complications and reduced size of brain limbic structures in familial schizophrenia. Schizophrenia Bulletin 14: 185-191.

DeLisi L (1987) Nongenetic etiological factors group report. Biological Perspectives of Schizophrenia. (eds.) H. Helmchen and FA Henn, pp. 162 - 184, John Wiley and Sons Limited, S Bernhard, Dahlem Konferenzen, 1987.

DeMyer MK, Gilmor RL, Hendrie HC, DeMyer WE, Augustyn GT, Jackson RK (1988) Magnetic resonance brain images in schizophrenic and normal subjects: Influence of diagnosis and education. Schizophrenia Bull 14: 21-32.

Dobyns WB (1987) Developmental aspects of lissencephaly and the lissencephaly syndromes. Birth Defects: Original Article Series, Volume 23, Number 1, pp. 225 - 241.

Dom R, de Saedeler J, Bogerts B, Hopf A (1981) Quantitative cytometric analysis of basal ganglia in catatonic schizophrenics. In: Perris et al. (eds) Biological Psychiatry, Elsevier, Amsterdam, pp 723-726.

Early TS, Reiman EM, Raichle ME, et al (1987) Left globus pallidus abnormality in never-medicated patients with schizophrenia. Proc Nat Acad Sci USA 84: 561-563.

Falkai P, Bogerts B (1986) Cell loss in the hippocampus of schizophrenics. Eur Arch Psychiatr Neurol Sci 236: 154-161.

Falkai P, Bogerts B, Rozumek M (1988a) Cell loss and volume reduction in the entorhinal cortex of schizophrenics. Biol Psychiatry 24: 515-521.

Falkai P, Bogerts B, Roberts GW, Crow TJ (1988b) Measurement of the alpha-cell-migration in the entorhinal region: a marker for developmental disturbances in schizophrenia? Schizophrenia Res 1: 157-158.

Falkai P, Bogerts B (1989) Morphometric evidence for developmental disturbances in brains of some schizophrenics. Schizophrenia Res 2 (1-2):99.

Falkai P, Bogerts B (1991) Is schizophrenia a neurodevelopmental disorder? A qualitative assessment of heterotopic pre-alpha-cell clusters in the entorhinal cortex of schizophrenic patients. J Psychopharmacology (submitted).

Flor-Henry P (1969) Psychosis and temporal lobe epilepsy: a controlled investigation. Epilepsia 10: 363 - 395.

Friede RL (1989) Some Features of Basic Reactions Characteristic for Immature Nervous Tissue. in: Developmental Neuropathology (ed.) RL Friede, chapter 2, p. 22.

Friede RL (1989 a) Dyplasias of Cerebral Cortex. in: Developmental Neuropathology (ed.) RL Friede, chapter 27, pp. 339 - 340.

Friede RL (1989 b) Peroxisomal Diseases. in: Developmental Neuropathology (ed.) RL Friede, chapter 38, pp. 484 - 485.

Fisman M (1975) The brain stem in psychosis. Brit J of Psychiatry 126: 414 - 422

Fünfgeld E (1925) Pathologisch-anatomische Untersuchungen bei Dementia praecox mit besonderer Berücksichtigung des Thalamus opticus. Z Ges Neurol Psychiat 95: 411 - 463.

Geraud G, Arne-Bes MC, Guell A, Bes A (1987) Reversibility of hemodynamic hypofrontality in schizophrenia. Journal of Cerebral Blood Flow and Metabolism 7: 9 - 12.

Galaburda AM, Sherman GF, Rosen GD, Aboitiz F, Geschwind N (1985) Developmental dyslexia: four consecutive patients with cortical anomalies. Ann Neurol 18: 222-233.

Geraud G, Arne-Bes MC, Guell A, Bes A (1987) Reversibility of hemodynamic hypofrontality in schizophrenia. Journal of Cerebral Blood Flow and Metabolism 7: 9 - 12.

Gill M, Taylor C, Murray RM (1989) Schizophrenia Research: attempting to integrate genetics, neuro-development and nosology. International Review of Psychiatry 1(4): 277 - 287.

Greenwood R, Bhalla A, Gordon A, Roberts J (1983) Behavior disturbances during recovery from herpes simplex encephalitis. Journal of Neurology, Neurosurgery and Psychiatry 46: 809 - 17.

Gross G, Huber G (1972) Sensorische Störungen bei Schizophrenien. Arch Psychiatr Nervenkr 216: 119 - 130.

Gross G, Huber G, Schüttler R (1982) Computerized tomography studies on schizophrenic diseases. Arch Psychiatr Nervenkr 231: 519 526.

Günther W (1990) Hirnfunktionsstörungen und Corpus-callosum Befunde bei Schizophrenen, gemessen mit EEG-Mapping, regionaler Hirndurchblutung und Kernspintomographie. in: Heinrich K, Bogerts B "Pathophysiologische lund pathomorphologische Aspekte bei schizophrenen Psychosen" pp. 97 - 113.

Gur RE, Resnick SM, Alavi A, et al (1987a) Regional brain function in schizophrenia. I. A positron emission tomography study. Arch Gen Psychiat 44: 119-125.

Gur RE, Resnick SM, Gur RC, et al (1987b) Regional brain function in schizophrenia. II. Repeated evaluation with positron emission tomography. Arch Gen Psychiat 44: 126-129.

Heckers S, Heinsen H, Heinsen Y, Beckmann H (1990a) Morphometry of the parahippocampal gyrus in schizophrenics and controls. Some anatomical considerations. J Neural Transm 80: 151-155.

Heckers S, Heinsen H, Heinsen YC, Beckmann H (1990b) Limbic structures and lateral ventricle in schizophrenia. Arch Gen Psychiatry 47: 1016-1022.

Hillbom E (1951) Schizophrenia-like psychoses after brain trauma. Acta Psychiat Neurol Scand 60: 36-47.

Hopf A (1954) Orientierende Untersuchung zur Frage pathoanatomischer Veränderungen im Pallium und Striatum bei Schizophrenie. J Hirnforschung 1: 97 - 145.

Huber G (1957) Die coenaesthetische Schizophrenie. Fortschr Neurol Psychiatr 25: 491 - 520.

Illowski BP, Juliano AM, Bigelow LB et al (1988) Stability of CT scan findings in schizophrenia: results of an eight-year follow-up study. JNNP 51:209-213.23.

Ingvar DH, Franzen G (1974) Abnormalities of cerebral blood flow distribution in patients with chronic schizophrenia. Acta Psychiatrica Scandinavica 50: 425-462.

Jakob J, Beckmann H (1986) Prenatal developmental disturbances in the limbic allocortex in schizophrenics. J Neural Transmiss 65: 303-326.

Jeste DV, Lohr JB (1989) Hippocampal pathologic findings in schizophrenia. Arch Gen Psychiatry 46: 1019 - 1024.

Johnstone EC, Owens DGC, Crow TJ, Frith CD, Alexandropolis K, Bydder G, Colter N (1989) Temporal lobe structure as determined by nuclear magnetic resonance in schizophrenia and bipolar affective disorder. J Neurol Neurosurg Psychiat 52: 736-741.

Kelsoe JR, Cadet JL, Pickar D, Weinberger DR (1988) Quantitative neuroanatomy in schizophrenia: a controlled magnetic resonance imaging study. Arch Gen Psychiatry 45: 533 - 41.

Kemali D, Maj M, Galderisi S et al (1985) Clinical and neurophysiological correlates of cerebral ventricular enlargement in schizophrenia. J Psychiatr Res 19: 587 - 596.

Kirkpatrick B and Buchanan RW (1990) The neural basis of the deficit syndrome of schizophrenia. J Nervous and Mental Disease 178(9): 545-555.

Kling AS, Metter EJ, Riege WH, et al (1986) Comparison of PET measurement of local brain glucose metabolism and CAT measurement of brain atrophy in chronic schizophrenia and depression. Am J Psychiat 143: 175-180.

Kovelmann JA, Scheibel AB (1984) A neurohistological correlate of schizophrenia. Biol Psychiatry 19: 1601-1621.

Laroche JL (1984) Malformations of the nervous system. In: Adams JM et al (eds.) Greenfield's Neuropathology. Edward Arnold, London, pp. 385 - 403.

Laroche JL (1984 a) Malformations of the nervous system. In: Adams JM et al (eds.) Greenfield's Neuropathology. Edward Arnold, London, pp. 393 - 395.

Laroche JL (1984 b) Malformations of the nervous system. In: Adams JM et al (eds.) Greenfield's Neuropathology. Edward Arnold, London, pp. 406 - 408.

Lesch A, Bogerts B (1984) The diencephalon in schizophrenia: Evidence for reduced thickness of the periventricular grey matter. Eur Arch Psychiatr Neurol Sci 234: 212-219.

Leonhard K (1952) Die Klinik des Thalamus opticus. Nervenarzt 21: 200 - 208.

Lohr JB, Jeste DV (1988) Locus ceruleus morphometry in aging and schizophrenia. Acta Psychiat Scand 77: 689-97.

Luchins DL, Metz JT, Marks RC and Cooper MD (1989) Basal ganglia glucose metabolism asymmetry during a catatonic episode. Biol. Psychiatry 26, 725 - 728.

Luchins DL (1990) A possible role of hippocampal dysfunction in schizophrenic symptomatology. Biol Psychiatry 28: 87 - 91.

Malamud M (1967) Psychiatric disorder with intracranial tumors of the limbic system. Arch Neurol 17: 113-123.

Marks RC, Luchins DJ (1990) Relationship between brain imaging findings in schizophrenia and psychopathology. In: Andreasen NC (ed) Schizophrenia: Positive and negative symptoms and syndromes. Karger, Basel pp. 89-123.

Mathew RJ, Barr DL, Weinman ML, Barr DL (1982) Regional blood flow in schizophrenia. Arch Gen Psychiatry 39: 1121 - 1124.

Mathew RJ, Wilson WH, Tant SR, Robinson L, Prakash R (1988) Abnormal resting regional blood flow patterns and their correlates in schizophrenia. Arch Gen Psychiatry 45: 542 - 549.

Mathew PJ, Partaïn CL, Prakash R, Kulkarni MV, Logan TP, Wilson WH (1985) A study of the septum pellucidum and corpus callosum in schizophrenia with MR imaging. Acta Psychiatr Scand 72 (5): 414 - 421.

McCarley RW, Faux SF, Shenton M, LeMay M, Cane M, Ballinger R, Duffy FH (1989) CT abnormalities in schizophrenia. A preliminary study of their correlations with P300/P200. Electrophysiological features and positive/negative symptoms. Arch Gen Psychiatry 46: 698 - 708.

McKenna PJ (1987) Pathology, phenomenology and the dopamine hypothesis of schizophrenia. Brit J of Psychiatry 151: 288-301.

McLardy T (1974) Hippocampal zinc and structural deficits in brains from chronic alcoholics and some schizophrenics. J Orthomol Psychiatry 4: 32-36.

Meltzer HY, Stahl SM (1976) The dopamine hypothesis of schizophrenia: A review. Schizophrenia Bull 2: 19 - 76.

Mesulam MM (1986) Patterns in behavioral neuroanatomy: association areas, the limbic system, and hemispheric specialization. In: Mesulam MM (Hrsg) Principles of behavioral neurology. Davis, Philadelphia, pp 1-70.

Mulder DW, Daly D (1952) Psychiatric symptoms associated with lesions of the temporal lobe. JAMA 150: 173-176.

Nasrallah HA, Andreasen NC, Coffman JA, Olson SC, Dunn VD, Ehrhardt JC, Chapman SM (1986) A controlled magnetic resonance imaging study of corpus callosum thickness in schizophrenia. Biol Psychiat 21: 274-282.

Nasrallah HA, McCalley-Whitters M, Rauscher FP et al (1983 a) A histological study of the corpus callosum in chronic schizophrenia. Psych Res 8: 151-160.

Nasrallah HA, Kuperman S, Hamra B, McCalley-Whitters M (1983 b) Clinical differences between schizophrenic patients with and without large cerebral ventricles. J Clin Psychiat 44: 407 - 409.

Nieto D, Escobar A (1972) Major psychoses. In Minkler J (ed) Pathology of the nervous system. McGraw-Hill, New York pp 2654-2665.

Oyanagi K, Yoshida Y, Icuta F (1986) Die chronology of lesion repair in the developing rat brain. Virchows Arch (Path Anat) pp. 347 - 359.

Pakkenberg B (1987) Post-mortem study of chronic schizophrenic brains. Brit J Psychiatry 151: 744-752.

Pakkenberg B (1990) Pronounced reduction of total neuron numbers in mediodorsal thalamic nucleus and nucleus accumbens in schizophrenics. Arch Gen Psychiatry 47: 1023 - 1028.

Raine A, Harrison GN, Reynolds GP, Sheard C, Cooper JE, Medley I (1990) Structural and functional characteristics of the corpus callosum in schizophrenics, psychiatric controls and normal controls. Arch Gen Psychiatry 47: 1060 - 1064.

Reske-Nielsen E, Christensen AL, Nielsen J (1982) A neuropathological and neuropsychological study of Turner's syndrome. Brain 18(2): 181 - 90.

Reveley AM (1987) Genetics as an approach to etiology. Biological Perspectives of Schizophrenia. (eds.) H. Helmchen, FA Henn , John Wiley and Sons Limited, S Bernhard, Dahlem Konferenz, pp. 72 - 82.

Roberts GW, Colter N, Lofthouse R, Bogerts B, Zech M, Crow TJ (1986) Gliosis in schizophrenia: A survey. Biol Psychiatry 21: 1043 - 1050.

Roberts GW, Colter N, Lofthouse R, Johnstone EC, Crow TJ (1987) Is there gliosis in schizophrenia? Investigation of the temporal lobe. Biol Psychiatry 22: 1459 - 1468.

Roberts GW, Crow TJ (1987) The neuropathology of schizophrenia - a progress report. Brit Med Bulletin 43 (3): 599-615.

Roberts GW and Bruton C (1990) Annotation. Notes from the graveyard: neuropathology and schizophrenia. Neuropathology and Applied Neurobiology 16: 3 - 16.

Roberts GW, Done DJ, Bruton C, Crow TF (1990) A "Mock up" of schizophrenia: temporal lobe epilepsy and schizophrenia-like psychosis. Biol Psychiatry 28: 127-143.

Rosenthal R and Bigelow LB (1972) Quantitative brain measurements in chronic schizophrenia. Brit J Psychiatry 121: 259 - 264.

Rossi A, Stratta P, Gallucci M, Passarellio R, Cassachia M (1989) Quantification of corpus callosum and ventricles in schizophrenia with nuclear magnetic resonance imaging: a pilot study. Am J Psychiat 146: 99-101.

Rossi A, Stratta P, D'Albenzio L, Tartaro A, Schiazza G, di Michele V, Bolino F, Casacchia M (1990) Reduced temporal lobe areas in schizophrenia: preliminary evidences from a controlled multiplanar magnetic resonance imaging study. Biol Psychiatry 27: 61 - 68.

Scheibel AB, Kovelman JA (1981) Disorientation of the hippocampal pyramidal cells and its processes in the schizophrenic patient. Biol Psychiat 16: 101-102.

Schulz SC, Koller MM, Kishore PR, Hamer RR, Gehl JJ., Friedel RO (1983) Ventricular enlargement in teenage patients with schizophrenia spectrum disorder. Am J Psychiatry 140:1592 - 1594.

Shelton RC, Weinberger DR (1986) X-ray computerized tomography studies in schizophrenia: a review and synthesis. In Nasrallah HA, Weinberger DR (eds) The neurology of schizophrenia. Elsevier, New York, pp 207-250.

Sheppard G, Gruzelier J, Manchanda R, Hirsch SR (1983) 15-0 positron emission tomographic scanning in predominantly never treated acute schizophrenic patients. Lancet II: 1448 - 52.

Stevens JR (1982) Neuropathology of schizophrenia. Arch Gen Psychiat 39: 1131-1139.

Stevens JR (1986) Clinicopathological correlations in schizophrenia. Arch Gen Psychiat 43: 715-716.

Stevens JR and Casanova MF (1988) Is there a neuropathology of schizophrenia ? Biol Psychiat 24: 123 - 128.

Stevens CD, Altshuler LL, Bogerts B, Falkai P (1988) Quantitative study of gliosis in schizophrenia and Huntington's chorea. Biol Psychiatry 24: 697 - 700

Stewart RM, Richman DP, Caviness VS (1975) Lissencephaly and Pachygyria. Acta neuropath.(Berl.) 31: 1 - 12.

Suddath RL, Christison GW, Torrey EF, Casanova MF, Weinberger DR (1990) Anatomical abnormalities in the brains of monozygotic twins discordant for schizophrenia. The New England Journal of Medicine 322 (12): 62 - 67.

Suddath RL, Casanova MF, Goldberg TE, Daniel DG, Kelsoe J, Weinberger DR (1989a) Temporal lobe pathology in schizophrenia: a quantitative magnetic resonance imaging study. Am J Psychiatry 146: 464-472.

Szechtman H, Nahmias C, Garnett S, et al (1988) Effect of neuroleptics on altered cerebral glucose metabolism in schizophrenia. Arch Gen Psychiat 45: 523-532.

Tandon R, Greden JF (1990) Cholinergic hyperactivity and negative schizophrenic symptoms. Arch Gen Psychiatry 46: 745 - 753.

Treff WM and Hempel KJ (1958) Die Zelldichte bei Schizophrenen und klinisch Gesunden. J Hirnforschung 4: 314 - 369.

Uematso M, Kaiya H (1988) The morphology of the corpus callosum in schizophrenia: an MRI study. Schizophr Res 1: 391 - 398.

Warkentin S, Nilsson A, Risberg J, et al (1990) Regional cerebral blood flow in schizophrenia: repeated studies during a psychotic episode. Psychiatry Res: Neuroimag 35: 27-38.

Weinberger DR (1987) Implications of normal brain development for the pathogenesis of schizophrenia. Arch Gen Psychiatry 44: 660-669.

Weinberger DR, Berman KF, Zec RF (1986) Physiological dysfunction of dorsolateral prefrontal cortex in schizophrenia. I. regional cerebral blood flow (rCBF) evidence. Arch Gen Psychiatry 43: 114-125.

Woods BT and Wolf J (1983) A reconsideration of the relation of ventricular enlargement to duration of illness in schizophrenia. Am J Psychiatry 140: 1564 - 1570.

Woods BT, Yurgelun-Todd D, Benes FM, Frankenburg FR, Pope HG, McSparren J (1990) Progressive ventricular enlargement in schizophrenia: comparison to bipolar affective disorder and correlation with clinical course. Biol Psychiatry 27: 341 - 352.

Zubin J, Spring B (1977) Vulnerability - a new view of schizophrenia. J Abnorm Psychol 86: 103 - 126.

OBSTETRICAL EVENTS AND ADULT SCHIZOPHRENIA

Karen L. Dykes, Sarnoff A. Mednick, Tyrone D. Cannon, and Christopher E. Barr

Social Science Research Institute
University of Southern California
Los Angeles, California

INTRODUCTION

In June, 1939, the dissertation of Barney Katz, "The etiology of the deteriorating psychoses of adolescence and early adult life" was approved by the Faculty of the University of Southern California. Barney Katz' study was the first empirical test of the hypothesis that obstetrical factors are important in the etiology of schizophrenia. Thirty-one years later, based upon data collected from the Danish high-risk study (Mednick & Schulsinger, 1965), Mednick (1970) hypothesized that genetic predisposition and perinatal complications interact to produce damage to the hippocampus which in turn may elevate risk for schizophrenia (1970). Since that time, many studies have been published examining links between genetic predisposition, obstetrical complications, and schizophrenia. This chapter examines three etiological models which include obstetrical complications as a factor.

Model 1

OCs could be the "sole" cause of schizophrenia if they were the phenotypic expression of the genetic predisposition. With this formulation the genetic condition would predispose to serious OCs which would then be sufficient to cause schizophrenia. Despite the demonstrated importance of genetic factors in schizophrenia, this possibility seems very unlikely. Too many infants who do not become schizophrenic are born with OCs just as severe as any observed in schizophrenics and there is a sizable subgroup of schizophrenics and individuals at high risk (HR) for schizophrenia who have apparently not experienced severe OCs (Cannon, Mednick, & Parnas, 1990a; Cannon, Mednick, & Parnas, 1990b).

Developmental Neuropathology of Schizophrenia
Edited by S.A. Mednick *et al.*, Plenum Press, New York, 1991

Model 2

A second suggested model hypothesizes that some cases of schizophrenia are caused solely or mainly by genetic factors while other cases are caused solely or mainly by OCs (Lewis & Murray, 1987). This model has grown from the results of some studies which have reported that schizophrenics with a familial psychiatric history evidence no OCs, while those schizophrenics with OCs evidence no family history of mental illness (Cazullo, Vita, & Sacchetti, 1989; Schwarzkopf, Nasrallah, Olson, & Coffman, 1989; Reveley, Reveley, & Murray, 1984).

However, these studies suffer from a methodological weakness: the obstetrical history and the family psychiatric history are usually obtained by interview with the schizophrenic or the parents of the schizophrenic 20-30 years after the birth. Aside from the fact that the schizophrenic could not personally remember the birth and the parent (usually the mother) is hardly an objective observer, the substantial amount of time elapsed since the event and the problem of separating a single child's OCs from those of other children in the family, may make this method of data acquisition less than ideal (Mednick & Shaffer, 1963; Mednick and Hefner, 1969). Murray and his colleagues (Murray, Reveley, & Lewis, 1988) also explored the fact that some families try to develop an explanation as to why their child became schizophrenic. One possible family theory might involve a psychotic grandparent and purposefully exclude other interpretations; another family might concentrate upon a complicated pregnancy and delivery.

In addition to these problems, McNeil (1988) has demonstrated empirically that parental recall of the obstetrical history of their adult psychiatrically hospitalized children is woefully incomplete. While Murray et al. (1988) point out that recall after 20-30 years could be an advantage in that only the important OCs are remembered, it would be more advantageous to use prospective data gathered by professionals at the time of the pregnancy and delivery.

Genetic factors may not be suited to be a sole cause of schizophrenia, even for a subgroup of schizophrenics. Since many identical twins are discordant for schizophrenia, some environmental factors must combine or interact with genetic predisposition to increase the risk for the affected twins (Gottesman, & Shields, 1982).

Given these considerations, it is difficult to see how either genetics alone or OCs alone could be responsible for schizophrenia.

Model 3

A third model, favored by the authors, is a two-hit approach which handles some of the logical difficulties mentioned above. It suggests that during a critical period of gestation the high risk fetus suffers a genetically predisposed (or teratogenic) disruption of fetal neural development. This maldevelopment would make the fetus especially susceptible to damage from OCs. Therefore, an infant with a strong genetic predisposition and who suffers severe OCs has a very high risk of succumbing to schizophrenia. (We do not mean to suggest that this causal pattern fits all schizophrenics. See Cannon, Mednick, & Parnas, 1990b).

OCs AND PSYCHOTIC DISORDERS

McNeil has provided the field with thoughtful and complete reviews of the literature relating to the obstetrical experiences of schizophrenics (McNeil, 1988; McNeil & Kaij, 1978). Following is a summary based on these reviews as well as the presentation of the findings of some more recent studies. Afterward, we will present our interpretation of the data.

OCs and Childhood Psychoses

It is not certain that studies of childhood psychotics are relevant to adult schizophrenia. It should be recalled, however, that a large percentage of childhood psychotics manifest schizophrenia as adults. Table 1 summarizes the results of the 12 studies we found in the literature. Nearly all of the studies relied on parent interview for the OC information; as we indicated earlier, this poses certain methodological difficulties. These parental reports were, however, often supplemented by birth certificates or hospital records and are consistent in finding a higher level of OCs in the childhood psychotics than in the controls. Four studies in Table 1 found a significant excess of both pregnancy and delivery complications. Three studies report significantly more delivery complications while the Hinton (1963) and Torrey and Hersch (1975) studies only found an excess of pregnancy complications. Terris, LaPouse, and Monk (1964) and Zitrin, Ferber, and Cohen (1964) observed no significant OC differences between childhood psychotics and normals. The data for these last two studies were restricted to birth certificates.

A recent study of autistic children noted that they were characterized by an abnormality of the vermis which the authors attribute to a failure of fetal neural development due to genetic or teratogenic influences during the pregnancy (Courchesney, Yeung-Courchesne, Press, Hesselink, & Jernigan, 1988).

In summary, there is evidence indicating that childhood psychosis is associated with an excessive level of OCs.

Table 1. Results of Studies Comparing Obstetrical Complications of Childhood Psychotics and Normal Subjects

Study	Affected Group	Type of Complications
Vorster (1960)	Childhood Psychotics	More PCs and DCs
Knobloch & Pasamanick(1962)	Childhood Psychotics	More PCs and DCs
Hinton (1963)	Childhood Psychotics	More PCs
Taft & Goldfarb (1964)	Childhood Psychotics	More PCs and DCs
Zitrin, Ferber & Cohen (1964)		No difference
Terris, LaPouse, & Monk (1964)		No difference
Whittam, Simon & Mittler (1966)	Childhood Psychotics	More DCs
Rutt & Offord (1971)	Childhood Psychotics	More DCs
Bender (1973)	Childhood Psychotics	More DCs
Mura (1974)	Childhood Psychotics	More PCs and DCs
Torrey & Hersch (1975)	Childhood Psychotics	More PCs

OCs and Adult Schizophrenics

Table 2 lists the studies which ascertained OCs for adult schizophrenics and controls. Katz (1939), mentioned in the introduction, examined the birth records for 100 individuals suffering schizophrenia and dementia praecox as well as 100 matched controls. He found that the schizophrenics evidenced significantly more prematurity and suffered a longer labor. Woerner, Pollack, and Klein (1971) reported that the schizophrenics in their study had significantly more OCs than their normal siblings but not significantly more than their abnormal siblings. Eagles et al. (1990) and DeLisi et al. (1988) found schizophrenics to have significantly more OCs than their healthy siblings. DeLisi and her colleagues, using data from MRI scans, reported a weak correlation among schizophrenic siblings in the size of some limbic structures, suggesting that neither OCs alone nor genetics alone can account for the structural brain anomalies. Lane and Albee (1966) and Woerner, Pollack & Klein (1973) also utilized sibling controls, both finding that the birth certificates of the schizophrenics showed them to have been six ounces lighter at birth than their sibs. Owen et al. (1988) examined the CT scans of schizophrenics with and without OCs. They found that those with OCs were more likely to have large VBRs accompanied by widening of cortical fissures and sulci. The study by Pollack et al. (1966) found no difference between the schizophrenics and their sibs. Their data source, however, was maternal interviews. Nimgaonkar (1988) compared schizophrenics with and without a family history of the illness and found no differences in OCs between the two groups. In this study the OC information was obtained through interviews and case-records.

Table 2. Studies Comparing Obstetrical Complications of Schizophrenics and Normal Subjects

Study	N	Findings
Katz (1939)	100 Schizophrenics 100 Controls	Schizophrenics: More OCs
Lane & Albee (1966)	52 Schizophrenics 115 Siblings	Schizophrenics: Lower birth weight
Pollack et al. (1966)	33 Schizophrenics 33 Siblings	No difference
Woerner et al. (1971)	34 Schizophrenics 42 Siblings	Schizophrenics: Lower birth weight
Woerner et al. (1973)	46 Schizophrenics 37 Normal Siblings 17 Abnormal siblings	Schizophrenics: More PCs & DCs than normal siblings
McNeil & Kaij (1978)	54 Process Schizo. 46 Psychotics 100 Controls	Process Schiz.: More PCs & DCs
Jacobsen & Kinney (1980)	63 Schizophrenics 63 Controls	Schizophrenics: More frequent & severe DCs
Parnas et al. (1982)	12 Schizophrenics 25 Schizotypals 55 High Risk Controls	Schizopht: Worse OCs Schizotypals: Least OCs
Lewis & Murray (1987)	955 Psychiatric Patients	Schizophrenics: More OCs than other psychiatric patients
Owen et al. (1988)	61 Schizophrenics	Large VBR with widened cortical sulci and fissures more common in those with OCs
DeLisi et al. (1988)	11 Schizo. Sib pairs 2 Schizophrenics 18 controls	Schizophrenics: More OCs No differences between schizophrenics with and without BCs
Nimgaonkar et al. (1988)	18 "familial" 30 "non-familial" Schizophrenics	No Difference
Eagles et al. (1990)	27 Schizophrenics 27 Siblings	Schizophrenics: More OCs

The three Scandinavian studies (Parnas et al., 1982; McNeil & Kaij, 1978; and Jacobsen & Kinney, 1980) utilized hospital and midwife records of OCs produced at the time of the pregnancy and delivery. All three show the schizophrenics as having suffered more numerous and more severe OCs than controls. The large study by Lewis and Murray (1987) found that the mothers of the schizophrenics report a greater frequency of OCs than do the mothers of other psychiatric patients.

Influenza During Gestation

To date, four studies have been conducted which investigate the relationship between exposure to a major influenza epidemic during fetal development and later rates of adult schizophrenia. The first study examined subjects exposed to the 1957 Type A2 influenza epidemic in Helsinki (Mednick et al., 1988). Those exposed to the epidemic during their second trimester of fetal development had significantly increased rates of schizophrenia. This result held independently for males and females and for each of the several mental hospitals in greater Helsinki. The association was not found for other mental illnesses.

Barr, Mednick, and Munk-Jorgensen (1990) analyzed a data set consisting of the following information for each of the 480 months from 1910-1950: 1) the number of people born in Denmark; 2) the number of those born each month who later were diagnosed schizophrenic in a Danish psychiatric hospital; 3) the number of cases of influenza reported to the Danish Ministry of Health in each month; 4) the population of Denmark during this 40-year period. The data set includes over 7500 schizophrenics which makes it possible to examine a window of vulnerability somewhat narrower than a trimester. Barr et al. noted that unusually high levels of influenza occurring during the sixth month of gestation was associated with unusually high rates of future adult schizophrenics being born.

Torrey, Rawlings, and Waldman (1988) report inconsistent results in their examination of the relationship between fetal exposure to viral epidemics and adult schizophrenia in Connecticut (CN) and Massachusetts (MA). One possible reason for these mixed results was that Torrey et al. could not determine the place of birth of their samples. Given the immigration and mobility rates in the United States, some considerable number of their schizophrenics (perhaps 50%) were very likely born in states or nations other than CN or MA. For these subjects, the viral disease frequencies and timing data for the states of MA and CN may be irrelevant. Because of this, the results of this study must be viewed with considerable caution.

Kendell and Kemp (1989) report a significant increase in adult schizophrenia for Edinburgh residents who were exposed to the 1957 influenza epidemic during the sixth month of gestation. However, the number of cases in this study is rather small (five index vs. one control). Kendell and Kemp also report on the rates of adult schizophrenia for all of those in Scotland who were exposed to the 1957 epidemic. Unfortunately, their data suffer from the same problem as the Torrey et al. data set: They do not have information on place of birth of their subjects. Additionally, they point out that a large number of Scottish males emigrated during the period of the study and may have been diagnosed schizophrenic in other countries. The data for the females is, therefore, more reliable. From data presented by Kendell and Kemp for Scotland (their Table 3), we examined the rates of female adult schizophrenia for each trimester of exposure to the 1957 influenza epidemic. The schizophrenia rates for exposure in trimesters 1, 2 and 3, respectively, were 1.62, 2.70, and 1.28, per 1,000 live born Scottish females. Females exposed in the second trimester evidenced a significantly greater rate of schizophrenia than females exposed in the first or third trimesters (Chi square (2) = 7.23, $p<.01$). In view of the difficulties with this data set, this finding must be interpreted with caution.

Kendell and Kemp mention that there were very severe influenza epidemics in 1918 and 1919 and reason that they would expect to see corresponding elevations in the rates of schizophrenia among those who, as fetuses, were exposed to these epidemics. They use a Scottish national psychiatric register for this study which, for many cases, does not include the date of birth of the schizophrenics; it only includes the schizophrenic's statement of age at time of admission. Based on inspection of the data (rather than statistical analysis) they concluded there was no increase in births of future schizophrenics in 1918 and 1919. By completing a trend analysis of the data they present in their Table 3, however, we found that the number of schizophrenics born in 1919 was significantly greater than would be predicted from the schizophrenic rates of previous years.

It is difficult to determine the implications of the Torrey et al. (1988) study for the viral hypothesis of schizophrenia because of the serious problems in their data sources. However, the Kendell and Kemp data (as analyzed above) do offer modest support for the viral hypothesis and the Finnish and Danish studies can be interpreted as suggesting that disturbances in fetal neural development may increase the risk of adult schizophrenia.

Other Teratogens

Other forms of prenatal insult have also been suggested as increasing the risk for schizophrenia. Otake and Schull (1984) demonstrated an increased incidence of psychosis in subjects who were exposed during their second trimester of gestation to the radiation from the atomic explosions in Nagasaki and Hiroshima. Studies of these individuals have noted disturbed patterns of cell migration in the brains of these subjects (Rakic, 1991). Also, a convincing argument has been presented by Lohr and Bracha (1989) for the possibility that prenatal exposure to alcohol could increase the risk of schizophrenia. While there is some evidence that these disruptions of fetal neural development may contribute to adult schizophrenia, it is not yet known exactly how these factors interrupt brain development. Two possibilities are discussed below.

Lyon et al. (1989) provide a summary of the first possibility, proposed by Rakic. Rakic proposed a model of cortical development involving two waves of cell migration (1984). During the first wave, radial glial fibers to the cortex are formed. The second wave of cells originates at the ventricular surface and migrates along the radial glial fibers toward the outer surface of the cortex, stacking up in reverse order of arrival. Thalamocortical projections, which could determine how far outward the second wave of cells migrates, grow during the second trimester. This is the same time frame in which fetal influenza exposure increase the risk for schizophrenia. Based on Rakic's theory, partial cell migration would be reflected in groups of cells remaining along the projection path or at their ventricular origin. In support of this, Rakic found that in animals that underwent an early migration disturbance, caused by ionizing radiation, many ectopic cells remained along the ventricle borders, in the region from which they originate (1988). Post-mortem evidence from schizophrenic brains also supports this theory. Bogerts (1991) found cells lying beneath the surface of the entorhinal cortex to which they normally migrate. Roberts reported at the Fetal Neural Development Conference that he had found similar results in the schizophrenic brains he had studied in England (Lyon et al., 1989).

This theory also could account for a lack of ventricular volume change in some schizophrenics. This divergent migration could occur without a great loss of cellular material. The cells would just not be in their proper location. At this same conference, Weinberger (1987) pointed out that this developmental abnormality would probably not lead to postnatal progressive ventricular enlargement, supporting his findings of relatively stable ventricular width. Overall, this theory could explain how influenza or radiation exposure during the second trimester increases the risk for brain abnormalities.

A review by Bogerts (1991) revealed a lack of gliosis in the limbic structures of the temporal lobe. This is considered to be consistent with an early acquired anomaly due to disturbed brain development, not to a degenerative disorder or viral infection later in life.

<u>OCs in Twins</u>

The study of the case histories of MZ twins discordant for schizophrenia

Table 3. Studies Comparing Obstetrical Complication Rates of Schizophrenics and their Co-twins

Study	**N**	**Findings**
Pollin & Stabenau (1968)	100 Discordant MZ twins	Schizophrenic twin: Lower birth weight
Gottesman & Shields (1972)	82 Discordant twin pairs	No difference
McNeil & Kaij (1978)	39 Discordant twin pairs	Schizophrenic twin: More DC's
Reveley, et al. (1983)	21 Schizophrenic MZ pairs 18 MZ controls	Schizophrenics with family history: No OCs. Schizophrenics: fewer OCs than controls

enables us to isolate environmental factors, including OC differences, which may be involved in the etiology of schizophrenia. Although twin pairs share many delivery conditions, the twin born first typically suffers fewer DCs and one twin usually has a lower birth weight. Table 3 summarizes the findings of these studies, all of which utilized maternal interview as their source of OC information.

Pollin and Stabenau (1968) noted that the schizophrenic twin of the pair had a significantly lower birth weight. However, Gottesman and Shields (1972) reported no difference in birth weight. When McNeil and Kaij (1978) reexamined the Gottesman and Shields data they found a significantly higher level of DCs for the schizophrenic twin. Reveley, Reveley, and Murray (1984) found that if a schizophrenic twin pair reported a familial psychiatric history they tended to report a surprisingly low level of OCs. Twins with a negative family history reported a high number of OCs. While this supports the theory that schizophrenia is caused by genetics in some cases and by OCs in the other cases, it should be emphasized that several studies have not found a dissociation between OCs and family history (reviewed in McNeil, 1988).

OCs in Children at HR for Schizophrenia

Systematic studies of children at high-risk (HR) for schizophrenia began in the early 60s in an attempt to observe and record characteristics of schizophrenics before their special life conditions (drug treatment, failures, long-term hospitalization, isolation, etc.) obscured their premorbid characteristics and warped the memories of their experiences. One other important advantage of HR studies is that, "if a low-risk control group is included in the design, then it is possible to evaluate whether a given environmental stressor affects the HR and LR groups differently. In other words the design encourages the examination of gene environment interactions in the etiology of the illness" (Mednick, & Silverton, 1987, p. 544). If such an interaction were discovered, careful study might shed light on the nature of the phenotypic expression of the genetic predisposition for schizophrenia.

A number of reports have noted interaction effects involving genetic predisposition for schizophrenia and OCs. The first of these reports (Mednick, Mura, Schulsinger and Mednick, 1974) presented at a meeting of the Society for Social Biology, studied the pregnancies and deliveries of all the children born to schizophrenic parents (N=83) in a Copenhagen birth cohort which had been the subject of an intensive perinatal investigation. They note that "low birth weight in the children born to schizophrenics is associated with developmental abnormalities in their one-year examination. Children born with identical low birth weights in the other two (Control) groups show no evidence of such effects at one year" (p. 112). Fish (1971) suggested that the developmental retardation and the eventual schizophrenia are both produced by the same genetic condition; low birth weight is simply another manifestation of the genetically-determined growth retardation. Goodman (1988) supports this theory, using as evidence the abnormal neuronal organization found in schizophrenic brains. He argues that if this abnormality can cause psychosis in adulthood and behavioral abnormalities in childhood, then certainly it could cause OCs in the prenatal and neonatal periods. The HR method offers a test of the differences in interpretation of these findings.

If genetic factors are responsible for obstetrical problems then we would hypothesize that offspring at higher genetic risk would experience a higher level of OCs than would controls. If the occurrence of OCs are independent of genetic background for schizophrenia then HR subjects would not be expected to evidence elevated levels of OCs.

Several studies (Mirdal et al., 1974; Marcus, et al., 1981; Hanson et al. 1976) and two reviews by McNeil (McNeil & Kaij, 1978; McNeil, 1988) which examined the research in this area concluded that OCs are <u>not</u> significantly elevated among those at genetically-defined HR for schizophrenia. This suggests that genetic factors are not responsible for OCs, but are more likely responsible for a special susceptibility to OCs when they do occur. (It should be noted that there are a few reports of increased anomalies for HR subjects during gestation. These will be discussed later.)

Another instance of a gene-perinatal interaction was noted by Rieder et al. (1977). These investigators examined the perinatal records and IQ test scores (at age seven) of subjects in the Boston sample of the Collaborative Study of Mental Retardation and Cerebral Palsy (Broman, Nichols & Kennedy, 1975). They identified the schizophrenic parents in the cohort and correlated obstetrical events with the IQ test scores for both the HR and LR children. Vaginal bleeding, edema, and conduction anesthesia explained 34% of the variance in IQ scores in the offspring of "continuous schizophrenics" (i.e, chronic, borderline and chronic schizoaffective schizophrenics, N=45); the same obstetrical factors did not relate to IQ in the Controls or in a group with acute schizophrenia in their parents. The authors point out that it is possible to interpret these results as showing that a common genetic liability is responsible for the obstetrical complications, IQ deficit and schizophrenia. This interpretation, however, would require that HR children have generally lower IQs than LR children, which has not been observed (Mednick, & Schulsinger, 1965). As the authors themselves state, the interaction interpretation better explains their findings.

Marcus and his colleagues(1985) studied the perinatal history and neuro-integrative functioning of 58 Jerusalem-born HR infants. They found that in "every case, low to low-normal birth weight in an infant of a schizophrenic was associated with poor performance during the first year" (p. 710). No such relationship was observed in the controls, prompting the authors to suggest "a genetically determined vulnerability of fetal brains of offspring of schizophrenics" (p. 710).

The Copenhagen HR study has followed a group of 207 HR and 104 LR subjects for the past 26 years. In 1972, 15 of the HR offspring were diagnosed schizophrenic (Schulsinger, 1976). These 15 schizophrenics had significantly elevated levels of perinatal complications while the LR subjects with equivalent levels of perinatal complications did not evidence schizophrenia (Parnas et al. 1982). The HR subjects who had become schizophrenic evidenced significantly wider third ventricles and larger ventricle-brain ratios (VBRs) than non-schizophrenic HR subjects; obstetrical complications were significantly related to both schizophrenia and ventricle measures (Schulsinger et al., 1984). The interaction between degree of genetic risk and birth complications accounted for 56% of the variance in the ventricular measurements (Cannon, Mednick, & Parnas, 1989).

Minor Physical Anomalies

A brief summary and description of minor physical anomalies (MPAs) appears in Guy et al. (1983). MPAs are slight physical defects (e.g., low-seated ears, curved fifth finger) that develop during gestation. They are caused by a disruption of fetal development due to either genetic or teratogenic factors. Because MPAs and the CNS develop from the same germinal layer (ectoderm), observable MPAs may serve as evidence for nonobservable CNS abnormalities. Additionally, it is believed that many MPAs have their origins in the first trimester (Waldrop et al., 1968), which is a critical time for CNS development. Bracha has reported an elevation in dermatoglyphic anomalies among schizophrenics and indicates that this suggests a second trimester developmental disruption (1991). This time frame coincides with the critical period for exposure to influenza.

There have been a number of studies examining the incidence of MPAs in schizophrenia. The consensus seems to be that there is a higher incidence of MPAs among schizophrenics than among the normal population (Guy et al., 1983; Gualtieri et al., 1982). Further, a higher number of MPAs has been associated with an earlier onset of schizophrenia (Green et al., 1987; Green et al., 1989). These results provide evidence for some type of developmental disruption during gestation within the schizophrenic population. They also suggest that there may have been a disruption of CNS development for these individuals.

Our interpretation of these data

In this review we have noted several strands of evidence which implicate a disturbance in fetal neural development in the etiology of adult schizophrenia.

1. Low birth weight and prematurity at birth have been shown to be more characteristic of schizophrenics than controls. These findings imply that some disturbance during the gestation of schizophrenics interferes with normal growth.
2. The elevated frequency of MPAs in schizophrenics may be interpreted as indicating genetic or teratogenic disturbances during gestation.
3. Finnish and Danish epidemiological studies suggest that an influenza epidemic may disrupt the growth of the fetal brain in the second trimester and may increase the risk for schizophrenia.
4. Recent neuropathological findings in schizophrenics have been interpreted as being caused by disruptions in neuronal migration, perhaps in the second trimester of gestation.

The origin of the hypothesized neural developmental disturbance may be due to genetic factors which have been found to be quite potent in producing neuronal migration disruption in laboratory animals (Nowakowski, 1991). Genetic factors can distort the organization of brain structures or functional systems by producing perturbations in the generation or migration of young neurons.

Models of adult syndromes of schizophrenia

We hypothesize that fetal neural developmental disturbance may be a critical part of the phenotypic expression of the genetic predisposition to schizophrenia. A teratogenic agent (such as a viral infection) striking during a critical period of brain development might mimic the genetic disturbance. The developmental disturbance may predispose the fetus to experience severe DCs. In our HR project we noted a significant elevation of DCs among the schizophrenics. As is reflected in the high level of DC score variance, about half of the schizophrenics had either very minor delivery complications or none at all. Those HR subjects who had suffered severe DCs evidenced large VBRs and widening of their third ventricles (Cannon, Mednick, & Parnas, 1989; Silverton, Finello, Mednick, & Schulsinger, 1985). This suggests that DCs and enlarged ventricles may be involved in the etiology of a particular type of schizophrenia or a subgroup of schizophrenics. We have conducted several analyses of the Copenhagen HR project data bank in order to characterize the nature of this subgroup.

Third ventricle widening attracted our special attention since it is the most commonly reported CT-scan anomaly in schizophrenics and because of our long interest in the role of the autonomic nervous system (ANS) in the etiology of schizophrenia (Mednick, 1958). The most important excitatory centers of the ANS border on the third ventricle (Wang, 1964; Barr, 1979). Based on this, we hypothesized that widening of the third ventricle (and not of the lateral cerebral ventricles) is associated with damage to one or more of these ANS centers. We have found that widening of the third ventricle is significantly associated with non-responding of the ANS, both for electrodermal and heart rate responsiveness (Cannon et al. 1988; Cannon, et al., in press). This suggests that perhaps damage to these excitatory ANS centers (such as the anterior hypothalamus) may seriously dampen sympathetic nervous system activity and result in deficient emotional and motivational responsiveness, including anergia, often a part of the pattern of negative symptoms observed in schizophrenics. This series of findings and interpretations led us to the prediction that genetic risk, DCs and ANS non-responsiveness increase the risk for schizophrenia with predominantly negative symptoms.

We used the Copenhagen HR study data to test this model. On the basis of the interview data, we prepared scales measuring degree of negative and positive symptoms in the HR sample. Using these scales with 15 diagnosed schizophrenics in 1972, we found that seven of the schizophrenics had severe negative symptoms and weak or absent positive symptoms. We tested the three hypothesized factors, severe DCs, ANS non-responding, and genetic risk expressed at two levels: Super-HR (schizophrenic mother and schizophrenia spectrum father) and HR (schizophrenic mother only), to see how well they distinguished these seven negative symptom schizophrenics from the other HR subjects.

The rate of predominantly negative-symptom schizophrenia in the HR sample is 4% and increases to 11% in the Super HR population. Furthermore, if the individual has experienced above-average DCs then the rate of negative symptom schizophrenia is 35%. If (in 1962) these individuals were also ANS nonresponders, the rate of negative-symptom schizophrenia is 86%; 131 HR subjects (including eight schizophrenics with predominantly positive symptoms) are classified by this model as NOT having negative-symptom schizophrenia. Only one of these 131 cases was diagnosed as a negative symptom schizophrenic, yielding a false-positive rate of only .008.

In this framework, Super-HR status implies an extremely high risk that a genetically-determined disruption in fetal neural development will occur during the second trimester of gestation. We have found possible signs of this disruption of development in specific defects in cognitive performance which distinguish the Super-HR from the HR and LR subjects. (These defects include signs noted by Fini Schulsinger when the subjects were first interviewed in 1962: clouded consciousness, incoherence, disorientation, and impaired train of associations, as well as indices of word association disturbance and poor performance on standardized IQ tests). We propose that the developmental disruption which may be responsible for these cognitive deficits is a critical part of the etiological background of schizotypal personality disorder, a condition genetically related to schizophrenia. Schizotypal personality disorder may be the basic "genetic" disorder of the schizophrenia spectrum. In this framework, schizophrenia-proper is a derivative condition whose likelihood is increased by the action of certain environmental agents (such as OCs).

If gestational and perinatal disturbance are related to schizophrenia, why does this illness first manifest itself in early adulthood? There are a few possible explanations for this. In most cases professionals have little access to information regarding the premorbid state of adult schizophrenics. It is possible that in many cases adult decompensation does not represent a major change in symptoms or behavior. In the Copenhagen high-risk study we have noted distinct premorbid behaviors associated with schizophrenia exhibited as far back as early adolescence (Cannon et al., 1990) and even infancy (Parnas et al., 1982). These premorbid behaviors could be the age-specific equivalents or manifestations of adult schizophrenia.

Another explanation suggests that the schizophrenic has a nonprogressive brain lesion long before schizophrenia becomes obvious (Weinberger, 1987; Benes, 1989). The disease progresses to a manifest level when the areas involved in the lesion site become more active due to normal maturation. Weinberger (1987) implicates the dopaminergic tracts between the brain stem, limbic structures, and dorsolateral prefrontal cortex. Not only do these pathways increase their activity during late adolescence, they are also activated during periods of stress. This explanation may be useful to help understand the onset of schizophrenia in males in late adolescence and early adulthood. It may fail, however, to help us understand the later onset of schizophrenia in females. Benes (1989) notes that myelination of the associative cortical areas does not occur until adolescence. She suggests that this later myelination may play a role in the manifestation of schizophrenic symptoms.

The two explanations offered are complementary and could explain both the premorbid behavior and later exacerbation of schizophrenic symptoms. Both would expect early signs of deviance due to early neurodevelopmental problems. They also suggest that neurodevelopmental changes during adolescence may exacerbate existing deviance.

SUMMARY

1. Epidemiological and neuropathological studies suggest that the phenotypic expression of the genetic predisposition for schizophrenia may consist of a susceptibility to disruption of brain development during a critical period of gestation. The genetic predisposition may be mimicked by teratogens during the critical period.

2. The evidence strongly supports the role of OCs in the etiology of schizophrenia.

3. The weight of the evidence indicates that OCs are most strongly associated with schizophrenia in individuals at high genetic risk.

4. In genetically vulnerable individuals, DCs increase the risk for periventricular tissue damage and later schizophrenia.

5. The genetics-DCs interaction may help explain schizophrenia with predominantly negative symptoms.

6. Schizophrenia may not suddenly appear in early adulthood. Longitudinal, prospective studies have reported early behavioral analogues of adult schizophrenia symptoms. The manifest symptomatic behavior may occur in response to the stress engendered by role transition (the assumption of occupational responsibility or parental responsibilities) or by neurodevelopmental changes in adolescence.

ACKNOWLEDGEMENTS

This research was supported by National Institute of Mental Health Grants 5RO1 MH37692, 1RO1 MH46014, and MH44188, a Grant from the Scottish Rite Foundation, and an All-University Merit Fellowship from the University of Southern California to K.L. Dykes.

REFERENCES

Barr, C. E., Mednick, S. A., & Munk-Jorgensen, P. (1990). Exposure to influenza epidemics during gestation and adult schizophrenia: A 40 year study. Archives of General Psychiatry, 47(9), 869-874.

Barr, M. L. (1979). The human nervous system (3rd ed.). Hagerstown, Maryland: Harper & Row.

Bender, L. (1973). The life course of children with schizophrenia. American Journal of Psychiatry, 130, 783-786.

Benes, F. M. (1989). Myelination of cortical-hippocampal relays during late adolescence. Schizophrenia Bulletin, 15(4), 585-593.

Bogerts, B. (1991). The neuropathology of schizophrenia: Pathophysiological and neurodevelopmental implications. In S. Mednick, T. Cannon, C. Barr & M.

Lyon (Eds.), Fetal Neural Development and Adult Schizophrenia. (pp. 153-173). Cambridge: Cambridge University Press.

Bracha, S. Personal Communication, 1991.

Broman, S. H., Nichols, P. I., & Kennedy W. A. (Eds.). (1975). Preschool IQ: Prenatal and Early Developmental Correlates. New York: Halstead Press.

Cannon, T. D., Fuhrmann, M., Mednick, S. A., Machon, R. A., Parnas, J., & Schulsinger, F. (1988). Third ventricle enlargement and reduced electrodermal responsiveness. Psychophysiology, 25, 153-156.

Cannon, T. D., Mednick, S. A., & Parnas, J. (1989). Genetic and perinatal determinants of structural brain abnormalities in schizophrenia. Archives of General Psychiatry, 46, 883-889.

Cannon, T. D., Mednick, S. A. & Parnas, J. (1990a). Two pathways to schizophrenia in children at risk. In L. Robins & M. Rutter (Eds.), Straight and devious pathways from childhood to adulthood. (pp. 328-350). Cambridge: Cambridge University Press.

Cannon, T. D., Mednick, S. A., & Parnas, J. (1990b). Antecedents of predominantly negative and predominantly positive symptom schizophrenia in a highrisk population. Archives of General Psychiatry, 47, 622-632.

Cannon, T. D., Raine, A., Herman, T. M., Mednick, S. A., Parnas, J., & Schulsinger, F. (in press). Third ventricle enlargement and reduced heart rate levels in a high-risk sample. Psychophysiology.

Cazullo, C. L., Vita, A. & Sacchetti, E. (1989). Cerebral ventricular enlargement in schizophrenia: Prevalence and correlates. In S. C. Schulz & C. A. Tamminga (Eds.), Schizophrenia: Scientific progress. (pp. 195-206). New York: Oxford University Press.

Courchesney, E., Yeung-Courchesne, R., Press, G. A., Hesselink, J. R., & Jernigan., T. L. (1988). Hypoplasia of cerebellar vermal lobules VI and VII in autism. New England Journal of Medicine, 318, 1349-54.

DeLisi, L.E., Dauphinais, I.D., & Gershon, E.S. (1988). Perinatal complications and reduced size of brain limbic structures in familial schizophrenia. Schizophrenia Bulletin, 14(2), 185-191.

Eagles, J.M., Gibson, I., Bremner, M.H., Clunie, F., Ebmeier, K.P. & Smith, N.C. (1990). Obstetric complications in DSM-III schizophrenics and their siblings. The Lancet, 335, 1139-1141.

Fish, B. (1971). Discussion: Genetic or traumatic developmental deviation. Social Biology, 18, S117-S119.

Goodman, R. (1988). Are complications of pregnancy and birth causes of schizophrenia? Developmental Medicine and Child Neurology, 30, 391-406.

Gottesman, I. I. & Shields, J. (1972). Schizophrenia and genetics: A twin study vantage point. New York: Academic Press.

Gottesman, I. I., & Shields, J. (1982). Schizophrenia: The epigenetic puzzle. Cambridge, England: Cambridge University Press.

Green, M.F., Satz, P., Soper, H.V. & Kharabi, F. (1987). Relationship between physical anomalies and age at onset of schizophrenia. American Journal of Psychiatry, 144(5), 666-667.

Green, M.F., Satz, P., Gaier, D.J., Ganzell, S. & Kharabi, F. (1989). Minor physical anomalies in schizophrenia. Schizophrenia Bulletin, 15(1), 91-99.

Gualtieri, C.T., Adams, A., Shen, C.D. & Loiselle, D. (1982). Minor physical anomalies in alcoholic and schizophrenia adults and hyperactive and autistic children. American Journal of Psychiatry, 139(5), 640-643.

Guy, J.D., Majorski, L.V., Wallace, C.J. & Guy, M.P. (1983). The incidence of minor physical anomalies in adult male schizophrenics. Schizophrenia Bulletin, 9(4), 571-582.

Hinton, G. G. (1963). Childhood psychosis or mental retardation: A diagnostic dilemma. II. Paediatric and neurological aspects. Canadian Medical Association, 89, 1020-1024.

Hanson, D. R., Gottesman, I. I., & Heston, L. L. (1976). Some possible childhood indicators of adult schizophrenia inferred from children of schizophrenics. British Journal of Psychiatry, 129, 142.

Jacobsen B. & Kinney, D. K. (1980). Perinatal complications in adopted and non-adopted schizophrenics and their controls: preliminary results. Acta Psychiatrica Scandinavia, Supplement, 285(62), 337-351.

Katz, B. (1939). The etiology of the deteriorating psychoses of adolescence and early adult life. Unpublished doctoral dissertation, University of Southern California.

Kendell R.E., & Kemp I.W. (1989). Maternal influenza in the etiology of schizophrenia. Archives of General Psychiatry, 46, 878-882.

Knobloch, H. and Pasamanick, B. (1962, September). Etiologic factors in "early infantile autism" and "childhood schizophrenia. Paper presented at the 10th International Congress of Paediatry, Lisbon.

Lane, E. A. & Albee, G. W. (1966). Comparative birth weights of schizophrenics and their siblings. Journal of Psychology, 64, 227-231.

Lewis, S. W., & Murray, R. M. (1987). Obstetric complications, neurodevelopmental deviance, and risk of schizophrenia. Journal of Psychiatric Research, 21, 413-421.

Lohr, J.B. & Bracha, H.S. (1989). Can schizophrenia be related to prenatal exposure to alcohol? Some speculations. Schizophrenia Bulletin, 15(4), 595603.

Lyon, M., Barr, C.E., Cannon, T.D., Mednick, S.A. & Shore, D. (1989). Fetal neural development and schizophrenia. Schizophrenia Bulletin, 15(1), 149-161.

Marcus, J., Hans, S. L., Mednick, S. A., Schulsinger, F., & Michelsen, N. (1985). Neurological dysfunctioning in offspring of schizophrenics in Israel and Denmark: A replication analysis. Archives of General Psychiatry, 42, 753-761.

Marcus J., Auerback, J. Wilkinson, L., & Burack, C. M. (1981). Infants at risk for schizophrenia. The Jerusalem Infant Development Study. Archives of General Psychiatry, 38, 703-713.

McNeil, T. F. (1988). Obstetric factors and perinatal injuries. In M. T. Tsuang & J. C. Simpson (Eds.), Handbook of schizophrenia. (pp. 319-344). Amsterdam: Elsevier.

McNeil, T. F., & Kaij, L. (1978). Obstetric factors in the development of schizophrenia: Complications in the births of preschizophrenics and in reproduction by schizophrenic parents. In L. C. Wynne, R. L. Cromwell, & S. Matthysse (Eds.), The nature of schizophrenia: New approaches to research and treatment (pp. 401-429). New York: John Wiley and Sons

Mednick, S.A. (1970). Breakdown in individuals at high risk for schizophrenia: Possible predispositional perinatal factors. Mental Hygeine, 54(1), 50-63.

Mednick, S. A. (1958). A learning theory approach to research in schizophrenia. Psychological Bulletin, 55, 316-327.

Mednick, S.A. & Hefner, T. (1969). Reliability of developmental histories. Pediatrics Digest, 11, 28-39.

Mednick, S.A., Mura, E., Schulsinger, F., Mednick, B. (1974). Perinatal conditions and infant development in children with schizophrenic parents. In S.A. Mednick, F. Schulsinger, J. Higgins, B Bell, B., (Eds.), Genetics, Environment, and Psychopathology, (pp. 231-248). North Holland, Amsterdam: Elsevier.

Mednick, S. A. & Schulsinger, F. (1965). A longitudinal study of children with a high risk for schizophrenia: A preliminary report. In S. Vandenberg (Ed.), Methods and goals in human behavior genetics (pp. 255-296). New York: Academic Press.

Mednick, S. A. & Shaffer, J. (1963). Mother's retrospective reports in child rearing research. American Journal of Orthopsychiatry, 33, 451-461.

Mednick, S. A., Machon, R. A., Huttunen, M. O., & Bonett, D. (1988).Adult schizophrenia following prenatal exposure to an influenza epidemic. Archives of General Psychiatry, 45, 189-192.

Mednick, S. A. & Silverton, L. (1987). High-risk studies of the etiology of schizophrenia. In M. T. Tsuang & J. C. Simpson (Eds.), Handbook of schizophrenia, vol. 3: Nosology, epidemiology and genetics. Amsterdam: Elsevier.

Mirdal G. K. M., Mednick, S. A., Schulsinger, F., & Fuchs F. (1974). Perinatal complications in children of schizophrenic mothers. Acta Psychiatrica Scandinavia, 50, 553-568.

Mura, E. L. (1974). Perinatal differences: a comparison of child psychiatric patients and their siblings. Psychiatric Quarterly, 48, 239-255.

Murray, R. M., Reveley, A. M. & Lewis, S. W. (1988). Family history, obstetric complications and cerebral abnormality in schizophrenia. In M. T. Tsuang & J. C. Simpson (Eds.), Handbook of schizophrenia, vol. 3: nosology, epidemiology, and genetics. (pp. 563-578). Amsterdam: Elsevier.

Nimgaonkar, V.L., Wessely, S. & Murray, R.M. (1988). Prevalence of familiality, obstetric complications, and structural brain damage in schizophrenic patients. British Journal of Psychiatry, 153, 191-197.

Nowakowski, R. S. (1991). Genetic disturbances of neuronal migration: Some examples from the limbic system of mutant mice. In S. Mednick, T. Cannon, C. Barr & M. Lyon (Eds.), Fetal Neural Development and Adult Schizophrenia. (pp. 153-173). Cambridge: Cambridge University Press.

Otake, M. & Schull, W.I. (1984). In utero exposure to A-bomb radiation and mental retardation: A reassessment. British Journal of Radiology, 57, 409414.

Owen, M.J., Lewis, S.W. & Murray, R.M. (1988). Obstetric complications and schizophrenia: A computed tomographic study. Psychological Medicine, 18, 331-339.

Parnas, J., Schulsinger, F., Teasdale, T. W., Schulsinger, H., Feldman,P. M., & Mednick, S. A. (1982). Perinatal complications and clinical outcome within the schizophrenia spectrum. British Journal of Psychiatry, 140, 416-420.

Pollack, M., Woerner, M. G., Goodman, W., & Greenberg, I. M. (1966). Childhood development patterns of hospitalized adult schizophrenic and nonschizophrenic patients and their siblings. American Journal of Orthopsychiatry, 36, 510.

Pollin W. & Stabenau, J. R. (1968). Biological, psychological and historical differences in a series of monozygotic twins discordant for schizophrenia. In D. Rosenthal, S. S. Kety (Eds.), The Transmission of Schizophrenia, pp. (317-332). London: Pergamon Press.

Rakic, P. (1988). Specification of cerebral cortical areas. Science, 241, 170-176.

Rakic, P. Personal Communication, March 8, 1991.

Reveley, A. M., Reveley, M. A., & Murray, R. M. (1984). Cerebral ventricular enlargement in non-genetic schizophrenia: A controlled twin study. British Journal of Psychiatry, 144, 89-93.

Rieder, R. O., Broman, S. H., Rosenthal, D. (1977). The offspring of schizophrenics. II. Perinatal factors and IQ. Archives of General Psychiatry, 34, 789.

Rutt, C. N. & Offord D. R. (1971). Prenatal and perinatal complications in childhood schizophrenics and their siblings. Journal of Nervous and Mental Disease, 152, 324-331.

Schulsinger, F., Parnas, J., Petersen, E. T., Schulsinger, H., Teasdale, T. W., Mednick, S. A., Moller, L., & Silverton, L. (1984). Cerebral ventricular size in the offspring of schizophrenic mothers. Archives of General Psychiatry, 41, 602-606.

Schulsinger, H. (1976). A ten year follow-up of children of schizophrenic mothers: Clinical assessment. Acta Psychiatrica Scandinavica, 53, 371-386.

Schwarzkopf, S.B., Nasrallah, H.A.. Olson, S.C. & Coffman, J. A. (1989). Relationship of perinatal complications and genetic loading in schizophrenia. Psychiatry Research, 27, 233-239.

Silverton, L., Finello, K. M., Mednick, S. A., & Schulsinger, F. (1985). Low birth weight and ventricular enlargement in a high-risk sample. Journal of Abnormal Psychology, 94, 405-409.

Taft, L. T., & Goldfarb, W. (1964). Prenatal and perinatal factors in childhood schizophrenia. Developmental Medicine and Child Neurology, 6, 32-43.

Terris, M. LaPouse, R. & Monk, M. A. (1964). The relation of prematurity and previous fetal loss to childhood schizophrenia. American Journal of Psychiatry, 121, 476-481.

Torrey, E. F., & Hersch, S. P. (1975). Early childhood psychosis and bleeding during pregnancy: A prospective study of gravid women and their offspring. Journal of Autism and Childhood Schizophrenia, 5,(4), 287-297.

Torrey E. F., Rawlings R., & Waldman P. (1988). Schizophrenic births and viral diseases in two states. Schizophrenia Research, 1, 73-77.

Vorster, D. (1960). An investigation into the part played by organic factors in childhood schizophrenia. Journal of Mental Science, 106, 494-522.

Waldrop, M.F., Pederson, F.A. & Bell, R.Q. (1968). Minor physical anomalies and behavior in preschool children. Child Development, 39, 391-400.

Wang, G. H. (1964). Neural control of sweating. Madison, Wisconsin: University of Wisconsin Press.

Weinberger, D.R. (1987). Implications of normal brain development for the pathogenesis of schizophrenia. Archives of General Psychiatry, 44, 660-669.

Whittam H., Simon, G. B., & Mittler, P. J. (1966). The early development of psychotic children and their sibs. Developmental Medicine and Child Neurology, 8, 552-560.

Woerner M. G., Pollack, M., & Klein, D. F. (1971). Birth weight and length in schizophrenics, personality disorders, and their siblings. British Journal of Psychiatry, 118, 461-464.

Woerner, M. G., Pollack, M., & Klein, D. F. (1973). Pregnancy and birth complications in psychiatric patients: A comparison of schizophrenic and personality disorder patients with their siblings. Acta Psychiatrica Scandinavia, 49, 712-721.

Zitrin, A., Ferber P., & Cohen, D. (1964). Pre- and paranatal factors in mental disorders of children. Journal of Nervous and Mental Disease, 121, 357-361.

STRUCTURAL BRAIN MEASUREMENTS ON MRI SCANS IN SCHIZOPHRENIA: EVIDENCE OF NEURODEVELOPMENTAL PATHOLOGY

Henry A. Nasrallah, Steven B. Schwarzkopf, and
Stephen C. Olson,

Department of Psychiatry, Ohio State University
Columbus, Ohio

INTRODUCTION

There now exists a substantial body of evidence suggesting that the schizophrenia syndrome is associated with both genetic and environmental factors (Tsuang and Simpson, 1988). The genetic evidence comes from family (Guze et al., 1983), twin (Kendler, 1983), and adoption (Kety, 1983) studies. Evidence of environmental influence comes from the reports of prenatal (Mednick et al., 1988) (intrauterine environment), neonatal (McNeil and Kaij, 1978) (obstetric complications) and postnatal brain insults (Wilcox and Nasrallah, 1987), all of which suggest that the biological environment during development may play a critical role in brain development leading to psychotic brain disorders labeled as schizophrenia, and may be additive to genetic factors (Mednick and Silverton, 1988).

Over the past few years, a large body of literature has emerged which points to atrophic structural brain changes in schizophrenic patients (Nasrallah and Weinberger, 1986). Within the computed tomography (CT) literature, a few reports have suggested that a large ventricular to brain ratio (VBR) in schizophrenia is associated with family history (Nasrallah et al., 1983; Owens et al., 1985; Delisi et al., 1985). While several other studies suggest that ventriculomegaly is related to perinatal complications (Reveley et al., 1984; Turner et al., 1988; Lewis and Murray, 1989), some have used this evidence to propose a genetic-sporadic dichotomy as a research strategy in schizophrenia (Lewis et al., 1987).

Developmental Neuropathology of Schizophrenia
Edited by S.A. Mednick *et al.*, Plenum Press, New York, 1991

We previously reported a magnetic resonance imaging (MRI) study of schizophrenia (Andreasen et al., 1986), in which smaller cerebral and cranial midsagittal areas were found in schizophrenic patients compared to controls. We suggested that there may be an early developmental impairment of normal brain development in schizophrenia. The possible contributions of genetic and perinatal factors to smaller brain size were not addressed in that report.

We present here an MRI study of the brain in a new sample of patients in which we examined the effects of genetic history versus perinatal complications to the measures of the cranium, cerebrum and lateral ventricles in schizophrenia. We have previously reported that perinatal complications occur more frequently in schizophrenics without family history (Schwarzkopf et al., 1989). Our pre-hoc hypothesis was that a history of perinatal complications is associated with smaller cerebral and larger ventricular size.

METHOD

Schizophrenic and schizoaffective patients (n=35) living in the community (i.e. not chronically institutionalized) were consecutively admitted to the study after signing informed consent. Inclusion criteria included: 1) males and females age 20 to 50 years with onset of illness before age 45 years, 2) fulfilling DSM-IIIR criteria for schizophrenia or schizoaffective disorder, and 3) have the ability to give informed consent. Exclusion criteria included: 1) serious and or debilitating medical illness including seizure disorder, 2) past history of penetrating head injury or neurosurgery, 3) metallic implants in the body, and, 4) past or present history of severe substance abuse or dependence.

A structured diagnostic interview (SCID-R) was used to document the diagnosis. Family history of schizophrenia (FH-RDC) was obtained by interviews with the parents, or if not available, another close family member. Perinatal history was obtained through a self-administered questionnaire from the mother, and if not available, from the father or other relatives. Perinatal complications variables are shown on Table 1.

Midsagittal MRI scans were obtained on a General Electric 1.5 tesla scanner using an inversion recovery pulse sequence (TI=800 MS, TR=1500 MS). Eight scans per subject were obtained with a slice thickness of 3mm and an inter-slice distance of 1mm. The midsagittal slice was selected for demonstration of the smallest corpus callosum image and least inclusion of cerebral white matter.

Table 1. Perinatal Complication Variables

-Premature delivery
-Postmature delivery
-Prolonged labor (MD report)
-Breech presentation
-Forceps delivery
-Cord around neck
-Blue at birth
-Bradycardia at birth
-Apneic at birth
-Jaundice
-Infant "jittery"
-Required 02 at birth
-Needed transfusions
-Required incubator
-Multiple births

The scans were magnified to normal head size, traced, and the following measurements made with computerized planimetry:

1. Cranial area
2. Cerebral area
3. Frontal area (defined as the cerebral cortical area anterior to a line drawn perpendicular to the midpoint of the maximum length of the corpus callosum)
4. Ventricular to brain ratio (defined as the ratio of the midsagittal ventricular area to the midsagittal cerebral area)

The reliability of the midsagittal MRI measurements has been described elsewhere.

The schizophrenic patients were classified as family history positive (FH-POS) based on the presence of a first or second degree relative who was hospitalized for either schizophrenia or a major affective disorder, or has had a completed suicide. Absence of such history was considered as family history negative (FH-NEG).

With regards to perinatal complications, schizophrenic patients were classified as "perinatally damaged" (PC+) if they had two or more events from Table 1, and "perinatally undamaged" (PC-) if they had none of those events.

Table 2. Demographic Variables

VARIABLE	Schizophrenia/Schizoaffective Patients Males	Females	TOTAL Sample
MEAN AGE (years)	29.8	33.7	31.2
MEAN HEIGHT (cm)	177.3	162.8	172.1
MEAN WEIGHT (Kg)	84.7	70.1	79.5
ILLNESS DURATION (years)	10.0	10.3	10.1
EDUCATION (years)	13.5	13.8	13.6

Table 3. MRI Brain Measurements in Perinatally Damaged (PC+) and Undamaged (PC-) Schizophrenics (Males and Females, N=26)*

	PC+(N=7)		PC-(N=9)		
MEASURE	MEAN	(SD)	MEAN	(SD)	P-VALUE
CRANIAL AREA	165.84	(14.92)	160.38	(10.73)	.31
CEREBRAL AREA	75.04	(6.35)	72.00	(7.28)	.52
FRONTAL AREA	35.70	(2.12)	34.70	(3.63)	.50
VBR	0.0325	(0.02)	0.0320	(0.02)	.94

*Perinatal data were not available for the entire sample.

Table 4. MRI Brain Measurements in Family History Positive (FH-POS) and Family History Negative (FH-NEG) Schizophrenics (Males and Females, N=35)

	FH + Pos (N=6)		FH - Neg (N=19)		
MEASURE	MEAN	(SD)	MEAN	(SD)	P-VALUE
CRANIAL AREA	156.48	(8.33)	165.33	(13.68)	.030
CEREBRAL AREA	71.16	(5.30)	75.49	(7.31)	.055
FRONTAL AREA	33.28	(2.69)	35.67	(3.39)	.029
VBR	0.033	(0.02)	0.037	(0.02)	.574

The mean MRI measurements of the two groups were compared using analysis of variance (ANOVA).

RESULTS

Table 2 shows the demographic variables of the schizophrenic sample, total and by gender.

Table 3 shows a comparison of the PC + VS PC- schizophrenic subjects. No significant differences emerged between the two groups. Similarly, no significant differences emerged when the schizophrenic males or females were examined separately.

Table 4 shows a comparison of schizophrenic subjects divided into FH-POS and FH-NEG groups. Significant differences emerged in cranial and frontal areas with a strong trend for cerebral area, all in the direction of a smaller brain measurement in the FH-POS schizophrenic group. No difference in VBR was found.

DISCUSSION

The results clearly do not support the hypothesis of small brain measurements (cranial, cerebral, frontal) in schizophrenics with a history of perinatal complications compared to their counterparts without such history. In fact, the cranial, cerebral, frontal and callosal means in the PC+ group are actually <u>larger</u> than in the PC- group.

As for the relationship of family history to MRI brain measurements, our findings suggest a strong link between family history of psychosis and reduced brain size in schizophrenia, which has now been reported in several studies (Roberts, 1990). The data can be interpreted as: 1) that genetic factors in schizophrenia are associated with smaller brain measurements in the familial group, or 2) that FH-Neg patients, where perinatal complications tend to cluster (Schwarzkopf et al., 1989) have larger brains than FH-Pos group, possibly because of adverse neurodevelopmental events. Based on the trends we are observing so far in an age-, sex-, and education-match control groups, it appears that the PC+ groups are closer to control values, while the FH-Pos group appear to be significantly smaller than normal controls. This suggests that a genetic influence, rather than perinatal complications is the more critical factor in smaller brain size (hypoplasia?) in schizophrenia. However, the effect of perinatal complications may be more evident at the cellular level (Falkai et al., 1988).

Finally, this study points to the importance of controlling for family history and perinatal history in the conduct of brain imaging studies in schizophrenia. It also suggests that one or more of those factors may have an important association with brain plasticity in utero (Nasrallah, 1990), postnatally or even during adolescence (Feinberg et al., 1983).

REFERENCES

Andreasen NC, Nasrallah HA, Dunn V et al.: Structural abnormalities in the Frontal System in Schizophrenia. A magnetic Resonance Imaging Study. Archives of General Psychiatry 43: 136-144, 1986.

Coffman JA, Schwarzkopf SB, Olson SC, Nasrallah HA: Cerebral anatomy by magnetic resonance imaging: The importance of slice position and thickness. Schizophrenia Research 2:287-294, 1989.

Delisi LE, Goldin LR, Hamovit JR et al.: Is Cerebral Ventricular Enlargement a Genetic Marker for Schizophrenia. Psychopharmacology Bulletin 21: 365-367, 1985.

Delisi LE, Goldin LR, Hamovit JR et al.: A Family Study of the Association of Increased Ventricular Size in Schizophrenia. Archives of General Psychiatry 43: 48-52, 1986.

Falkai P, Bogerts B, Roberts GW, Crow TJ: Measurement of the alpha cell migration in the entorhinal region: A marker for the developmental disturbances in schizophrenia? Schizophrenia Research 1: 157-158, 1988.

Feinberg I: Schizophrenia: Caused by a Fault in Programmed Synaptic Elimination during Adolescence? Journal Psychiatric Research 17: 315-344, 1983.

Guze SB, Cloninger CR, Martin RL et al.: A Follow-up and Family Study of Schizophrenia. Archives of General Psychiatry 1273-1776, 1983.

Kendler KS: Twin Studies in Schizophrenia, a Current Perspective. American Journal of Psychiatry 140: 1413-1419, 1983.

Kety SS: Observations on Genetic and Environmental Inferences in the Etiology of Mental Disorders from Studies on Adoptees and Their Families. In Genetics of Neurological and Psychiatric Disorders. SS Kety, LP Rowland, RL Sedman, and SW Matthysse, (Editors) Raven Press, New York 1983 pp. 105-114.

Lewis SW, Reveley AM, Reveley MA et al.: The familial/Sporadic Distinction as a Strategy in Schizophrenia Research. British Journal of Psychiatry 151: 306-310, 1987.

Lewis SW, Murray RM: Obstetric Complications, Neurodevelopmental deviance and Risk of Schizophrenia. Journal of Psychiatric Research 21: 413-421, 1987.

McNeil TF, Kaij L: Obstetric Factors in the Development of Schizophrenia. Wynne LC, Cromwell RL, Mathysses (Editors) The Nature of Schizophrenia, Wiley, New York, 1978, pp 401-429.

Mednick SA, Machon RA, Huttunen MO et al.: Adult Schizophrenia Following Prenatal Exposure to an Influenza Epidemic. Archives of General Psychiatry 45: 189-192, 1988.

Mednick SA, Silverton L: High-risk Studies of the Etiology of Schizophrenia. The Handbook of Schizophrenia (HA Nasrallah, Series Editor) Volume III, Nosology, Epidemiology and Genetics of Schizophrenia (MT Tsuang and JC Simpson Volume Editors), Elsevier, Amsterdam, 1988, pp 543-562.

Nasrallah HA: Brain structure and function in Schizophrenia: Evidence for fetal neurodevelopmental impairment. Current Opinion in Psychiatry 3: 75-78, 1990.

Nasrallah HA, Kuperman S, Hamra BJ et al.: Clinical Differences between Schizophrenic Patients With and Without Large Cerebral Ventricles. Journal of Clinical Psychiatry 44: 407-409, 1983.

Nasrallah HA, Weinberger DR (Editors): The Handbook of Schizophrenia (HA Nasrallah, Series Editor) Volume I. The Neurology of Schizophrenia, Elsevier, Amsterdam, 1986.

Owens DGC, Johnstone EC, Crow TJ et al.: Lateral Ventricular Size in Schizophrenia: Relationship to the Disease Process and its Clinical Manifestations. Psychological Medicine 15 27-41, 1985.

Reveley AM, Reveley MA, Murray RM: Cerebral Ventricular Enlargement in Non-Genetic Schizophrenia: A Controlled Twin Study. British Journal of Psychiatry 144: 89-92, 1984.

Roberts GW: Schizophrenia: The Cellular Biology of a Functional Psychosis. Trends in Neuroscience 13: 207-211, 1990.

Schwarzkopf SB, Nasrallah HA, Olson SC, Coffman JA: Relationship of Perinatal Complications and Genetic Loading in Schizophrenia. Psychiatry Research 27: 233-239, 1989.

Schulsinger F, Parnas J, Petersen ET et al.: Cerebral Ventricular Size in the Offspring of Schizophrenic Mothers. Archives of General Psychiatry 41: 602-605, 1984.

Tsuang MT, Simpson JC (Editors): The Handbook of Schizophrenia (HA Nasrallah, Series Editor) Volume III, Nosology, Epidemiology and Genetics of Schizophrenia, Elsevier, Amsterdam, 1988.

Turner SW, Toone BK, Brett-Jones JR: Computerized Tomographic Scan Changes in Early Schizophrenia. Psychological Medicine 16: 219-224, 1988.

Wilcox JA, Nasrallah HA: Childhood Head Trauma and Schizophrenia. Psychiatry Research 10: 303-306, 1987.

THE POSSIBLE NEURODEVELOPMENTAL SIGNIFICANCE OF STRUCTURAL IMAGING FINDINGS IN SCHIZOPHRENIA

Tyrone D. Cannon

University of Southern California
Los Angeles, California, United States of America

INTRODUCTION

The notion that brain abnormalities may underlie cognitive impairment and other "deficit" symptoms of schizophrenia was emphasized in early formulations of the disorder. Kraepelin (1919) viewed these deficits as reflecting a deteriorating brain disease of early adult onset, as indicated by his use of term dementia praecox. Pneumoencephalographic studies carried out in the middle part of this century tended to support this view. The most common finding was subtle cerebral pathology, as evidenced by enlargement of the hollow, fluid-filled spaces in the brain, particularly in the region of the third ventricle, or diencephalon, and particularly in those patients with intellectual and emotional deficits (e.g., Haug, 1962; Huber, 1957; Storey, 1966). These studies were limited by several methodological weaknesses, however, including the questionable reliability of pneumoencephalography, inadequate or unspecified diagnostic criteria and procedures, and inadequate controls (Weinberger et al., 1983).

Modern imaging studies

The advent of the modern brain imaging technologies in the last two decades has provided more reliable and less invasive means by which to assess structural pathology of the brain. Both early and recent uses of these technologies (i.e., computed tomography [CT] and magnetic resonance imaging [MRI]) have confirmed the presence of brain abnormalities in schizophrenic patients (see Cannon, 1991; Raz and Raz, 1990, for recent reviews).

In the typical study, a sample of schizophrenics and a sample of medical or normal volunteer controls are recruited and undergo brain scanning. Axial slices showing the third and lateral ventricles and cerebral sulci at their largest are obtained for each subject. The most common measure of the lateral ventricles is ventricle-brain ratio, or VBR, which is the area of the lateral ventricles divided by the total intracranial area multiplied by 100. The third ventricle and cortical sulci are most often measured at their maximum widths.

When this is done, schizophrenics are usually found to evidence significantly larger third and lateral ventricles and cortical sulci than controls. In about 85% (24/28) of the studies appearing before January of 1990, schizophrenics were reported to show enlargement of the third ventricle; in 79% (55/72) of the studies schizophrenics were reported as having enlarged lateral ventricles or VBRs; and in 61% (19/31) of the studies schizophrenics were reported to have greater cortical sulcal prominence (see Cannon, 1991, for a complete list of the references used to obtain these figures). Abnormalities have been observed in a number of other brain regions, including the cerebellum, but these are less well replicated than the ventricular and cortical abnormalities.

Two perspectives on brain imaging findings

There are two main perspectives on the significance of structural brain abnormalities in schizophrenia. First, some or all of the brain changes may be associated with the etiology of schizophrenia. Evidence supporting an etiological role includes the finding of brain anomalies in young, never-treated patients (e.g., Schulz et al., 1983a), correlations between brain abnormalities, obstetric complications, and genetic risk for schizophrenia (e.g., Cannon et al., 1989), and relationships between brain abnormalities and indices of impaired premorbid functioning (e.g., Erel et al., 1991). Second, some of the brain changes may be consequences of aging or illness processes, psychiatric treatments, or other brain abnormalities. Evidence supporting a secondary, nonpathogenic, or epiphenomenal role includes, respectively, correlations between brain abnormalities and age and psychiatric treatments (e.g., Tanaka et al., 1981), the failure to find a consistent deficit present in all schizophrenics or in all schizophrenics of a particular subtype (e.g., Cazullo et al., 1989), and the finding of similar brain abnormalities in other disorders and in normal aging (e.g., Barron et al., 1976; Pearlson & Veroff, 1981).

Thus, the success of the modern brain imaging studies in uncovering organic aspects of schizophrenia has been qualified by a lack of understanding of the roles of the abnormalities in the etiology and phenomenology of the disease and by the lack of specificity of the abnormalities to schizophrenia.

Goals of this chapter

This chapter will first consider the evidence concerning the possibility that third and lateral ventricular enlargement and cortical sulcal prominence are consequences of subject, treatment, and illness factors; it will then examine studies which have investigated the association between ventricular enlargement and genetic and perinatal sources; finally, data from the Copenhagen schizophrenia high-risk project will be presented which suggests a possible relationship between CT scan abnormalities and genetic and perinatal antecedent factors.

CONTRIBUTIONS OF SUBJECT, TREATMENT, AND ILLNESS FACTORS

Table 1 provides a tabulation of studies which did and did not find significant relationships between three indices of structural brain damage (i.e., lateral ventricular enlargement, third ventricle enlargement, cortical sulcal prominence) and several subject, treatment, and illness factors (see Cannon, 1991, for a complete list of references).

Subject variables

As can be seen from Table 1, neither gender nor race was found to be significantly related to third and lateral ventricular enlargement and cortical sulcal prominence in most studies. In addition, history of substance abuse and head injury were not reliably associated with ventricular or cortical abnormalities. In contrast, age was significantly associated with the three types of brain abnormalities in varying fractions of studies. The contribution of aging to the findings of structural imaging studies of schizophrenics will be considered in greater detail below (see Illness effects).

Treatment effects

Only a few studies found associations between ventricular enlargement and hospitalization, neuroleptic therapy, and ECT (see Table 1). In the few studies which did find correlations between the brain abnormalities and the treatment factors, never treated subjects were still found to evidence the abnormalities (e.g., Johnstone et al., 1976; 1978; Weinberger et al., 1979a).

Illness effects

Age and duration of illness were the only factors which showed a trend toward correlation with ventricular and sulcal enlargement in schizophrenics across studies. However, neither factor was significantly correlated with any of the brain measures in a majority of studies.

Age and duration of illness have been suggested as a possible basis of structural brain pathology in schizophrenia. If this is correct, one would expect not to find reliable differences between schizophrenics and controls using very young

Table 1. Tabulation of CT and MRI studies reporting significant and nonsignificant associations between three brain regions and twelve subject, illness, and treatment factors.[1]

Subject, Illness, or Treatment Factor Significantly Correlated With:

	Lateral Ventricular Enlargement		Third Ventricular Enlargement		Cortical Sulcal Prominence	
Factor	Yes	No	Yes	No	Yes	No
Age	16	46	7	15	5	21
Gender	0	20	1	5	1	5
Race	0	7	0	0	0	2
Substance Abuse	1	8	1	2	0	4
Head Injuries	1	4	0	1	0	1
Age at Onset	2	25	1	7	0	9
Duration of Illness	5	40	4	9	0	16
Length of Hospitalization	1	31	1	8	0	8
Medications	1	26	1	7	0	7
ECT	1	9	0	5	1	3
Leukotomy	1	0	0	0	1	0
Insulin Coma	0	2	0	0	0	1

[1] Multiple publications using the same samples were counted only once in the tabulations. See Cannon (1991) for a complete list of references.

patients. To examine this implication, ten studies were located which examined ventricular enlargement in teenage psychotics, first episode schizophreniform patients, and schizophrenics within 1 to 2 years of the onset of psychosis (Benes et al., 1982; Cazullo et al., 1989; Iacono et al., 1988; Nyback et al., 1982, 1983; Obiols et al., 1986; Reiss et al., 1983; Schulz et al., 1982, 1983a, 1983b; Turner et al, 1986; Weinberger et al., 1982; Woods & Wolf, 1983). Only one out the these ten studies failed to find significantly larger ventricles in the patient group (Benes et al., 1982).

Since age and duration of illness have not been found to be significantly correlated with cortical sulcal prominence and ventricular enlargement in a majority of studies, and since the abnormalities have been observed in the majority of studies examining very young patients, age and duration of illness probably do not <u>explain</u> the finding of ventricular enlargement in schizophrenia. It is still possible, however, that age and duration of illness (or factors associated with them) <u>contribute</u> to ventricular enlargement in schizophrenic samples. It is well known that in normals ventricular size increases with age, particularly after age 50 (Barron et al., 1976). There is no reason to believe that aging processes do not also affect ventricular size in older schizophrenics. However, it is not known if aspects of the schizophrenic disease process are also capable of influencing ventricular size. It would be useful to know how much of the variance in ventricular enlargement is accounted for by these two factors in order to determine the relative contributions of the various possible causal agents.

<u>Progression of brain abnormalities</u>

Duration of illness tends to correlate positively with exposure to physical therapies and length of hospitalization and presumably with any progressive aspects of the disease process in schizophrenia. As a temporal measure, however, duration of illness also tends to be highly correlated with age. Interestingly, in four of the five studies which reported significant associations between lateral ventricular enlargement and duration of illness, there was also a significant correlation between lateral ventricular enlargement and age (Andreasen et al., 1982; Mathew et al., 1985; Naber et al., 1985; Shima et al., 1985). This result suggests that the association between ventricular enlargement and duration of illness is <u>not</u> independent of age. Two studies examined this implication statistically and found that duration of illness made a negligible and nonsignificant contribution to ventricular size once age was controlled (Andreasen et al., 1982; Mathew et al., 1985).

<u>Meta-analysis</u>

Analyses similar to those reported in the preceding paragraph were conducted to summarize the relationships between age, duration of illness, length of hospitalization, and VBR at the level of sample means (that is, the correlations between the mean values of these variables across all studies which reported such values) (see Cannon, 1991, for a complete list of references). There was a significant and substantial relationship between VBR and age in the schizophrenic samples ($r = .60$, $n = 66$, $p < .0001$). The mean VBR of the schizophrenic samples was also significantly correlated with their mean duration of illness ($r = .46$, $n = 47$, $p < .001$) and mean length of hospitalization ($r = .78$, $n = 20$, $p < .0001$). After controlling for the relationship between VBR and age, the correlation between VBR and duration of illness was reduced and became nonsignificant ($r = .09$, $n = 47$, ns). (This analysis effectively controls for the overlap between age and duration of illness since the confounding of these two variables is only of interest vis-a-vis their mutual association with VBR.) In contrast, the partial correlation between VBR and length of hospitalization (i.e., controlling for age) remained significant ($r = .47$, $n = 20$, $p < .04$). This pattern of findings is consistent with the interpretation that larger VBRs are associated with increasing severity but not duration of illness (e.g., Pandurangi et al., 1987). The mean age and VBR of the control samples were also significantly correlated, to about the same degree as in the schizophrenic samples ($r = .55$, $n = 50$, $p < .0001$).

It is important to note that relationships between variables at the level of sample means do not necessarily reflect relationships between those variables at the level of individuals. Nevertheless, the findings reported above are consistent with the results of similar analyses conducted on individual data (Andreasen et al., 1982; Mathew et al., 1985). Together, the results suggest that 1) age may account for about one-third of the variance in the VBRs of both schizophrenic and control samples, and 2) duration of illness may make a negligible contribution to schizophrenics' VBRs once aging variance is controlled.

Summary

In view of these considerations, the ventricular abnormalities in schizophrenia are probably not a consequence of the illness or its treatment. In addition, because the correlations between age and VBR were about the same in the schizophrenic and control samples, ventricular enlargement in schizophrenia is probably not progressive beyond that associated with normal aging processes.

GENETIC AND PERINATAL FACTORS

If the structural abnormalities are not a secondary phenomenon, perhaps they are associated with the etiology of schizophrenia. It has already been indicated that the abnormalities are present at or before the onset of schizophrenia, which is probably a necessary condition if ventricular enlargement contributes to the onset of the disorder. However, the strongest evidence for an etiological role is based on the relationships between ventricular enlargement and genetic and perinatal factors.

Two etiological perspectives

There are two main perspectives on how genetic and perinatal factors may contribute to the brain abnormalities in schizophrenia. First, genetic and perinatal factors may interact in the determination of brain pathology and eventual schizophrenia (e.g., Cannon et al., 1989, 1990). Second, birth complications may lead to brain pathology and later schizophrenia only in those individuals without genetic predisposition to schizophrenia (e.g., Kendler & Hays, 1982; Lewis et al., 1987). Studies examining genetic and perinatal contributions to structural brain abnormalities (primarily ventricular enlargement) in schizophrenia have used designs that are not equally suited to test genetic and perinatal effects. They can be divided into two types: 1) studies using inter- and intrafamilial designs (i.e., comparisons among schizophrenics and their non-ill twins or siblings and unrelated controls), and 2) studies comparing unrelated samples of schizophrenics and controls in terms of family history and birth history.

Familial comparisons

Four studies have appeared which compared brain imaging findings among schizophrenics and their non-ill twins or siblings and normal controls.

DeLisi et al. (1986) examined the contributions of birth and family variables to ventricular enlargement in 26 schizophrenics and 10 non-ill siblings from 12 different families and 20 unrelated normal controls. In this study, birth complications were assessed by a standard checklist filled out by the subjects' mothers. Birth complications accounted for about one-third of the variance in ventricular size, but family membership was significantly related to VBR even after controlling for birth complications, age and head injuries. These findings suggest that there is a significant relationship between ventricular enlargement and schizophrenia within families even after the contributions of several environmental factors have been partialled out. Unfortunately, the interaction of birth complications and family membership was not assessed.

In a study by Reveley et al. (1982), there was a high heritability rate for ventricular area in both normal MZ twins and in MZ twins discordant for schizophrenia. However, the schizophrenics had significantly larger ventricles than their non-ill twins, which must reflect differential environmental conditions, since their genetic compositions are identical.

Weinberger et al. (1981) found that both schizophrenics and their non-ill sibs had larger ventricles than normal controls, probably reflecting a genetic component to increased ventricular size; the schizophrenics also had larger ventricles than their non-ill sibs, which could reflect a higher genetic loading, or differential environmental conditions, or both.

Suddath et al. (1990) examined MRI measurements of the ventricles and hippocampi in 15 pairs of MZ twins discordant for schizophrenia and 5 pairs of normal MZ twins. In nearly all of the discordant twin pairs, the schizophrenic twin could be identified by visual inspection to have larger third and lateral ventricles and smaller left hippocampi than their unaffected co-twins. These results suggest a strong environmental component to the morphological findings. Unfortunately, there was no attempt to determine heritability coefficients for the brain measures employed, and there were no comparisons in brain morphology between the unaffected co-twins of the schizophrenics and the normal MZ twins. Such analyses may have revealed effects related to genetic factors.

Non-familial comparisons

A number of other investigations have been carried out relating family history and birth history to ventricular abnormalities in unrelated samples of schizophrenics and controls. The results of these studies are mixed. Three studies found that ventricular enlargement was negatively related to family history (Cazullo et al, 1989; Reveley et al., 1983; Turner et al., 1986); two found that ventricular enlargement was positively related to family history (Kaija et al., 1989; Nasrallah et al., 1983); and eight found no relationship (Campbell et al., 1979; Farmer et al., 1987; Nasrallah et al., 1988; Nimgaonkar et al., 1988; Owen et al; 1988a; Pandurangi et al., 1986; Pearlson et al, 1985; 1989). Several other studies were not evaluated in this context since they failed to specify the diagnostic procedures and/or the definition of a positive family history. Studies examining ventricular enlargement in relation to birth history are divided about evenly into those which did (Lewis & Murray, 1987; Owen et al., 1988b; Pearlson et al., 1985, 1989; Turner et al., 1986) and did not (Nasrallah et al., 1988; Nimgaonkar et al., 1988; Oxenstierna et al., 1984; Reveley et al., 1983, 1984) find a positive correlation between an abnormal birth history and increased ventricular size in the schizophrenic samples. In three studies there was a dissociation between family history and birth history (Cazullo et al., 1989; Nasrallah et al., 1988; Reveley et al., 1983). Several other studies were not evaluated because they failed to specify how obstetric complications were assessed and/or how positive OC histories were defined.

Methodological considerations

The mixed results of the studies reviewed in the previous section probably reflects the fact there their methodologies are limited by several factors. In the family history studies, family history is usually assessed only by interview of the patient or his or her parents. No studies conducted diagnostic interviews of the affected relatives to determine familial risk. Another problem with this method is that many individuals who have increased genetic risk are not detected due to a small family size or failure of expression of genetic vulnerability in the family members (DeLisi et al., 1986). In addition, many studies are also vulnerable to an excessive rate of false positive, since positive family histories were defined as the presence of any major psychiatric disorder in the family, which is a dubious basis from which to infer genetic risk for schizophrenia.

The birth history studies are limited primarily by the use of retrospective, nonuniform, and nonstandardized assessment procedures. Some of the studies assessed birth complications only by interview of the patient. The major limitation with respect to the dissociation between family history and birth history is that the sources of the two types of information are usually the same, which opens the possibility for selective or biased recall or reporting based on "pet" hypotheses of the cause of illness or explanations which exonerate the reporter from blame. This practice could systematically and artifactually dissociate family and birth history in view of the fact that the subject's mother is most frequently the source of the family and birth information.

Summary

Studies using designs comparing brain abnormalities among schizophrenics, their unaffected relatives, and unrelated controls found evidence consistent with a significant genetic contribution to increased ventricular size in schizophrenia. All of these studies also pointed to a substantial role of environmental contributions, including perinatal complications. Unfortunately, none of these studies examined the possibility of an interaction between genetic and environmental disturbances. In contrast, studies using family and birth history variables in unrelated samples of schizophrenics and controls obtained mixed results, but can not be considered very reliable in view of a number of methodological problems.

BRAIN DEFICITS IN HIGH-RISK SUBJECTS

Two types of structural abnormalities in schizophrenia

An important issue in understanding the sources of the various types of brain abnormalities in schizophrenia is their degree of intercorrelation or independence. In one of the early CT studies, Weinberger and coworkers (1979b) found that lateral ventricular enlargement was unrelated to signs of cortical atrophy, which suggested that "more than one pathological event or etiology may be involved in producing these abnormalities." Several subsequent reports have supported the lack of association between ventriculomegaly and cortical atrophy, while others have found evidence that the two deficits are related. The number of overlapping cases is, however, small, indicating that ventricular enlargement and cortical damage often occur independently of each other. Thus, there may be at least partially independent etiologic processes underlying these deficits.

A theoretical framework

This chapter has referred to two primary sources of brain abnormalities in schizophrenia: genetic factors and perinatal complications. We have proposed that one aspect of the genetic predisposition to schizophrenia may be a disruption of fetal neural development, perhaps centered in the second trimester of gestation (Mednick et al., 1988; Cannon et al., 1989). Several postmortem studies of the brains of schizophrenics have found evidence of ectopic cells in the hippocampal formation and other regions (e.g., Falkai et al., 1988; Jacob & Beckmann, 1986; Kovelman & Scheibel, 1984; McLardy, 1974). In several studies these neuronal aberrations were said to be consistent with disruption of cell migration and positioning in the second trimester of gestation (Jacob & Beckmann, 1986; Kovelman & Scheibel, 1984). The same types of neuronal migratory and positioning disturbances in these same locations have been linked to genetic factors in inbred strains of mice (e.g., Nowakowski, 1991a). Another line of investigation which bears on this issue is the association between viral exposure during pregnancy and the risk for later schizophrenia. Mednick and colleagues (1988) found that individuals exposed to severe influenza epidemic in second trimester of pregnancy later evidenced significantly higher rates of schizophrenia than individuals exposed during the first or third trimesters. These findings have recently been confirmed by Barr et al. (1991). In this study, there was a significant association between exposure to viral epidemics in the sixth month of gestation and later risk for schizophrenia over a 40-year period in Denmark.

The viral work may be most significant for defining the window of vulnerability in which genetic or teratogenic factors may disturb fetal neural development resulting in a predisposition to schizophrenia. What is the significance of fetal neural developmental disruption in the second trimester? Genetic or teratogenic effects occurring in this window could disrupt the migration and positioning of cells as they proliferate from the periventricular germinal matrix (Nowakowski, 1991b). In other words, there is a cellular layer surrounding the ventricular system from which cells targeted for the neocortex and other areas proliferate and begin their migratory pathways following radial glial fibers. There is a heightened risk for hemorrhage into the germinal matrix at end of second trimester, when brain growth increases dramatically (Brann, 1985). Developmental disturbances to the ventricular zone germinal matrix may result in structural and/or vascular vulnerabilities which increase the risk for even greater periventricular tissue damage secondary to anoxia and other complications at delivery. A similar effect has been observed in preterm and low-birth weight infants who show elevated levels of periventricular and intraventricular bleeding (Sinha et al., 1985).

Hypotheses

Based on this series of observations, we suggest two hypotheses concerning the possible roles of genetic and perinatal factors in the brain abnormalities in schizophrenia:

1. Genetic risk for schizophrenia may be associated with developmental brain deficits at many different sites.

2. Complications at birth and genetic risk for schizophrenia may interact in producing ventricular enlargement.

A preliminary test

These hypotheses were put to a preliminary empirical test using a subsample of subjects from the Copenhagen schizophrenia high-risk project (Mednick & Schulsinger, 1965). In this study, 207 children of schizophrenic mothers were first identified in 1962 and were later followed-up to determine their psychiatric status (Schulsinger, 1976). As part of the initial examination in 1962, we collected and coded the original midwife reports on the pregnancy and births of the subjects. It is important to note that the birth data were recorded at the time of the subjects' births and were coded prospectively, before any of the subjects became ill. From these midwife reports we derived two obstetric scales: one reflecting the number of pregnancy complications and one reflecting the number of delivery complications. Birth weight was not included in either scale and was entered as a separate factor in the analyses.

A subsample of 34 high-risk subjects underwent CT scanning in 1980 (Schulsinger et al., 1984). This subsample included 10 schizophrenics, 10 individuals with schizotypal personality disorder, and 14 individuals with no mental illness. Our CT scan measures were relatively crude: they included measures of the sylvian and interhemispheric fissures, cortical sulci, cerebellar vermis, lateral ventricles, and third ventricle.

Since all of the subjects in this subsample had schizophrenic mothers, the major source of genetic variability is contributed by the diagnostic status of their fathers. We interviewed the subjects' biological fathers and assigned each a psychiatric diagnosis (Parnas, 1985). These diagnoses were then coded as being in the schizophrenia spectrum or as not being in the schizophrenia spectrum. Gottesman and Shields (1982) have termed individuals with two schizophrenic or schizophrenia spectrum parents "super high-risk." With respect to our hypotheses, those individuals with both a schizophrenic mother and a schizophrenia spectrum father were considered to be at super high-risk for multisite developmental brain deficits.

Factor analysis of CT measurements

To test our hypotheses, we first conducted a factor analyses of the six CT scan measures. This analysis yielded two significant factors. The first factor reflected multisite brain deficits as indicated by abnormality of the cerebellar vermis and widening of the sylvian and interhemispheric fissures and cortical sulci. The second factor reflected periventricular damage as indicated with widening of the third and lateral ventricles (Cannon et al., 1989).

Sources of two types of structural damage

We then asked what factors contributed to the two types of brain deficits. To examine this, we conducted a set of stepwise regression analyses in which pregnancy complications, delivery complications, birth weight, genetic risk status (i.e., fathers' schizophrenia spectrum diagnoses), and the interactions of these factors, were included as possible predictors.

In the first analysis, the factor score for multisite developmental brain deficits was the dependent variable. Genetic risk for schizophrenia was the only significant predictor of the multisite neural developmental deficits factor scores (Cannon et al., 1989).

In the second analysis, the factor score for periventricular damage was the dependent variable. The interaction of genetic risk for schizophrenia and delivery complications entered the prediction on the first step, accounting for almost half of the variance in the periventricular damage scores of the subjects. Birth weight entered the equation on the second step, predicting negatively, and accounting for an additional ten percent of the variance in the periventricular damage scores. Another way of expressing the interaction effect mentioned above is that ventricular enlargement was highly correlated with delivery complications in the subjects who were at super high-risk for schizophrenia (the correlation was .71), but not in the subjects with a moderate risk (the correlation was .08). That is, the individuals who were at super high-risk for schizophrenia evidenced greater ventricular enlargement if they suffered delivery complications (Cannon et al., 1989).

Diagnostic comparisons

The next question we asked is what relevance do the two types of brain deficits have for schizophrenia. To examine this question, we first compared the multisite deficits factors scores of the schizophrenics, schizotypals, and non-mentally ill subjects. There were no significant differences between the three groups (Cannon et al., 1989). This result was expected since all subjects with the genetic predisposition to schizophrenia would be expected to evidence the multisite deficits, not just the schizophrenics.

We then compared the periventricular damage factors scores of the three diagnostic subgroups. The schizophrenics evidenced significantly larger periventricular damage scores than the schizotypals and non-mentally-ill subjects. The latter two groups did not differ significantly from each other (Cannon et al., 1989).

Summary

We tentatively interpret these results as supporting a gene-environment interaction perspective. This is, the genetically-based multisite neural developmental deficits may constitute a vulnerability or sensitivity to delivery complications. Among individuals with this vulnerability, those who experience severe complications during delivery may be at greater risk for periventricular damage, which in turn may increase the risk for overt schizophrenia.

REFERENCES

Andreasen, N. Andreason, C., Olsen, S. A., Dennert, J. W., & Smith, M. R. (1982). Ventricular enlargement in schizophrenia: Relationship to positive and negative symptoms. American Journal of Psychiatry, 139, 297-302.

Barr, C. E., Mednick, S. A., & Munk-Jorgensen, P. (1990). Exposure to influenza epidemics during gestation and adult schizophrenia: A 40-year study. Archives of General Psychiatry, 47, 869-874.

Barron, S. A., Jacobs, L., & Kinkel, W. R. (1976). Changes in size of normal lateral ventricles during aging determined by computerized tomography. Neurology, 26, 1011-1013.

Benes, F., Sunderland, P., Jones, B. D., LeMay, M., Cohen, B. M., & Lipinski, J. F. (1982). Normal ventricles in young schizophrenics. British Journal of Psychiatry, 141, 90-93.

Brann, A. W. (1985). Factors during neonatal life that influence brain disorders. In J. M. Freeman (Ed.), Prenatal and perinatal factors associated with brain disorders (pp. 263-358). Washington D.C.: National Institutes of Health.

Campbell, R., Hays, P., Russel, D. B., & Zacks, D. J. (1979). CT scan variants and genetic heterogeneity in schizophrenia. American Journal of Psychiatry, 136, 722-723.

Cannon, T. D. (1991). Sources and correlates of structural brain abnormalities in schizophrenia. In S. A. Mednick, T. D. Cannon, C. E. Barr, & M. Lyon (Eds.), Fetal neural development and adult schizophrenia (pp. 174-198). Cambridge: Cambridge University Press.

Cannon, T. D., Mednick, S. A., & Parnas, J. (1989). Genetic and perinatal determinants of structural brain deficits in schizophrenia. Archives of General Psychiatry, 46, 883-889.

Cannon, T. D., Mednick, S. A., & Parnas, J. (1990). Antecedents of predominantly negative and predominantly positive symptom schizophrenia in a high-risk population. Archives of General Psychiatry, 47, 662-632.

Cazullo, C. L., Vita, A., & Sacchetti, E. (1989). Cerebral ventricular enlargement in schizophrenia: Prevalence and correlates. In S. C. Schulz & C. A. Tamminga (Eds.), Schizophrenia: Scientific Progress (pp.195-206). New York: Oxford University Press.

DeLisi, L. E., Goldin, L. R., Hamovit, J. R., Maxwell, E., Kurtz, D., & Gershon, E. S. (1986). A family study of the association of increased ventricular size with schizophrenia. Archives of General Psychiatry, 43, 148-153.

Erel, O., Cannon, T. D., Hollister, M., Mednick, S. A., & Parnas, J. (1991). Ventricular enlargement and premorbid deficits in school-occupational attainment in a high-risk sample. Schizophrenia Research, 4, 49-52.

Falkai, P., Bogerts, B., Roberts, G. W., & Crow, T. J. (1988). Measurement of the alpha-cell-migration in the entorhinal region: A marker for developmental disturbances in schizophrenia? Schizophrenia Research, 1, 157-158.

Farmer, A., Jackson, R., McGuffin, P., & Storey, P. (1987). Cerebral ventricular enlargement in chronic schizophrenia: Consistencies and contradictions. British Journal of Psychiatry, 150, 324-330.

Gottesman, I. I., & Shields, J. (1982). Schizophrenia: The epigenetic puzzle. New York: Cambridge University Press.

Haug, J. O. (1962). Pneumoencephalographic studies in mental disease. Acta Psychiatrica Scandinavica, 38, 1-115.

Huber, G. (1957). Pneumoencephalographische und psychopathologische bilder bei endogen psychosen. Berlin: Springer-Verlag.

Iacono, W. G., Smith, G. N., Moreau, M., Beiser, M., Fleming, J. A. E., Lin, T., & Flak, B. (1988). Ventricular and sulcal size at the onset of psychosis. American Journal of Psychiatry, 145, 820-824.

Jakob, H., & Beckmann, H. (1986). Prenatal-developmental disturbances in the limbic allocortex in schizophrenia. Biological Psychiatry, 1181-1183.

Johnstone, E. C., Crow, T. J., Frith, C. D., Husband, J., & Kreel, L. (1976). Cerebral ventricular size and cognitive impairment in chronic schizophrenia. Lancet, 924-926.

Johnstone, E. C., Crow, T. J., Frith, C. D., Stevens, M., Kreel, L., & Husband, J. (1978). The dementia of dementia praecox. Acta Psychiatrica Scandinavica, 57, 305-324.

Kaija, H., Uematsu, M., Ofuji, M., Nishida, A., Morikiyo, M., & Adachi, S. (1989). Computerized tomography in schizophrenia: Familial versus non-familial forms of illness. British Journal of Psychiatry, 155, 444-450.

Kendler, K. S., & Hays, P. (1982). Familial and sporadic schizophrenia: A symptomatic, prognostic and EEG comparison. American Journal of Psychiatry, 139, 1557-1562.

Kovelman, J. A., & Scheibel, A. B. (1984). A neurohistological correlate of schizophrenia. Biological Psychiatry, 19, 1601-1621.

Kraepelin, E. (1919). Dementia praecox and paraphrenia. Edinburgh, Scotland: Livingston.

Lewis, S. W., & Murray, R. M. (1987). Obstetric complications, neurodevelopmental deviance, and risk of schizophrenia. Journal of Psychiatric Research, 21, 413-421.

Lewis, S. W., Reveley, A. M., Reveley, M. A., Chitkara, B., & Murray, R. M. (1987). The familial-sporadic distinction as a strategy in schizophrenia research. British Journal of Psychiatry, 151, 306-313.

Mathew, R. J., Partain, C. L., Rakash, R., Kulkarni, M. V., Logan, T. P., & Wilson, W. H. (1985). A study of the septum pellucidum and corpus callosum in schizophrenia with MR imaging. Acta Psychiatrica Scandinavica, 72, 414-421.

McLardy, T. (1974). Hippocampal zinc and structural deficit in brains from chronic alcoholics and some schizophrenics. Journal of Orthopsychiatry, 4(1), 32-36.

Mednick, S. A., & Schulsinger, F. (1965). A longitudinal study of children with a high risk for schizophrenia: A preliminary report. In S. Vandenberg (Ed.), Methods and goals in human behavior genetics (pp. 255-296). New York: Academic Press.

Mednick, S. A., Machon, R. A., Huttunen, M. O., & Bonett, D. (1988). Adult schizophrenia following prenatal exposure to an influenza epidemic. Archives of General Psychiatry, 45, 189-192.

Naber, D., Albus, M., Burke, H., Muller-Spahn, F., Munch, U., Reinertshofer, T., Wissman, J., & Akenheil, M. (1985). Neuroleptic withdrawal in chronic schizophrenia, CT and endocrine variables relating to psychopathology. Psychiatry Research, 16, 207-219.

Nasrallah, H. A., Kuperman, S., Hamra, B. J., & McCalley-Whitters, M. (1983). Clinical differences between schizophrenic patients with and without large cerebral ventricles. Journal of Clinical Psychiatry, 44, 407-409.

Nasrallah, H. A., Schwarzkopf, S. B., Coffman, J. A., & Olson, S. C. (1988). A magnetic resonance imaging study of genetic vs perinatal factors and brain measurements in schizophrenia. Paper presented at the NIMH conference on Fetal Neural Development and Schizophrenia, Washington D. C., May 30, 1988.

Nimgaonkar, V. L., Wessely, S., & Murray, R. M. (1989). Prevalence of familiality, obstetric complications and structural brain damage in schizophrenic patients. Psychological Medicine.

Nowakowski, R. S. (1991a). Genetic disturbances of neuronal migration: Some examples from the limbic system of mutant mice. In S. A. Mednick, T. D. Cannon, C. E. Barr, & M. Lyon (Eds.), Fetal neural development and adult schizophrenia (pp. 69-95). Cambridge: Cambridge University Press.

Nowakowski, R. S. (1991b). Some basic concepts of the development of the central nervous system. In S. A. Mednick, T. D. Cannon, C. E. Barr, & M. Lyon (Eds.), Fetal neural development and adult schizophrenia (pp. 17-39). Cambridge: Cambridge University Press.

Nyback, H., Berggren, B.-M., Hindmarsh, T., Sedvall, G., & Wiesel, F.-A. (1983). Cerebroventricular size and cerebrospinal fluid monoamine metabolites in schizophrenic patients and healthy volunteers. Psychiatry Research, 9, 301-308.

Nyback, H., Wiesel, F.-A., Berggren, B.-M., & Hindmarsh, T. (1982). Computed tomography of the brain in patients with acute psychosis and in healthy volunteers. Acta Psychiatrica Scandinavica, 65, 403-414.

Obiols L. J. E., Ruscalleda, J., & Masferrer, M. (1986). Ventricular enlargement in young chronic schizophrenics. Acta Psychiatrica Scandinavica, 73, 42-44.

Owen, M. J., Lewis, S. W., & Murray, R. M. (1988a). Family history and cerebral ventricular enlargement in schizophrenia: A case control study. British Journal of Psychiatry.

Owen, M. J., Lewis, S. W., & Murray, R. M. (1988b). Obstetric complications and schizophrenia: A computed tomographic study. Psychological Medicine, 18, 331-339.

Oxenstierna, G., Bergstrand, G., Bjerkenstedt, L., Sedvall, G., & Wik, G. (1984). Evidence of disturbed CSF circulation and brain atrophy in cases of schizophrenic psychosis. British Journal of Psychiatry, 144, 654-661.

Pandurangi, A. K., Dewan, M. J., Boucher, M., Levy, B., Ramachandran, T., Bartell, K., Bick, P. A., Phelps, B. H., & Major, L. (1986). A comprehensive study of chronic schizophrenic patients: II. Biological, neuropsychological, and clinical correlates of CT abnormality. Acta Psychiatrica Scandinavica, 73, 161-171.

Parnas, J. (1985). Mates of schizophrenic mothers: A study of assortative mating from the American-Danish high-risk study. British Journal of Psychiatry, 146, 490-497.

Pearlson, G. D., & Veroff, A. E. (1981). Computerized tomographic scan changes in manic-depressive illness. Lancet, p. 470.

Pearlson, G. D., Garbacz, D. J., Moberg, P. J., Ahn, H. S., & DePaulo, J. R. (1985). Symptomatic, familial, perinatal, and social correlates of computerized axial tomography (CAT) changes in schizophrenics and bipolars. Journal of Nervous and Mental Disease, 173, 42-50.

Pearlson, G. D., Kim, W. S., Kubos, K. L., Moberg, P. J., Jayaram, G., Bascom, M. J., Chase, G. A., Goldfinger, A. D., & Tune, L. E. (1989). Ventricle-brain ratio, computed tomographic density, and brain area in 50 schizophrenics. Archives of General Psychiatry, 46, 690-697.

Raz, S., & Raz, N. (1990). Structural brain abnormalities in the major psychoses: A quantitative review of the evidence from computerized imaging. Psychological Bulletin, 108, 93-108.

Reiss, D., Feinstein, C., Weinberger, D. R., King, R., Wyatt, R. J., & Brallier, D. (1983). Ventricular enlargement in child psychiatric patients: A controlled study with planimetric measurements. American Journal of Psychiatry, 140, 453-456.

Reveley, A. M., Reveley, M. A., & Murray, R. M. (1983). Enlargement of cerebral ventricles in schizophrenia is confined to those without known genetic predisposition. Lancet, 2, 525.

Reveley, A. M., Reveley, M. A., & Murray, R. M. (1984). Cerebral ventricular enlargement in nongenetic schizophrenia: A controlled twin study. British Journal of Psychiatry, 144, 89-93.

Reveley, A. M., Reveley, M. A., Clifford, C. A., & Murray, R. M. (1982). Cerebral ventricular size in twins discordant for schizophrenia. Lancet, 1, 540-541.

Schulsinger, H. (1976). A ten-year follow-up of children of schizophrenic mothers: Clinical assessment. Acta Psychiatrica Scandinavica, 53, 371-386.

Schulsinger, F., Parnas, J., Petersen, E. T., Schulsinger, H., Teasdale, T. W., Mednick, S. A., Moller, L., & Silverton, L. (1984). Cerebral ventricular size in the offspring of schizophrenic mothers. Archives of General Psychiatry, 41, 602-606.

Schulz, S. C., Koller, M. M., Kishore, P. R., Hamer, R. M., Gehl, J. J., & Friedel, R. O. (1983a). Ventricular enlargement in teenage patients with schizophrenia spectrum disorder. American Journal of Psychiatry, 140, 1592-1595.

Schulz, S. C., Sinicrope, P., Kishore, P., & Friedel, R. O. (1983b). Treatment response and ventricular enlargement in young schizophrenic patients. Schizophrenia Bulletin, 19, 505-509.

Schulz, S. C., Koller, M., Kishore, P. R., Hamer, R. M., & Friedel, R. O. (1982). Abnormal scans in young schizophrenics. Psychopharmacology Bulletin, 18, 163-164.

Shima, S., Kanba, S., Masuda, Y., Tsukomo, T., Kitamura, T., & Asai, M. (1985). Normal ventricles in chronic schizophrenics. Acta Psychiatrica Scandinavica, 71, 25-29.

Sinha, S. K., Davies, J. M., Sims, D. G., & Chiswick, M. L. (1985). Relation between periventricular hemorrhage and ischemic brain lesions diagnosed by ultrasound in very preterm infants. Lancet, 2, 1154-1156.

Storey, P. B. (1966). Lumbar air encephalography in chronic schizophrenia: A controlled experiment. British Journal of Psychiatry, 112, 135-144.

Suddath, R. L., Christison, G. W., Torrey, E. F., Casanova, M. F., & Weinberger, D. R. (1990). Anatomical abnormalities in the brains of monozygotic twins discordant for schizophrenia. New England Journal of Medicine, 322, 789794.

Tanaka, Y., Hazama, H., Kawahara, R., & Kobayashi, K. (1981). Computerized tomography of the brain in schizophrenic patients. Acta Psychiatrica Scandinavica, 63, 191-197.

Turner, S. W., Toone, B. K., & Brett-Jones, J. R. (1986). Computerized tomographic scan changes in early schizophrenia - preliminary findings. Psychological Medicine, 16, 219-225.

Weinberger, D. R., DeLisi, L. E., Perman, G. P., Targum, S., & Wyatt, R. J. (1982). Computed tomography in schizophreniform disorder and other acute psychiatric disorders. Archives of General Psychiatry, 39, 778-783.

Weinberger, D. R., DeLisi, L. E., Neophytides, A. N., & Wyatt, R. J. (1981). Familial aspects of CT scan abnormalities in chronic schizophrenic patients. Psychiatry Research, 4, 65-71.

Weinberger, D. R., Torrey, E. F., Neophytides, A. N., & Wyatt, R. J. (1979a). Lateral cerebral ventricular enlargement in schizophrenia. Archives of General Psychiatry, 36, 735-739.

Weinberger, D. R., Torrey, E. F., Neophytides, A. N, & Wyatt, R. J. (1979b). Structural abnormalities of the cerebral cortex in chronic schizophrenic patients. Archives of General Psychiatry, 36, 935-939.

Weinberger, D. R., Wagner, R. L., & Wyatt, R. J. (1983). Neuropathological studies of schizophrenia: A selective review. Schizophrenia Bulletin, 9, 193-212.

Woods, B. T., & Wolf, J. (1983). A reconsideration of the relation of ventricular enlargement to duration of illness in schizophrenia. American Journal of Psychiatry, 140, 1564-1570.

MORPHOLOGIC MARKERS OF NEURODEVELOPMENTAL PATHS TO SCHIZOPHRENIA

Robert M. Bilder and Gustav Degreef

Hillside Hospital, Long Island Jewish Medical Center and
Department of Psychiatry, Albert Einstein College of Medicine
Glen Oaks, New York

INTRODUCTION

The most widely studied cerebral morphologic abnormalities in schizophrenia may be classified as indications of: 1. medial fronto-limbic system defects; 2. periventricular damage; and 3. cerebral specialization abnormalities. The existing literature supports the independence of these morphologic abnormalities and suggests that they may reflect different pathologic processes. We hypothesize that these pathologic dimensions may be accompanied by distinguishable developmental courses and psychopathologic evolutions. An outline of these hypothetical paths to schizophrenia is presented as a heuristic for understanding heterogeneity of the cerebral morphological, neuropsychological, and clinical features of the schizophrenic syndrome.

A major goal of schizophrenia research is to subdivide the syndrome along pathophysiologic lines. History, symptoms, neuropsychological (NP) function, and brain morphology offer partially independent windows on possible pathologic processes. Insight into plausible pathologic processes may be maximized by combining these measures, and identifying multidimensional constructs with high concurrent validity. Existing data support the convergent and divergent validity of at least three overlapping but distinguishable pathologic processes that may: (a) be reflected by different gross morphologic and cytoarchitectonic abnormalities; (b) have different functional manifestations over the course of neurodevelopment and later symptom expression; and (c) have distinct etiologic bases. Starting with a consideration of gross structural abnormalities, evidence is presented that supports the existence and independence of these pathologic processes.

Developmental Neuropathology of Schizophrenia
Edited by S.A. Mednick *et al.*, Plenum Press, New York, 1991

INDEPENDENCE OF STRUCTURAL ABNORMALITIES

The literature on structural abnormalities in the schizophrenic brain is remarkable for the sheer diversity of positive findings. Post-mortem pathology, computerized tomography (CT), and magnetic resonance (MR) imaging have revealed multiple abnormalities of cytoarchitectonic structure and gross morphology. Gross morphology offers a convenient starting point for inquiry into structural abnormality because: (a) abnormalities of gross anatomy might be expected to have more readily identifiable functional consequences; and (b) gross abnormalities can be observed readily with in vivo methods, enabling detailed clinico-anatomic correlation.

The best investigated abnormalities of gross morphology include: subarachnoid space or cortical sulcal enlargement; ventricular enlargement; and absence or reversals of normal hemispheral asymmetry. Most CT studies supported the independence of cortical sulcal and ventricular enlargement (of the lateral or third ventricles) in schizophrenia by showing that they were not significantly correlated (Weinberger, Torrey, Neophytides and Wyatt, 1979; Weinberger, DeLisi, Perman, Targum, and Wyatt, 1982; Nasrallah, Kuperman, Whitters-McCalley and Hamra, 1983; Tanaka, Hazama and Kobayashi, 1981; Boronow et al., 1985; Okasha and Madkour, 1982; Dewan et al., 1983; Iacono et al., 1988). There are only a few reports of modest association (Kling, Kurtz, Tachiki and Orzeck, 1982; Rieder, Mann, Weinberger, Van Kammen and Post, 1983; Pfefferbaum et al., 1988). A recent analysis of multiple cortical and ventricular regions demonstrated that "multisite" defects (including enlarged cortical sulci and fissures, and abnormalities of the cerebellar vermis) loaded together on a single factor that was independent from a ventricular enlargement factor (Cannon, Mednick and Parnas, 1989). Meta-analysis further supported the independence of ventricular and sulcal enlargement (Raz and Raz, 1990).

Absence or reversal of normal cortical asymmetry has also shown independence from both ventricular and subarachnoid space enlargements (Luchins and Meltzer, 1983; Luchins, Weinberger and Wyatt, 1982; Andreasen, Dennert, Olsen and Damasio, 1982). In some studies, absence of the normal pattern of hemispheral asymmetry was found specifically in patients without evidence of ventricular enlargement, subarachnoid space enlargement, or cerebellar abnormality (Luchins, Weinberger and Wyatt, 1979; Luchins, Weinberger and Wyatt, 1982). Several recent studies suggest further that overall brain size is not significantly correlated with ventricular size (Andreasen et al., 1990; Johnstone et al., 1989).

This evidence suggests that the three most studied classes of gross morphologic abnormality -- multisite cortical abnormalities, ventricular enlargement, and anomalous patterns of cerebral asymmetry (and possibly more general reductions in brain size) -- may represent independent pathologic dimensions. Unfortunately, there are few comprehensive studies of brain morphology in which all three types of abnormality were assessed in the same sample. The increased availability of high resolution magnetic resonance (MR) imaging, with multiplanar reconstruction capacities, should simplify direct tests of this suggestion using highly reliable volumetric measures of each pathologic dimension. Awaiting results from comprehensive studies, there is evidence that these different types of morphologic abnormality may have different functional correlates (i.e., that they may show divergent validity vis a vis functional measures). This evidence, while inconclusive, offers further insights into the possible consequences of abnormal cerebral morphology. A selective review of this evidence is provided below.

SYMPTOMATIC AND NEUROPSYCHOLOGICAL CORRELATES

Multiple attempts to relate symptoms to morphologic abnormalities have yielded conflicting and often equivocal results. A number of studies focused on the symptomatic correlates of ventricular enlargement or sulcal prominence, generally to test the hypothesis that these abnormalities are associated with either more "negative" or fewer "positive" symptoms. Some findings were seen as consistent with this hypothesis (Andreasen, Olsen, Dennert and Smith, 1982; Kemali et al., 1987; Luchins et al., 1984; Pearlson et al., 1984; Takahashi et al., 1981; Williams et al., 1985), but more studies have yielded equivocal, contradictory, or complex results suggesting that these morphologic features do not relate to the positive-negative symptom dimension in a straightforward way (Besson et al., 1987; Bishop et al., 1983; Boronow et al., 1985; DeLisi et al., 1986; Farmer et al., 1987; Johnstone et al., 1978; Johnstone et al., 1989; Keilp et al., 1988; Losonczy et al., 1986a; McCarley et al., 1989; Nasrallah, Jacoby, McCalley-Whitters and Kuperman, 1982; Nasrallah, Kuperman, Whitters-McCalley and Hamra, 1983; Nyman, Nyback, Wiesel, Oxenstierna and Schalling, 1986; Owens et al., 1985; Pandurangi, Bilder, Rieder, Mukherjee and Hamer, 1988; Pfefferbaum et al., 1988; Smith et al., 1983).

The failure to find clear relations between symptoms and abnormal brain morphology might reflect the absence of a real relation, but could just as easily reflect flaws in our definitions of relevant constructs. In a previous analysis of the construct validity of the positive-negative symptom distinction, we suggested that a major contribution to symptom variance was comprised by phenomena that reflect conceptual disorganization (Bilder, Mukherjee, Rieder and Pandurangi, 1985). Symptoms of formal thought disorder and bizarre behavior ("positive" symptoms) loaded together with attentional impairment and alogia ("negative" symptoms) on a single factor, violating the a priori definitions of positive and negative symptoms. Similar findings have been reported by others (Kulhara, Kota and Joseph, 1986; Liddle, 1987b; O'Leary, Andreasen, Arndt and Kesler, 1991). Some investigators found clear separation of positive and negative symptom constructs only after removing the contribution of "general" symptom severity factors (Kay and Opler,

1987). These findings indicate that the positive-negative symptom dichotomy does not capture adequately the full range of symptom expression; in particular the symptoms of conceptual disorganization may emerge as an independent symptom dimension. It has been suggested that this pattern of conceptual disorganization may merit separate syndromal status (Liddle, 1987a; Pandurangi and Bilder, 1988). In our studies, the symptoms of conceptual organization accounted for more variance than other symptom clusters, and were associated with more pervasive neuropsychological deficits (Bilder et al., 1985). Liddle (1987b) also reported that ". . . the most widespread and severe disturbance is associated with the disorganization syndrome" (p. 148). Thus, these conceptual disorganization symptoms may be both independent, and particularly important, contributors to behavioral morbidity.

The symptoms of conceptual disorganization do not appear to reflect either ventricular or sulcal enlargement. Several studies suggested that these symptoms might be related to a pathologic process that is at least independent of, and is perhaps negatively correlated with these morphologic abnormalities. We found that conceptual disorganization was most severe in patients who <u>did not</u> have ventricular or sulcal enlargement (Bilder, 1985; Pandurangi, Bilder, Rieder, Mukherjee and Hamer, 1988). Another study, sometimes cited as supporting the relation of ventricular enlargement with negative symptoms, actually showed only an increase of <u>bizarre behavior</u> (one of the disorganization symptoms) among patients with the <u>smallest</u> ventricles (Andreasen, Olsen, Dennert and Smith, 1982). While sparse, this evidence suggests that conceptual disorganization may be greater among patients with smaller ventricles and less prominent cortical sulci.

A clue to the pathologic process possibly underlying conceptual disorganization was found in the relations between symptoms and neuropsychological performance. The symptoms of conceptual disorganization were correlated strongly with a neuropsychological deficit pattern suggesting failure in the early development of basic linguistic and general cognitive competencies (Bilder et al., 1985). Like the symptoms of conceptual disorganization, these neuropsychological deficits were also most severe in patients <u>without</u> ventricular or sulcal enlargement (Bilder et al., 1988; Pandurangi et al., 1988). This led to an unexpected association of <u>better</u> functioning with <u>more</u> ventricular or sulcal enlargement. Others have replicated this apparently paradoxical positive correlation of ventricular enlargement with measures of premorbid neuropsychological ability -- that is, the patients with larger ventricles performed better on tests of general knowledge and/or vocabulary, which are considered resistant to deterioration (Nyman, Nyback, Wiesel, Oxenstierna and Schalling, 1986; Obiols, Marcos and Salamero, 1987; DeQuardo et al., 1990). These findings suggest the possibility that a pathologic process, unrelated to ventricular enlargement or sulcal prominence, may be associated with particularly poor early acquisition of neuropsychological abilities. This does not imply that ventricular and sulcal enlargement are not associated with neuropsychological deficits. In fact, neuropsychological deficits were correlated significantly with morphologic abnormalities in a number of studies (Adams, Jacisin, Brown, Boulos and Silk, 1984; Donnelly, Weinberger, Waldman and Wyatt, 1980; Golden et al., 1980; Golden et al., 1982; Keilp et al., 1988; Rieder, Donnelly, Herdt and Waldman, 1979; for a review, see Bilder, in press).

Resolution of this apparent paradox may be provided by the largest (N = 108) study of the relation between neuropsychological performance and ventricular size: an "inverted-U" relation was found, with poorest neuropsychological performance among patients with either largest or smallest ventricles (Owens et al., 1985). The finding of neuropsychological impairment in patients with large ventricles was expected. But this study shows that patients with the smallest ventricles also had deficits relative to patients with average ventricular size, and were at least as impaired as patients with the largest ventricles. In summary, these studies point to the possible existence of an additional pathologic process, causing significant neuropsychological morbidity, that is not reflected by either ventricular enlargement or sulcal prominence.

What aspect of cerebral morphology, which is independent of ventricular and sulcal enlargement, might be associated with failed early neurocognitive development, particularly the development of basic linguistic competence? As noted above, absence or reversal from the normal pattern of hemispheral asymmetry were found most frequently in patients without evidence of either ventricular or sulcal enlargement (Luchins, Weinberger and Wyatt, 1979; Luchins, Weinberger and Wyatt, 1982). The strongest clinical correlate of absent or reversed asymmetry was "poor quality of interview", interpreted as reflecting a dysfunction of language and communication abilities (Luchins and Meltzer, 1983). Possible impairment of basic language competence in patients with abnormal asymmetry was further supported by the finding that these patients had lower Verbal than Performance IQ (Luchins, Weinberger and Wyatt, 1979). These observations suggest that failure in the normal process of hemispheral specialization may underlie significant defects of language and general cognitive development, and that such defects may be manifest as symptoms of conceptual disorganization.

The foregoing discussion focused on what was not associated with ventricular or sulcal enlargement. It was already suggested that studies of relations between symptoms and these morphologic measures yielded equivocal results. Unfortunately few studies have assessed both ventricular and sulcal enlargement in the same sample, so it is difficult to determine whether each may have unique symptomatic correlates. There is some evidence, however, that ventricular and sulcal enlargement may differ in their neuropsychological correlates. In a computed tomography (CT) study of 57 chronic schizophrenic patients, we found that sulcal enlargement was predicted by deficits of executive and motor functions, while ventricular enlargement was predicted by memory deficits (Bilder et al., 1988)[1]. Our preliminary findings in a separate magnetic resonance (MR) imaging study of 24 first episode schizophrenic patients further support the association of total ventricular volume with deficits of memory, but not other neuropsychological functions (Bilder et al., 1989). In several other investigations, deficits on tests of new learning and memory were the most robust correlates of ventricular enlargement (Johnstone et al., 1989; Keilp et al., 1988; for a review, see Bilder, in press).

While further study is clearly necessary to enable firm conclusions, these findings point to a plausible discrepancy between the neuropsychological correlates of sulcal enlargement and periventricular damage. Executive and motor deficits are most frequently associated with dysfunction of anterior cortical systems. To the extent that sulcal prominence reflects compromise of these cortical territories, a relation with executive-motor dysfunction would be predicted. Deficits of new learning and memory, on the other hand, have been most strongly related to dysfunction of subcortical systems, specifically those mesiotemporal and diencephalic regions that surround the third ventricle and the temporal horns of the lateral ventricles.

PREMORBID FUNCTIONING AND DETERIORATION

There have been reports of association between ventricular enlargement and poor premorbid social adjustment (DeLisi et al., 1983), but few studies have assessed relations of social adjustment to other morphologic abnormalities. Using global ratings of social adjustment (NIMH Modification of the Premorbid Adjustment Scale), together with neuropsychological methods, we found that ventricular enlargement was associated more with poor social adjustment, while sulcal enlargement was associated more with deficits on neuropsychological tests sensitive to "anterior" cortical functioning (Bilder, 1985). More detailed temporal analyses of premorbid history suggested that ventricular enlargement was associated more with persistent deficits of social function, while sulcal enlargement was associated more with deterioration of academic functioning in late childhood (Mukherjee et al., 1989). These findings suggested possible differences in both the time course, and the types of maladjustment that occur prior to decompensation. While ventricular enlargement was related to social dysfunction, sulcal enlargement was tied more strongly to academic/intellectual deterioration.

Progressive cortical degeneration may be more likely than progressive ventricular enlargement. These abnormalities were dissociated in a sample of first episode schizophrenic patients; ventricular enlargement was present but sulcal

---

[1] In these analyses, neuropsychological deficit acquired significant predictive power only after controlling for the effects of estimated premorbid intellectual ability.

enlargement was not, suggesting that sulcal enlargement might occur later in the course of illness (Iacono et al., 1988). Sulcal enlargement also was related to patterns of NP deficit and social functioning that suggested a deteriorative process, although it appeared likely that this deterioration might precede the onset of overt symptoms (Bilder et al., 1988; Pandurangi et al., 1988). Several studies further suggested that NP deterioration may occur specifically in executive and response organization functions usually associated with anterior cortical systems (Bilder et al., 1988; Smith, 1964).

In contrast, deviations from the normal pattern of cerebral asymmetry may confer a protective advantage against progressive deterioration, such as that hypothetically associated with risk for tardive dyskinesia (TD)(Barr, Mukherjee, Degreef and Caracci, 1989). Patients with non-right-handedness and absence of the normal occipital asymmetry were less likely to have persistent TD than those with normal dominance and asymmetry patterns (Barr et al., 1989). Another study demonstrated that cognitive deterioration was associated with the emergence of TD (Waddington, Youssef and Kinsella, 1990). Taken together, these findings suggest that patients with more specialized patterns of cerebral organization may be more vulnerable to deteriorative processes. Such a pattern could help explain the high proportion of TD following neuroleptic treatment in syndromes that are less marked by conceptual disorganization, such as schizoaffective and affective psychoses. On the other hand, patients with failures in the normal program of cerebral specialization may have more profound deficits from the beginning. In such patients, failure to develop a normal neurocognitive repertoire might be reflected early if cognitive "milestones" are not passed on time. The persistence of immature neurobehavioral programs into adolescence and adulthood would become increasingly inappropriate, and an "early" or "gradual" onset may be documented. It is interesting in this respect that age of onset may be later in patients with ventricular enlargement (Andreasen, Olsen, Dennert and Smith, 1982; Jeste et al., 1982; Johnstone et al., 1989). These findings pose problems for the hypothesis that ventricular enlargement is a general index of a more severe "structural" pathology, but make sense if one postulates that a mechanism unrelated to ventricular enlargement, such as failure in cerebral specialization, is more conspicuous early in life.

INDEPENDENCE OF HYPOTHETICAL ETIOLOGIC FACTORS

The precise etiologies of different morphologic abnormalities remain unknown. To the extent that etiologic hypotheses have been advanced, these offer further support for the possible independence of different morphologic abnormalities. Moreover, the hypothetical etiologic mechanisms may serve to better organize additional pathologic findings into a smaller number of general pathologic trends.

Cannon and his colleagues provided evidence that multisite cortical defects and ventricular enlargement have different historical antecedents (Cannon, Mednick and Parnas, 1989). The multisite cortical defects were predicted by familial factors but not by birth complications. The authors argued that the familial (presumably genetic) factor underlying these defects is failed fetal neural development, probably during the second trimester of gestation.

Similar dysplastic processes, primarily failures in neuronal migration during the second trimester of gestation, may be suggested as the basis for cytoarchitectonic and morphologic abnormalities in hippocampus, cingulate gyrus, motor, and prefrontal cortex (Conrad and Scheibel, 1987; Jakob and Beckmann, 1986; Bogerts, Meertz and Schonfeld-Bausch, 1985; Benes, Davidson and Bird, 1986; Benes, 1987). The hippocampus, cingulate gyrus, and medial frontal cortices comprise archicortical, proisocortical, and isocortical divisions of a "dorsal" evolutionary cytoarchitectonic trend in the anterior brain (Sanides, 1969; Yeterian and Pandya, 1988). Posterior constituents of this trend include parahippocampal[2], dorsal striate cortex, and dorsal somatosensory regions (Yeterian and Pandya, 1988). The inter-relations of territories within this trend have been corroborated by studies of both intrinsic and long-range connectivity patterns (Yeterian and Pandya, 1988). We speculate here that a defect of cellular migration in this dorsal cytoarchitectonic trend (of which the hippocampus is the primordial cellular moiety) could underlie both the cytoarchitectonic anomalies and "multisite" cortical abnormalities.[3]

Ventricular enlargement, in contrast to multisite cortical abnormalities, has been predicted by a combination of familial factors and birth complications (Cannon et al., 1989; DeLisi et al., 1986). The link between ventricular enlargement and birth complications has been supported further by several independent investigations (see Lewis, Owen, and Murray, 1989). Cannon and his colleagues

---

[2] Although certain regions of the parahippocampal gyrus (TH, TF, TL, and prostriate regions) were considered part of the archicortical trend deriving from proisocortex of the ventral temporal region, its connectivity patterns suggest that it may be related more to the ventral paleocortical trend (Galaburda, 1984; Pandya and Yeterian, 1985; Sanides, 1972).

[3] Defects in migration might also affect the "ventral" (paleocortical) trend, and be associated with cytoarchitectonic abnormalities in insular, entorhinal, temporal polar, superior temporal, ventral parietal, and ventral frontal regions. Brown, et al. (1986) found no difference between affective and schizophrenic groups in the thickness of the insular-opercular region, but otherwise, abnormalities in the ventral trend have not been well studied. Further investigation of both dorsal and ventral components of frontal regions (i.e., Brodmann's areas 10, 8, and 6) and contrasts between medio-dorsal and latero-ventral areas would be informative. If there are different functional correlates of interhemispheric fissure enlargement (dorsal trend) from Sylvian fissure enlargement (ventral trend), as suggested by McCarley et al. (1989), this might support the independence of defects within dorsal and ventral cytoarchitectonic lines.

suggested that the genetic diathesis may comprise increased vulnerability to the potential anoxic and hemorrhagic consequences of delivery complications, perhaps through maldevelopment of the cerebrovasculature or periventricular structures. Even if the genetic factor is necessary, it is apparently not sufficient; an independent pathologic process, such as that posed by birth complications, is required to yield periventricular damage.

Cerebral asymmetries are probably regulated by a complex interaction of primary genetic and hormonal controls. Annet (1985) postulated that a "right shift" gene programs the normal pattern of cerebral asymmetries. Crow has argued that a defect in or near this gene (perhaps at the pseudoautosomal locus of the X chromosome) may underlie psychosis (Crow, 1988, 1989; Crow et al., 1989). Others have focused on the role of gonadal steroids in controlling the timing and rate of neuronal maturation; slow growing zones have been seen as more vulnerable to teratogenic influences, and more likely to fail in the competition to establish synapses, thereby becoming more vulnerable to cellular elimination (Geschwind and Galaburda, 1985a; 1985b; 1985c; 1984). There is still controversy surrounding the relative rates of hemispheral growth (see Witelson, 1988), and it may be that different regions within each hemisphere show different rates of maturation (Thatcher et al., 1987). A detailed discussion of these issues is beyond the scope of this brief presentation. Without considering the specific mechanisms, it is still possible to suggest that a mechanism involving regional hemispheral growth and cellular elimination has gross anatomic correlates with implications for understanding the functional defects of schizophrenia.

The best studied gross anatomic indices of cerebral hemispheral specialization are cortical "torque" (i.e., relative enlargement of the left posterior and right anterior hemispheres over their contralateral homologues), and the morphology of the corpus callosum. Most attention has been paid to the relations of these features with hand preference, although there is limited information also on their relations with measures of functional asymmetry and sex differences (see Witelson and Kigar, 1988). These data suggest that a process leading to ambiguous lateral preference (more non-right-handedness) and lack of the normal functional asymmetry, is associated with decreased cortical torque and larger cross-sectional area of the corpus callosum (Witelson, 1986; Witelson and Kigar, 1988). An increased frequency of non-right-handedness, absence or reversal of the normal torque, and increased callosal area, have all been documented in schizophrenia, although the prevalence of these abnormalities remains controversial. To the best of our knowledge, these different indices of functional and anatomic specialization have not yet been studied concurrently, so their co-occurrence remains unknown.

The process of cerebral specialization in man is not necessarily restricted to hemisphere differences; general growth and cellular elimination trends affect the development of tertiary isocortical fields in frontal and parietal cortices that underlie the most uniquely human cognitive capacities. Following the "temporal vulnerability" model, and due to their location with respect to main arterial supplies, these tertiary neocortical territories may have enhanced susceptibility to a range of teratogenic influences, including hypoxia. Overall volume reductions may characterize some schizophrenics (Andreasen et al., 1986; DeMyer et al., 1988), and be associated with relative neuropsychological deficits in both schizophrenia and healthy controls (Johnstone et al., 1989; DeMyer et al., 1988). More information is needed to determine whether these overall volume reductions relate to patterns of hemisphere-specific growth trends or represent an independent dimension of cerebral specialization. Because they share putative mechanisms involving general growth and cellular elimination, and because they have some similar implications for cognitive development, we provisionally classify hemispheral asymmetries, callosal pruning, and tertiary cortical growth trends together as possible morphologic indices of cerebral specialization.

SUMMARY AND "PATH" PROTOTYPES

We speculate that medial fronto-limbic system neuromigratory defects, periventricular damage, and general cerebral anatomic specialization failures may comprise dissociable pathologic processes contributing to behavioral morbidity in schizophrenia. The possibility remains, of course, that some primary factor could underlie the different types of abnormality by increasing vulnerability to different pathologic processes. A primary defect in the genetic program governing cellular migration, or an insult during critical periods of growth, could increase vulnerability to birth complications in periventricular zones, or lead to establishment of anomalous connectivity patterns that would in turn lead to excessive or incomplete neuronal regression, possibly on a hemisphere- or region-specific basis.

Even if the different abnormalities can be related to a single common defect, the obvious pleiotropy of such a defect must be acknowledged to account for the lack of association between different morphologic variants. A single basic defect might be found, but still fail to explain the heterogeneous course and symptoms of schizophrenia. For example, defects in hippocampal cytoarchitectonics might be necessary and sufficient to cause schizophrenia, but additional defects in the medial frontolimbic trend, periventricular damage, or cerebral specialization anomalies might affect the pre-onset characteristics, acute symptom presentation, and long-term outcome. By examining the unique contributions of different pathologic processes, even if these processes are "secondary", there is hope that we may understand better the complex range of functional impairment in the schizophrenia syndrome.

An overview of features hypothetically associated with the three pathologic processes is provided in the Table. "Prototype" presentations are used to illustrate the neurodevelopmental trajectories that would be predicted by this hypothesis, for cases in which the influence of one pathologic process predominates. It is assumed that "pure" cases may be relatively rare and overlapping pathologies frequent. Each prototype represents a set of features that are predicted to co-vary across heterogeneous samples, and thus comprises a framework for hypothesis testing. Following Ciompi (1989), events are outlined in three phases: Phase I - Premorbid Evolution; Phase II - Psychotic Decompensation; and Phase III - Post-psychotic Course.

Medial Fronto-Limbic Path

Phase I - Genetic and/or intra-uterine environmental effects, probably during weeks 16 to 24 of gestation, cause defects in the normal growth of elements comprising the medial paralimbic trend, which develops from the archicortical hippocampal moiety (Sanides, 1969; Conrad and Scheibel, 1987) (Pandya and Barnes, 1987; Yeterian and Pandya, 1988). "Multisite" defects may be observed in one or more of the elements of this complex functional system, including: hippocampal formation, (Kovelman and Scheibel, 1984; Falkai, Bogerts and Rozumek, 1988; Falkai, Bogerts, Roberts and Crow, 1988) cingulate (Benes, 1987), ventral striatum (Bogerts, Meertz and Schonfeld-Bausch, 1985; Early, Posner, Reiman and Raichle, 1989), and the medial and dorsal motor, premotor and prefrontal cortices (Benes, Davidson and Bird, 1986). If severe, early deficits of motor control or attention can be detected, specifically on tasks requiring response preparation and anticipation (Cornblatt and Erlenmeyer-Kimling, 1985; Neuchterlein and Dawson, 1984). If milder, deficits are not apparent until the later development of prefrontal neocortex (Weinberger, 1987), or until hormonal effects on mesiotemporal regions are prominent during adolescence (Bogerts, 1989; Saugstad, 1989).

Phase II - Individuals with these medial frontolimbic deficits are exquisitely sensitive to conflicting demands (intellectual or social) and the compromised system fails to modulate these stressors (Weinberger, 1987; Stevens, 1973). Overstressing this medial frontolimbic system may be a major common path to schizophreniform psychotic reactions through disregulation of dopaminergic/cholinergic balance in cortico-striato-pallido-thalamo-cortical loops (Early, Posner, Reiman and Raichle, 1989a; 1989b) which may be modified by neuroleptic and cholinergic treatments (Tandon and Greden, 1989). Decompensations are characterized by misattributions of intentions and significance, leading to ideas of reference, paranoid states, and other florid psychotic phenomena (Frith, 1987; Frith and Done, 1988; Douglas, 1967). Patients who have only this defect may respond well to neuroleptic treatment through reduction of mismatch between intentions and action (Frith, 1987; Frith and Done, 1988; Frith and Done, 1989). If untreated, accumulation of dopamine metabolites and free radical formation may have neurotoxic consequences (Cadet and Lohr, 1987).

Phase III - Neuropsychological exams following onset may reveal prominent

Table 1. Neurodevelopmental paths to schizophrenia and their correlates

	Medial Fronto-Limbic Defect	Periventricular Damage	Cerebral Specialization Failure
Hypothetical Mechanism	Faulty migration of elements in the dorsal cytoarchitectonic trend	Delivery complic's periventricular anoxia or hemorrhage	Failure of hemisphere specific or tertiary cortical growth and cellular "pruning"
Gross Morphologic Indices	Sulcal enlargement, volume reductions in anterior hippocampal formation	Ventricular enlargement	Absence or reversal of normal asymmetry, "thick" corpus callosum, small brain size?
Histopathologic Indices	Cytoarchitectonic variations in hippocampus, cingulate, and dorsomedial frontal cortex	Periventricular thinning	Altered asymmetry of planum temporale, frontal operculum, decreased relative volume of isocortical fields
Early Developmental "Markers"	If severe, attentional and motor disturbance	If severe, social withdrawal	Poor acquisition of language competence, early academic deficits
Pattern of Psychotic Decompensation	Florid, active, "paranoid"	Blunted, withdrawn, "flat"	Regressive, simple, "hebephrenic"
Response to Neuroleptics	Good	Fair/poor	Fair/poor
Deterioration?	Most likely	Possible	Least likely
Risk for TD	Highest	High?	Least likely
Neuropsychological Profile after Compensation	Executive and motor deficits; defects in response preparation and organization	Learning and memory deficits	Language deficits, "primitive" cognitive style; anomalous dominance
Psychophysiologic Abnormalities	Reduced CNV; alteration of "processing negativity"	Orienting response dysfunction; alteration of mismatch negativity?	???

executive and/or motor deficits in the context of adequate linguistic and symbolic abilities. This may lead to apparent left hemisphere hyperfunction with relative right hemisphere dysfunction (Gur, 1978; Gur, 1979; Early, Posner, Reiman and Raichle, 1989a; 1989b; Gruzelier, Seymour, Wilson, Jolley and Hirsch, 1988). Corollary information processing deficits will include "restriction of inputs" and "perseveration of outputs" (Gruzelier, Seymour, Wilson, Jolley and Hirsch, 1988; Shakow, 1962; Cromwell, 1972; Spohn, Lacoursiere, Thompson and Coyne, 1977). Psychophysiologic correlates of these defects in the preparedness to respond may be observed in reduction of the contingent negative variation or "processing negativity" potential (Pribram and McGuinness, 1975; Näätänen, 1988). MRI exams may reveal reduced volume of the anterior hippocampal formation (Bogerts et al., 1990), and/or "multisite" defects in cortical sulci, interhemispheric and sylvian fissures, or cerebellum (Bilder et al., 1988; McCarley et al., 1989; Cannon, Mednick and Parnas, 1989).

Periventricular Path

Phase I - Genetic controls combined with delivery complications lead to ventriculomegaly impacting the structures surrounding the ventricular system (Cannon et al., 1989; see also Lewis, Owen and Murray, 1989). Key brain-stem, hypothalamic, thalamic, and temporal lobe structures may be affected. Core-brain arousal controls may be affected early, and if so will be reflected primarily by social incompetencies and in some cases withdrawal (Weinberger, Cannon-Spoor, Potkin and Wyatt, 1980; DeLisi et al., 1983). Early academic progress may be normal. Subsequent hormonal and social stressors, however, lead to further dysregulation of autonomic controls and possible dysfunction in the hypothalamo-pituitary axis, accompanied by hypercortisolemia and possibly further ventricular enlargement (Weinberger, 1984; Kellner, Rubinow, Gold and Post, 1983).

Phase II - Acute decompensation may involve florid psychotic phenomena, but in most cases affective flattening, further social withdrawal, and avolition/apathy will be prominent (Crow, 1985). Neuroleptics will lead to improvement of florid psychotic phenomena and secondary negative symptoms, but affective flattening and social withdrawal may persist (Crow, 1985; Carpenter and Kirkpatrick, 1988).

Phase III - Neuropsychological tests will show prominent memory impairments, along with other attentional and intentional deficits depending on the severity of the pathology (Bilder et al., 1988; Johnstone et al., 1989). Psychophysiologic correlates may include defects in the "mismatch" negativity and/or orienting response abnormalities (Cannon et al., 1988; Näätänen, 1988). MRI exams reveal ventricular enlargement. Third ventricular enlargement may offer the best index of diencephalic involvement (Boronow et al., 1985). Temporal horn involvement may affect other mesiotemporal and limbic sites, leading to syndromal overlap with the medial fronto-limbic trend.

Cerebral Specialization Path

Phase I - Genetic, hormonal, and/or congenital factors lead to failure in the normal process of asymmetric cerebral specialization (Geschwind and Galaburda, 1987; Satz, 1972; Crow, 1988; Crow et al., 1989). In some cases specialization failures may limit the growth of widespread tertiary neocortical territories, including prefrontal and the posterior association cortices (Rakic and Goldman-Rakic, 1982; Goldman-Rakic 1987). This failure is manifest in faulty early cognitive development, especially of language and formal symbolic functions (Goldberg and Costa, 1981; Satz, 1973). Communication difficulties may be reflected early in scholastic performance, but may also lead to social incompetencies (Pandurangi, Bilder, Rieder, Mukherjee and Hamer, 1988; Merrin, 1984).

Phase II - Typical social, academic, and maturational stresses of adolescence are severe for these individuals, at least in part because they lack adequate coping strategies (Strauss, 1989). Schizophrenic decompensations take a regressive form, manifest in "hebephrenic" or "simple" evolutions (Kay and Singh, 1989). Prominent symptoms of cognitive disorganization may include alogia, attentional impairment, formal thought disorder, and bizarre behavior (Bilder, Mukherjee, Rieder and Pandurangi, 1985; Kulhara, Kota and Joseph, 1986; Liddle, 1987b; Manoach, Maher and Manschreck, 1988; Kay and Singh, 1979). Response to neuroleptic treatment is "partial" because elements of cognitive disorganization persist (Kay and Singh, 1989).

Phase III - Neuropsychological tests reveal "left hemisphere" impairment, primarily due to language impairments and lack of the normal right hand advantage on motor tests (Flor-Henry, 1983). Assessment of handedness reveals ambiguous or mixed lateral preference (Shan-Ming et al., 1985; Green, Satz, Smith and Nelson, 1989). Brain morphology may show an absence or reversal of asymmetry at cortical levels associated with a lack of sulcal prominence (Luchins, Weinberger and Wyatt, 1979; Luchins, Weinberger and Wyatt, 1982). MRI may reveal abnormalities of the corpus callosum (Nasrallah et al., 1986). The presence or absence of ventricular enlargement may relate to the etiology of dominance failure; in pure "genetic" variants ventricular size may be normal or small, while in "pathological" left handedness ventricular size would be enlarged (Katsanis and Iacono, 1989), leading to syndromal overlap with the periventricular path.

CONCLUDING COMMENT

This hypothesis about pathological processes in schizophrenia is offered as a simple heuristic for research on structure-function relations in schizophrenia. The hypothesis was derived to resolve some apparently paradoxical and conflicting findings, and to serve as a theoretical starting point for further investigations of relations between abnormal brain morphology and neuropsychological dysfunction in schizophrenia. We hope that in the process, new and more refined theories of the pathophysiologic processes underlying schizophrenia may be advanced.

ACKNOWLEDGEMENTS

The authors thank Richard Lewine for his comments on a previous draft of the manuscript, and Lauren Lipschutz-Broch and Regina Graham for their assistance in preparing the manuscript for publication. Preparation of this paper was supported by USPHS grants from the National Institute of Mental Health (MH-41646; MH-41960), and a Faculty Research Award (3-926) from Long Island Jewish Medical Center.

REFERENCES

Adams, K. M., Jacisin, J. J., Brown, G. G., Boulos, R. S., and Silk, S. D., 1984, Neurobehavioral deficit and computed tomographic abnormalities in three samples of schizophrenic patients, Perceptual and Motor Skills, 590:115-119.

Andreasen, N. C., Dennert, J. W., Olsen, S. A., and Damasio, A., 1982, Hemispheric asymmetries and schizophrenia, American Journal of Psychiatry, 139:427-430.

Andreasen, N. C., Ehrhardt, J. C., Swayze, V. W., Alliger, R. J., Yuh, W. T. C., Cohen, G., and Ziebell, S., 1990, Magnetic resonance imaging of the brain in schizophrenia, Archives of General Psychiatry, 47:35-44.

Andreasen, N. C., Nasrallah, H. A., Dunn, V., Olson, S. C., Grove, W. M., Ehrhardt, J. C., Coffman, J. A., and Crossett, J. H., 1986, Structural abnormalities in the frontal system in schizophrenia. A magnetic resonance imaging study, Archives of General Psychiatry, 43:136-144.

Andreasen, N.C., Olsen, S.A., Dennert, J.W. and Smith, M.R., 1982, Ventricular enlargement in schizophrenia: Relationship to positive and negative symptoms. American Journal of Psychiatry, 139:279-301.

Annett, M., 1985, "Left, right, hand and brain: The right shift theory," L.Erlbaum, London.

Barr, W. B., Mukherjee, S., Degreef, G., and Caracci, G., 1989, Anomalous dominance and persistent tardive dyskinesia, Biological Psychiatry, 25:826-834.

Benes, F. M., 1987, An analysis of the arrangement of neurons in the cingulate cortex of schizophrenic patients, Archives of General Psychiatry, 44:608-616.

Benes, F. M., Davidson, B., and Bird, E. D., 1986, Quantitative cytoarchitectural studies of the cerebral cortex of schizophrenics, Archives of General Psychiatry, 43:31-35.

Besson, J. A. O., Corrigan, G. R., Cherryman, G. R., and Smith, F. W., 1987, Nuclear magnetic resonance brain imaging in chronic schizophrenia, British Journal of Psychiatry, 150:161-163.

Bilder, R. M., in press, Structure-function relations in schizophrenia: Brain morphology and neuropsychology. Progress in Experimental Personality and Psychopathology Research.

Bilder, R. M., 1985, "Subtyping in chronic schizophrenia: Clinical, neuropsychological, and structural indices of deterioration," University Microfilms, Ann Arbor, MI.

Bilder, R. M., Bogerts, B., Degreef, G., Ashtari, M., Lieberman, J. A., Alvir, J., and Jody, D., 1989, Neuropsychological correlates of brain morphology in schizophrenia, Paper presented at the Annual Meeting of the Society for Research in Psychopathology, Coral Gables, Florida.

Bilder, R. M., Degreef, G., Pandurangi, A. K., Rieder, R. O., Sackeim, H. A., and Mukherjee, S., 1988, Neuropsychological deterioration and CT-scan findings in chronic schizophrenia, Schizophrenia Research, 1:37-45.

Bilder, R. M., Mukherjee, S., Rieder, R. O., and Pandurangi, A. K., 1985, Symptomatic and neuropsychological components of defect states, Schizophrenia Bulletin, 11:409-419.

Bishop, R. S., Golden, C. J., MacInnes, W. D., Chu, C. C., Ruedrich, S. L., and Wilson, J., 1983, The BPRS in assessing symptom correlates of cerebral ventricular enlargement in acute and chronic schizophrenia, Psychiatry Research, 9:225-231.

Bogerts, B., 1989, Limbic and paralimbic pathology in schizophrenia: Interaction with age- and stress-related factors, In: "Schizophrenia: Scientific Progress," Schulz, S. C., Tamminga, C. A., eds., Oxford University Press, New York, NY.

Bogerts, B., Ashtari, M., Degreef, G., Alvir, J. Ma.J., Bilder, R. M., and Lieberman, J. A., 1990, Reduced temporal limbic structure volumes in first episode schizophrenia, Psychiatry Research: Neuroimaging, 35:1-13.

Bogerts, B., Meertz, E., and Schonfeldt-Bausch, R., 1985, Basal ganglia and limbic system pathology in schizophrenia: A morphometric study of brain volume and shrinkage, Archives of General Psychiatry, 42:784-791.

Boronow, J., Pickar, D., Ninan, P. T., Roy, A., Hommer, D., Linnoila, M., and Paul, S. M., 1985, Atrophy limited to the third ventricle in chronic schizophrenic patients: report of a controlled series, Archives of General Psychiatry, 42:266-270.

Brown, R., Colter, N., Corsellis, N., Crow, T. J., Frith, C. D., Jagoe, R., Johnstone, E. C., and Marsh, L., 1986, Postmortem evidence of structural brain changes in schizophrenia, Archives General Psychiatry, 43:36-42.

Cadet, J. L., and Lohr, J. B., 1987, Free radicals and the developmental pathobiology of schizophrenic burnout, Integrative Psychiatry, 5:40-48.

Cannon, T. D., Fuhrmann, M., Mednick, S. A., Machon, R. A., Parnas, J., and Schulsinger, F., 1988, Third ventricle enlargement and reduced electrodermal responsiveness, Psychophysiology, 25:153-156.

Cannon, T. D., Mednick, S. A., and Parnas, J., 1989, Genetic and perinatal determinants of structural brain deficits in schizophrenia, Archives of General Psychiatry, 46:883-889.

Carpenter, Jr W. T., and Kirkpatrick, B., 1988, The heterogeneity of the long-term course of schizophrenia, Schizophrenia Bulletin, 14:645-652.

Ciompi, L., 1989, The dynamics of complex biological-psychosocial systems. Four fundamental psycho-biological mediators in the long-term evolution of schizophrenia, British Journal of Psychiatry, 155(suppl. 5):15-21.

Conrad, A. J., and Scheibel, A. B., 1987, Schizophrenia and the hippocampus: The embryological hypothesis extended, Schizophrenia Bulletin, 13:577-587.

Cornblatt, B. A., and Erlenmeyer-Kimling, L., 1985, Global attentional deviance as a marker of risk for schizophrenia: Specificity and predictive validity, Journal of Abnormal Psychology, 94:470.

Cromwell, R. L., 1972, Strategies for studying schizophrenic behavior, Psychopharmacologia (Berl), 24:121-146.

Crow, T. J., 1989, Pseudoautosomal locus for the cerebral dominance gene, Lancet, ii:339-340.

Crow, T. J., 1988, Sex chromosomes and psychosis. The case for a pseudoautosomal locus, British Journal of Psychiatry, 153:675-683.

Crow, T. J., 1985, The two-syndrome concept: Origins and current status, Schizophrenia Bulletin, 11:471-486.

Crow, T. J., Ball, J., Bloom, S. R., Brown, R., Bruton, C. J., Colter, N., Frith, C. D., Johnstone, E. C., Owens, D. G. C., and Roberts, G. W., 1989, Schizophrenia as an anomaly of development of cerebral asymmetry: a post-mortem study and a proposal concerning the genetic basis of the disease, Archives of General Psychiatry, 46:1145-1150.

DeLisi, L. E., Schwartz, C. C., Targum, S. D., Byrnes, S., Cannon-Spoor, E., Weinberger, D. R., and Wyatt, R. J., 1983, CT scan findings and outcome in acute schizophreniform disorder, Psychiatry Research, 9:169-171.

DeLisi, L. E., Golden, L. R., Hamovit, J. R., Maxwell, M. E., Kurtz, D. and Gershon, E.S., 1986, A family study of the association of increased ventricular size with schizophrenia, Archives of General Psychiatry, 43:148-153.

DeMyer, M. K., Gilmore, R. L., Hendrie, H. C., DeMyer, W. E., Augustyn. G.T., and Jackson, R. K., 1988, Magnetic resonance brain images in schizophrenic and normal subjects: Influence of diagnosis and education, Schizophrenia Bulletin, 14:21-37.

DeQuardo, J., Tandon, R., and Meador-Woodruff, J. H., 1990, VBR and neuropsychological findings in schizophrenia, Paper presented at the 143rd Meeting of the American Psychiatric Association, New York.

Dewan, M. J., Pandurangi, A. K., Lee, S. H., and et al, 1983, Cerebellar morphology in chronic schizophrenic patients: a controlled computed tomography study, Psychiatry Research, 10:97-103.

Donnelly, E. F., Weinberger, D. R., Waldman, I. N., and Wyatt, R. J., 1980, Cognitive impairment associated with morphological brain abnormalities on computed tomography in chronic schizophrenic patients, Journal of Nervous and Mental Disease, 168:305-308.

Douglas, R. J., 1967, The hippocampus and behavior, Psychological Bulletin, 67:416-442.

Early, T. S., Posner, M. I., Reiman, E., and Raichle, M. E., 1989a, Hyperactivity of the left striato-pallidal projection. Part I: Lower level theory, Psychiatric Developments, 2:85-108.

Early, T. S., Posner, M. I., Reiman, E.,and Raichle, M. E., 1989b, Left striato-pallidal hyperactivity in schizophrenia. Part II: Phenomenology and thought disorder, Psychiatric Developments, 2:109-121.

Falkai, P., Bogerts, B., and Rozumek, M., 1988, Cell loss and volume reduction in the entorhinal cortex of schizophrenics, Biological Psychiatry, 24:515-521.

Falkai, P., Bogerts, B., Roberts, G.W. and Crow, T.J., 1988, Measurement of alpha-cell-migration in the entorhinal region: A marker for the developmental disturbances in schizophrenia?, Schizophrenia Research, 1:157-158.

Farmer, A., Jackson, R., McGuffin, P., and Storey, P., 1987, Cerebral ventricular enlargement in chronic schizophrenia: Consistencies and contradictions, British Journal of Psychiatry, 150:324-330.

Flor-Henry, P., 1983, "Cerebral basis of psychopathology," John Wright, Boston, MA.

Frith, C. D., 1987, The positive and negative symptoms of schizophrenia reflect impairments in the perception and initiation of action, Psychological Medicine, 17:631-648.

Frith, C. D., and Done, D. J., 1989, Experiences of alien control in schizophrenia reflect a disorder in the central monitoring of action, Psychological Medicine, 19:359-363.

Frith, C. D., and Done, D. J., 1988, Towards a neuropsychology of schizophrenia, British Journal of Psychiatry, 153:437-443.

Galaburda, A. M., 1984, Anatomy of language; lessons from comparative anatomy, In: "Neurolinguistics," D. Kaplan, A. R. LeCours and J. Marshall, eds., MIT Press, Cambridge, MA.

Geschwind, N. and Galaburda, A. M., 1984, "Cerebral Dominance. The Biological Foundations," Harvard University Press, Cambridge, MA.

Geschwind, N., and Galaburda, A. M., 1985a, Cerebral lateralization. Biological mechanisms, associations, and pathology: I. A hypothesis and a program for research, Archives of Neurology, 42:428-459.

Geschwind, N., and Galaburda, A. M., 1985b, Cerebral lateralization. Biological mechanisms, associations, and pathology: II. A hypothesis and a program for research, Archives of Neurology, 42:521-552.

Geschwind, N., and Galaburda, A. M., 1985c, Cerebral lateralization. Biological mechanisms, associations, and pathology: III. A hypothesis and a program for research, Archives of Neurology, 42:634-654.

Geschwind, N. and Galaburda, A. M., 1987, "Cerebral Lateralization. Biological Mechanisms, Associations, and Pathology," MIT Press, Cambridge, MA.

Goldberg, E., and Costa, L. D., 1981, Hemisphere differences in the acquisition and use of descriptive systems, Brain and Language, 14:144-173.

Golden, C. J., Moses, J. A., Zelazowski, R., Graber, B., Zatz, L. M., Horvath, T. B., and Berger, P. A., 1980, Cerebral ventricular size and neuropsychological impairment in young chronic schizophrenics, Archives of General Psychiatry, 37:619-623.

Golden, C. J., MacInnes, W.D., Ariel, R.N., Ruedrich, S.L., Chu, C.C., Coffman, J.A., Graber, B., and Bloch, S., 1982, Cross-validation of the ability of the Luria-Nebraska Neuropsychological Battery to differentiate chronic schizophrenics with and without ventricular enlargement, Journal of Consulting and Clinical Psychology, 50:87-95.

Goldman-Rakic, P. S., 1987, Circuitry of primate prefrontal cortex and regulation of behavior by representational memory, In: "Handbook of Physiology," Plumm, F., Mountcastle, V., eds., American Physiological Society, Washington, DC.

Green, M. F., Satz, P., Smith, C., and Nelson, L., 1989, Is there atypical handedness in schizophrenia?, Journal of Abnormal Psychology, 98:57-61.

Gruzelier, J., Seymour, K., Wilson, L., Jolley, A., and Hirsch, S., 1988, Impairments on neuropsychologic tests of temporohippocampal and frontohippocampal functions and word fluency in remitting schizophrenia and affective disorders, Archives of General Psychiatry, 45:623-629.

Gur, R. E., 1979, Cognitive concomitants of hemispheric dysfunction in schizophrenia, Archives of General Psychiatry, 36:269-274.

Gur, R. E., 1978, Left hemisphere dysfunction and left hemisphere overactivation in schizophrenia, Journal of Abnormal Psychology, 87:226-238.

Iacono, W. G., Smith, G. N., Moreau, M., and et al, 1988, Ventricular and sulcal size at the onset of psychosis, American Journal of Psychiatry, 145:820-824.

Jakob, J., and Beckmann, H., 1986, Prenatal developmental disturbances in the limbic allocortex in schizophrenics, Journal of Neural Transmission, 65:303-326.

Jeste, D. V., Kleinman, J. E., Potkin, S. G., Luchins, D. J., and Weinberger, D. R., 1982, Ex uno multi: Subtyping the schizophrenic syndrome, Biological Psychiatry, 17(2): 199-222.

Johnstone, E. C., Crow, T. J., Frith, C. D., Stevens, M., Kreel, L., and Husband, J., 1978, The dementia of dementia praecox, Acta Psychiatrica Scandinavica, 57:305-324.

Johnstone, E. C., Owens, D. C. G., Bydder, G. M., Colter, N., Crow T.J., and Frith, C. D., 1989, The spectrum of structural brain changes in schizophrenia: Age of onset as a predictor of cognitive and clinical impairments and their cerebral correlates, Psychological Medicine, 19:91-103.

Katsanis, J., and Iacono, W. G., 1989, Association of left-handedness with ventricle size and neuropsychological performance in schizophrenia, American Journal of Psychiatry, 146:1056-1058.

Kay, S. R., and Opler, L. A., 1987, Positive and negative subtypes of schizophrenia, American Journal of Psychiatry, 144:1367.

Kay, S. R., and Singh, M. M., 1979, Cognitive abnormality in schizophrenia: A dual-process model, Biological Psychiatry, 14:155-175.

Kay, S. R., and Singh, M. M., 1989, The positive-negative distinction in drug-free schizophrenic patients, Archives of General Psychiatry, 46:711-718.

Keilp, J. G., Sweeney, J. A., Jacobsen, P., Solomon, C., St.Louis, L., Deck, M., Frances, A., and Mann, J. J., 1988, Cognitive impairment in schizophrenia: specific relations to ventricular size and negative symptomatology, Biological Psychiatry, 24:47-55.

Kellner, C. H., Rubinow, D. R., Gold, P. W., and Post, R. M., 1983, Relationship of cortisol hypersecretion to brain CT scan alterations in depressed patients, Psychiatry Research, 8:191-197.

Kemali, D., Maj, M., and Galderisi, S., 1987, Clinical, biological, and neuropsychological features associated with lateral ventricular enlargement in DSM-III schizophrenic disorder, Psychiatry Research, 21:137-149.

Kling, K. S., Kurtz, N., Tachiki, K., and Orzeck, A., 1982, CT scans in subgroups of chronic schizophrenics, Journal of Psychiatric Research, 17:375-394.

Kovelman, J. A., and Scheibel, A. B., 1984, A neurohistological correlate of schizophrenia, Biological Psychiatry, 19:1601-1621.

Kulhara, P., Kota, S. K., and Joseph, S., 1986, Positive and negative subtypes of schizophrenia, Acta Psychiatrica Scandinavica, 74:353-359.

Lewis, S. W., Owen, M. J., and Murray, R. M., 1989, Obstetric complications and schizophrenia: Methodology and mechanisms, In: "Schizophrenia: Scientific Progress," Schulz, S. C., Tamminga, C. A., eds., Oxford, New York, NY.

Liddle, P. F., 1987a, Schizophrenia syndromes, cognitive performance and neurological dysfunction, Psychological Medicine, 17:49-57.

Liddle, P. F., 1987b, The symptoms of chronic schizophrenia: A re-examination of the positive-negative dichotomy, British Journal of Psychiatry, 151:145-151.

Losonczy, M.F., Song, I.S., Mohs, R.C., Small, N.A., Davidson, M., Johns, C.A., and Davis, K.L., 1986, Correlates of lateral ventricular size in chronic schizophrenia. I. Behavioral and treatment response measures, American Journal of Psychiatry, 143:976-981.

Luchins, D., Lewine, R., and Meltzer, H., 1984, Lateral ventricular size, psychopathology and medication response in the psychoses, Biological Psychiatry, 19:29-44.

Luchins, D. J., and Meltzer, H. Y., 1983, A blind, controlled study of occipital asymmetry in schizophrenia, Psychiatry Research, 10:87-95.

Luchins, D. J., Weinberger, D. R., and Wyatt, R. J., 1982, Schizophrenia and cerebral asymmetry detected by computed tomography, American Journal of Psychiatry, 139:753-757.

Luchins, D. J., Weinberger, D. R., and Wyatt, R. J., 1979, Schizophrenia: Evidence of a subgroup with reversed cerebral asymmetry, Archives of General Psychiatry, 36:1309-1311.

Manoach, D. S., Maher, B. A., and Manschreck, T. C., 1988, Left-handedness and thought disorder in the schizophrenias, Journal of Abnormal Psychology, 1:97-99.

McCarley, R. W., Faux, S. F., Shenton, M., and et al, 1989, CT abnormalities in schizophrenia. A preliminary study of their correlations with P300/P200 electrophysiological features and positive/negative symptoms, Archives of General Psychiatry, 46:698-708.

Merrin, E., 1984, Motor and sighting dominance in chronic schizophrenia: relationship to social competence, age at first admission, and clinical course, British Journal of Psychiatry, 145:401-406.

Mukherjee, S., Reddy, R., and Schnur, D. B., 1989, A developmental model of negative syndromes in schizophrenia, In: "Negative Schizophrenic Symptoms: Pathophysiology and Clinical Aspects," Greden, J., Tandon, R., eds., American Psychiatric Press, Washington, DC.

Näätänen, R., 1988, Implications of ERP data for psychological theories of attention, Biological Psychiatry, 26:117-163.

Nasrallah, H. A., Andreasen, N. C., Coffman, J. A., Olson, S. C., Dunn, V. D., Ehrhardt, J. C., and Chapman, S. M., 1986, A controlled magnetic resonance imaging study of corpus callosum thickness in schizophrenia, Biological Psychiatry, 21:274-282.

Nasrallah, H. A., Jacoby, C. G., McCalley-Whitters, M., and Kuperman, S., 1982, Cerebral ventricular enlargement in subtypes of chronic schizophrenia, Archives of General Psychiatry, 39:774-777.

Nasrallah, H. A., Kuperman, S., Jacoby, C. G., McCalley-Whitters, M., and Hamra, B. J., 1983, Clinical correlates of sulcal widening in chronic schizophrenia, Psychiatry Research, 10:237-242.

Neuchterlein, K. H., and Dawson, M. E., 1984, Information processing and attentional functioning in the developmental course of schizophrenic disorders, Schizophrenia Bulletin, 10:160-202.

Nyman, H., Nybäck, H., Wiesel, F. A., Oxenstierna, G., and Schalling, D., 1986, Neuropsychological test performance, brain morphological measures and csf monoamine metabolites in schizophrenic patients, Acta Psychiatrica Scandinavica, 74:292-301.

Obiols, J. E., Marcos, T., and Salamero, M., 1987, Ventricular enlargement and neuropsychological testing in schizophrenia, Acta Psychiatrica Scandinavica, 76:199-202.

O'Leary, D. S., Andreasen, N. C., Arndt, S., and Kesler, M. I., 1991, Neuropsychological performance in schizophrenia: Relation to positive and negative symptoms, Journal of Clinical and Experimental Neuropsychology, 13:99.

Okasha, A., and Madkour, O., 1982, Cortical and central atrophy in chronic schizophrenia, Acta Psychiatrica Scandinavica, 65:29-34.

Owens, D. G. C., Johnstone, E. C., Crow, T. J., Frith, C. D., Jagoe, J. R., and Kreel, L., 1985, Lateral ventricular size in schizophrenia: relationship to the disease process and its clinical manifestations, Psychological Medicine, 15:27-41.

Pandurangi, A. K., and Bilder, R. M., 1988, The symptoms of chronic schizophrenia, British Journal of Psychiatry, 152:127.

Pandurangi, A. K., Bilder, R. M., Rieder, R. O., Mukherjee, S., and Hamer, R. M., 1988, Schizophrenic symptoms and deterioration: Relation to computed tomographic findings, Journal of Nervous and Mental Disease, 176:200-206.

Pandya, D. N., and Yeterian, E. H., 1985, Architecture and connections of cortical association areas, In: "Cerebral cortex: Association and auditory cortices", A. Peters and E. G. Jones, eds., Vol 4, Plenum Publishing Corp., New York.

Pandya, D. N., and Barnes, C. L., 1987, Architecture and connections of the frontal lobe, In: "The frontal lobes revisited," E. Perecman, ed., IRBN Press, New York, NY.

Pearlson, G. D., Garbacz, D. J., Breakey, W. R., Ahn, H. S., and DePaulo, J. R., 1984, Lateral ventricular enlargement associated with persistent unemployment and negative symptoms in both schizophrenia and bipolar disorder, Psychiatry Research, 12:1-9.

Pfefferbaum, A., Zipursky, R. B., Lim, K. O., Zatz, L. M., and Stahl, S. M. Jernigan, T.L., 1988, Computed tomographic evidence for generalized sulcal and ventricular enlargement in schizophrenia, Archives of General Psychiatry, 45:633-640.

Pribram, K. H., and McGuinness, D., 1975, Arousal, activation, and effort in the control of attention, Psychological Review, 82:116-149.

Rakic, P., and Goldman-Rakic, P. S., 1982, Development and modifiability of the cerebral cortex, Neuroscience Research Program Bulletin, 20:433-611.

Raz, S., and Raz, N., 1990, Structural brain abnormalities in the major psychoses: A quantitative review of the evidence from computerized imaging, Psychological Bulletin, 108:93-108.

Rieder, R. O., Donnelly, E. F., Herdt, J. R., and Waldman, I. N., 1979, Sulcal prominence in young chronic schizophrenic patients: CT scan findings associated with impairment on neuropsychological tests, Psychiatry Research, 1:1-8.

Rieder, R. O., Mann, L. S., Weinberger, D. R., Van Kammen, D. P., and Post, R. M., 1983, Computed tomographic scans in patients with schizophrenia, schizo-affective and bipolar affective disorder, Archives of General Psychiatry, 40:735-739.

Sanides, F., 1969, Comparative architectonics of the neocortex of mammals and their evolutionary interpretation, Annals of the NY Academy of Sciences, 167:404-423.

Sanides, F., 1972, Representation in the cerebral cortex and its areal lamination patterns. In: "The structure and function of nervous tissue," G.H. Bourne, ed., Vol 5, Academic Press, New York and London.

Satz, P., 1973, Left-handedness and early brain insult: An explanation, Neuropsychologia, 11:115-117.

Satz, P., 1972, Pathological left-handedness: An explanatory model, Cortex, 8:121-135.

Saugstad, L. F., 1989, Social class, marriage, and fertility in schizophrenia, Schizophrenia Bulletin, 15:9-43.

Shakow, D., 1962, Segmental set, Archives of General Psychiatry, 6:1-17.

Shan-Ming, Y., Flor-Henry, P., Dayi, C., Tiangi, L., Shuguang, Q., and Zenxiang, M., 1985, Imbalance of hemispheric functions in the major psychoses: A study of handedness in the People's Republic of China, Biological Psychiatry, 20:906-917.

Smith, A., Mental deterioration in chronic schizophrenia, 1964, Journal of Nervous and Mental Disease, 139:479-487.

Smith, R. C., Largen, J., Calderon, M., Schoolar, J., Shvartsburd, A., and Ravichandran, G. K., 1983, Morphological and neurological abnormalities as predictors of clinical response to psychotropic drugs - CT scans and neuropsychological tests as predictors of clinical response in schizophrenics, Psychopharmacology Bulletin, 19:505-509.

Spohn, H. E., Lacoursiere, R. B., Thompson, K., and Coyne, L., 1977, Phenothiazine effects on psychological and psychophysiological dysfunction in chronic schizophrenics, Archives of General Psychiatry, 34:633-644.

Stevens, J. R., 1973, An anatomy of schizophrenia, Archives of General Psychiatry, 29:177-189.

Strauss, J. S., 1989, Mediating processes in schizophrenia, British Journal of Psychiatry, 155:22-28.

Takahashi, R, Inaba, Y, Inanaga, K., Kato, N., Kumashiro, H., Nishimura, T., Okuma, T., Otsuki, S., Sakai, T., Sato, T., and Shimazono, Y., 1981, CT scanning and the investigation of schizophrenia, in: "Biological Psychiatry," Elsevier Science Publishers, Amsterdam.

Tanaka, Y., Hazama, H., and Kobayashi, K., 1981, Computerized tomography of the brain in schizophrenic patients, Acta Psychiatrica Scandinavica, 63:191-197.

Tandon, R., and Greden, J. F., 1989, Cholinergic hyperactivity and negative schizophrenic symptoms. A model of cholinergic/dopaminergic interactions in schizophrenia, Archives of General Psychiatry, 46:745-753.

Thatcher, R. W., Walker, R. A., and Giudice, S., 1987, Human cerebral hemispheres develop at different ages, Science, 236:1110-1113.

Waddington, J. L., Youssef, H. A., and Kinsella, A., 1990, Cognitive dysfunction in schizophrenia followed up over 5 years, and its longitudinal relationship to the emergence of tardive dyskinesia, Psychological Medicine, 20:835-842.

Weinberger, D. R., 1984, Computed tomography (CT) findings in schizophrenia: Speculation on the meaning of it all, Journal of Psychiatric Research, 18:477-490.

Weinberger, D. R., 1987, Implications of normal brain development for the pathogenesis of schizophrenia, Archives of General Psychiatry, 44:660-669.

Weinberger, D. R., Cannon-Spoor, H. E., Potkin, S. G., and Wyatt, R. J., 1980, Poor premorbid adjustment and CT scan abnormalities in chronic schizophrenia, American Journal of Psychiatry, 137:1410-1413.

Weinberger, D. R., DeLisi, L. E., Perman, G., Targum, S., and Wyatt, R. J., 1982, Computed tomography in schizophreniform disorder and other acute psychiatric disorders, Archives of General Psychiatry, 39:778-783.

Weinberger, D. R., Torrey, E. F., Neophytides, A. N., and Wyatt, R. J., 1979, Lateral cerebral ventricular enlargement in chronic schizophrenia, Archives of General Psychiatry, 36:735-739.

Williams, A. O., Reveley, M. A., Kolakowska, T., Ardern, M., and Mandelbrote, B. M., 1985, Schizophrenia and good and poor outcome II: Cerebral ventricular size and its clinical significance, British Journal of Psychiatry, 146:348-357.

Witelson, S. F., 1986, Wires of the mind: Anatomical variation in the corpus callosum in relation to hemispheric specialization and integration, In: "Two Hemispheres, One Brain. Functions of the Corpus Callosum. Neurology and Neurobiology," Lepore, F., Ptito, M., Jasper, H. H., eds.,

Witelson, S. F., and Kigar, D. L., 1988, Anatomical Development of the Corpus Callosum in Humans: A Review with Reference to Sex and Cognition, In: "Brain Lateralization in Children: Developmental Implications," Molfese, D. L., Segalowitz, S. J., eds., The Guilford Press, New York, NY.

Yeterian, E. H., and Pandya, D. N., 1988, Architectonic features of the primate brain: Implications for information processing and behavior, In: "Information processing by the brain," Markowitsch, H. J., ed., Hans Huber Publishers, Bern, Switzerland.

NEURODEVELOPMENT AND THE CHRONOLOGICAL CURIOSITIES OF SCHIZOPHRENIA

P.B. Jones and R. Goodman
Institute of Psychiatry, De Crespigny Park, London, Great Britain

M.J. Owen
Department of Psychological Medicine, University of Wales College of Medicine, Cardiff, Wales

S.W. Lewis
Department of Psychiatry, Charing Cross and Westminster Medical, London, Great Britain

R.M. Murray
Kings College Hospital and Institute, De Crespigny Park, London, Great Britain

INTRODUCTION

Several lines of evidence suggest that at least some cases of schizophrenia are a consequence of a structurally abnormal brain (Stevens, 1982). Although it is only now possible to study the cells of the brain and the genes controlling them, many of the most enduring findings in the field of schizophrenia research were established more than half a century ago and concern the timing of events. These findings include the excess of schizophrenics born in the late winter and spring (Tramer, 1929), the importance of the perinatal period in the development of psychopathology (Critchton-Browne, 1862), the association of early head trauma and psychosis (Tennent, 1937), and the earlier age of onset of schizophrenia in males (Bleuler, 1911 trans. 1950). Such findings have been widely replicated but for many years were not considered to be of fundamental importance to the understanding of schizophrenia. Instead, they were disregarded as mere chronological curiosities.

Cortical sulcal widening and enlarged cerebral ventricles in a proportion of schizophrenics have both been demonstrated frequently, and now appear to be consequent not upon a degenerative process but rather to be neurodevelopmental in origin (Murray & Lewis, 1987; Weinberger, 1987). In this chapter, we examine the relationship of the chronological epiphenomena of schizophrenia to the genetic and environmental determinants of this neurodevelopmental deviance.

WHEN DOES CEREBRAL ABNORMALITY ARISE?

Early Childhood

An association between schizophrenia and head injury in adulthood has been claimed (see Davidson & Bagley, 1969) but results from large series of individuals who have suffered head injury indicate that the rates of psychosis are similar to those in the general population (Achte, 1969; Feuchtwanger & Mayer-Gross, 1938). Furthermore, in those cases who become psychotic, some psychological abnormality often predates the head injury. However, when the head injury occurs at a young age, it does appear to be associated with a significant increase in the risk of schizophrenia. Wilcox and Nasrallah (1987) compared the prevalence of head injury in 200 schizophrenics, 325 manic depressives and 134 normal subjects. They found head injury to be most common in the schizophrenic group where almost all the injuries were received before 10 years of age; indeed, two thirds occurred before the age of 3. It seems that injury to the immature brain is more likely to be associated with schizophrenia than injury closer to the accepted age of presentation of the disorder, a conclusion echoing the results of earlier studies showing head injury as an age-dependent risk factor for psychosis (Achte et al., 1969).

Perinatal or Prenatal?

The notion that the process of birth can influence the psyche of the child is far from new (Critchon-Brown, 1862). A history of obstetric complications (OCs) seems to increase the risk of the later development of schizophrenia (McNeil, 1987), and is found especially commonly in those patients with poor premorbid functioning, and those with an early onset (Pollack et al., 1968; Owen et al. 1988; O'Callaghan et al., 1988). Some computerised tomographic (CT) studies have shown OCs and other early developmental hazards to be associated with increased ventricular size and cortical sulcal widening in adult schizophrenics (Murray et al., 1985, Turner et al., 1986; O'Callaghan, Larkin & Waddington, 1988; Owen, Lewis & Murray, 1988; Pearlson et al., 1989).

At first it was thought there was an analogy between head trauma and traumatic birth, the first resulting in direct brain injury, and the second in hypoxic brain damage (Rosanoff et al., 1934). In reality, the situation is likely to be more complex. The earliest studies found perinatal abnormalities to be more common than prenatal events (McNeil & Kaij, 1978) but this could be because the latter are more difficult to detect (McNeil, 1987). Furthermore, perinatal difficulties may be secondary to pre-existing abnormality in the fetus caused either by an earlier insult or by genetic predisposition (Owen et al., 1988; Goodman, 1988). This appears to be the case for cerebral palsy, another condition which shows an association with OCs (Lancet, 1989); Nelson and Ellenberg (1986) found that events during labour, delivery and the new born period did not identify many more cases of cerebral palsy than did abnormal characteristics identified prior to labour. Indirect evidence for a similar situation in schizophrenia comes from the excess of minor developmental physical abnormalities seen in schizophrenics. Once again, the latter are associated with poor premorbid adjustment and early age at onset (Guy et al., 1983; Green et al., 1987).

Prenatal influences can be isolated in studies of monozygotic twins where differences already present at birth must be due wholly to factors acting on the fetuses in utero. Some (Mosher et al., 1971) but not all (Kringlen, 1967), studies of monozygotic (MZ) twins discordant for schizophrenia have shown the pre-schizophrenic twin to have a lower birthweight. Lewis et al. (1987) studied birthweight in a subsample of psychotic MZ twins from the Maudsley Twin Regi-ster. They found that the mean difference in birthweight between two MZ twins later to become discordant for schizophrenia was more than four times greater than the intra-pair difference in twins concordant for schizophrenia, although it was not always the pre-psychotic twin in the discordant pairs who was lighter. Low birth weight (under 2 kilograms) was more common in the discordant pairs. These findings were interpreted as evidence for prenatal environmental factors being important in discordant MZ pairs, a conclusion supported by the comparative rarity of a family history of major psychiatric disorder in this group.

SEX DIFFERENCES IN AGE AT ONSET

Among schizophrenics, men tend to be younger than women when they experience their first episode of psychosis. This is a well replicated finding (Lewine, 1981; Loranger, 1984) and is not due to artefacts such as earlier identification or presentation in males (Hafner et al., 1989). Loranger (1984) has pointed out that the peak onset for both sexes is in the quinquenium 20-24 years and that the age distributions are not two isomorphic curves but that onset is somehow delayed in some but not all women. Viewed another way, these findings suggest that some factor may be accelerating the appearance of schizophrenia in males and leading to more frequent presentation in the immediate post-pubertal period. Rosenthal (1971) considers that this pattern of illness is more in accord with Kraepelin's original views of dementia praecox as an illness particularly affecting adolescent and young adult males.

Aylward et al. (1984) reviewed the evidence of intellectual impairment in schizophrenics and concluded that a deficit in premorbid IQ is found almost exclusively in males. Male schizophrenics show poorer premorbid social competance than females (Kokes et al., 1977; Foerster et al., 1990). The clinical picture also differs between the sexes; males show more affective flattening and fewer positive affective symptoms so that the stricter the diagnostic criteria, the greater the proportion of male cases becomes (Lewine et al., 1984). Males also show a poorer response to neuroleptics and a worse outcome as judged by clinical or social variables (Seeman, 1982; Castle & Murray, 1990).

Some studies of MZ twins suggest that concordance rates, an indicator of the strength of genetic effect, are lower in male than in female twins (Rosenthal, 1962; Kringlen, 1967). The suggestion that environmental factors may be of greater importance in males than in females was discussed as early as 1934 when Rosanoff and colleagues stated that "the proportion of cases with a probable traumatic or infectious aetiology seems to be higher in the male than the female sex. The most prominent factor here seems to be cerebral birth trauma." This stronger link between neurodevelopmental insult and schizophrenia in males than in females has been demonstrated in high genetic risk studies (Schulsinger et al., 1980) and in unselected series of schizophrenics (Pearlson et al., 1989; Wilcox and Nasrallah, 1987; Foerster et al., 1990). Since schizophrenics with a history of OCs are known to present earlier than other cases (Pollack et al., 1968) this may be an explanation of the earlier age at onset and greater severity of illness in males (Castle & Murray, 1990).

We examined the effect of family history and obstetric complications on age at onset in a group of 123 RDC schizophrenics, all of whom had CT head scans and in whom the age at first psychiatric presentation was known in all but one. Retrospective data on obstetric complications was available in 110 cases. This group was assembled from two Maudsley Hospital Series described in detail by Owen et al. (1988 and 1989, respectively). Those scanned after 50 years of age, and two subjects with gross ventriculo-megaly, were excluded in the present sample as we were originally concerned with analysis of VBR (vide infra).

Figure 1 shows that, as expected, males exhibited a significantly lower age at onset, defined as first contact with the psychiatric services. The presence of definite OC's was also associated with a lower age at onset whereas family history (of inpatient psychiatric care in a first degree relative) did not affect age of onset. When sex, family history and obstetric history were considered together (Figure 2), the conventional sex difference seen in the whole population persisted in the majority of cases who had neither a history of OC's nor an ill relative (male 22.9 yrs, n=35; female 25.2 yrs, n=20; n.s.) and also in those with only a positive family history (male 21 yrs n=21; female 25 yrs n=6; n.s.). However, in the group with severe OC's alone, males and females had a similarly young age at onset (male 19.2 yrs n=12; female 18.3 yrs n=3; n.s.). The numbers of subjects in some of these groups (especially females with OCs) are very small. However, if these findings

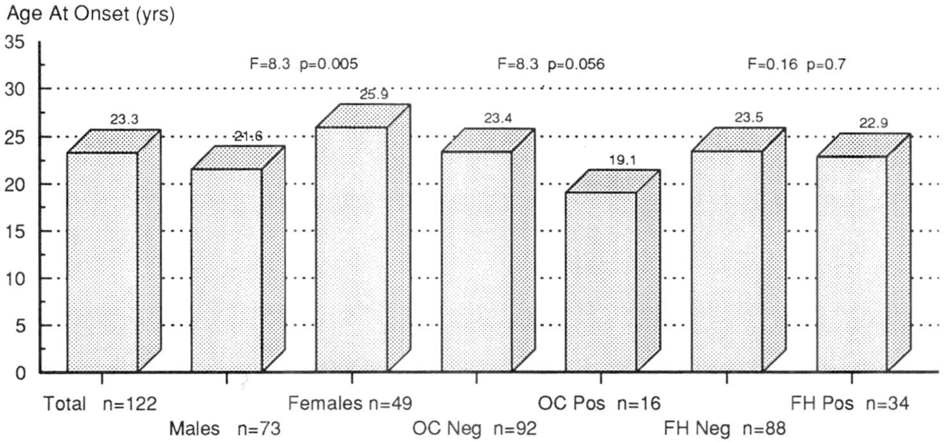

Figure 1. Age at onset by sex, family history and obstetric complications.

could be replicated in a larger sample, it would imply that it is the differential incidence or effect of early environmental hazards that leads to the sex difference in onset.

Why should pre- or perinatal hazards be more important in the aetiology of schizophrenia in males than females? Several possibilities come to mind. First, Amato et al. (1987) have shown that periventricular and intraventricular hemorrhage are more common in male than female premature infants even when there are no differences between the sexes in birthweight, gestational age or perinatal complications. The authors suggested that this greater vulnerability is due to the slower maturation of the cerebral vasculature in the male. Second, the brain parenchyma of the male fetus may be more susceptible to injury. Perhaps the relative delay in cerebral maturation of the male alters the consequences of potentially pathogenic events. Third, the functions of the cerebral hemispheres are less strongly lateralised in females who may therefore be less susceptible to damage to one hemisphere (Flor-Henry, 1978), an idea which is becoming increasingly appealing in schizophrenia research (Castle & Murray, 1990). There is, of course, considerable evidence implicating the left temporal lobe in schizophrenia. The left temporal lobe develops more slowly than the right and hence may be more susceptible to damage. For the reasons noted above, the male left temporal lobe may be especially vulnerable.

SEASON OF BIRTH

The majority of studies indicate that an excess of between 5 and 15% of schizophrenics are born in the late winter and spring (Bradbury & Miller, 1985). The methodology of these studies continues to be debated vigorously (Lewis, 1989,

1990) but the season of birth effect is a well replicated finding that requires explanation. This finding specifically suggests the existence of a seasonally varying aetiological factor whose effects are exerted early in life, perhaps before birth. More generally, it has implications for theories of causation such as the "two hit hypothesis" of Nowakowski (Lyon et al., 1989). Such a hypothesis predicts that if one "hit", or class of "hits", is constant throughout the year then any period associated with an excess of schizophrenic births should also be associated with an excess of the second "hit." More individuals will become ill and all these will show evidence of both "hits." If, however, schizophrenia can commonly result from one "hit" alone then the period of excess should be associated with an increased number of affected individuals with evidence of just one "hit." What could these hits consist of?

The "constitutional damage hypothesis" (Torrey, 1987) predicts that birth in the early months of the year is associated with an increased risk of environmentally mediated cerebral damage which predisposes to schizophrenia. If a single environmental "hit" of this type is sufficient to produce schizophrenia in a subgroup of patients, as proposed by Lewis et al. (1987), then schizophrenics with no obvious genetic predisposition should show more winter births than those at high genetic risk. Although we do not know which individuals constitute this excess, we can predict that the proportion of family history positive schizophrenics ought to be lower in the late winter and spring. However, if two "hits", environmental and genetic, are both necessary, then the proportion of family history positive individuals will remain constant throughout the year.

Kinney and Jacobson (1978) studied 34 schizophrenic adoptees and found a significant excess of low genetic risk patients born in the early months of the year. In a similarly small series, Zipursky and Schulz (1987) found winter born schizophrenics less likely to have a family history of psychosis. McNeil (1988) also reported a significant negative relationship between a family history of schizophrenia and birth in January to April among 70 schizophrenic patients. In a much larger series, Shur (1982) studied 975 schizophrenics and noted that those with schizophrenic relatives were born less often in the first quarter of the year by 29% compared to those without such relatives. More recently, Sacchetti et al. (1989) looked at morbidity risk in the relatives of 187 patients and found a risk 2.7 times smaller in the relatives of probands born in the winter and spring months compared to those born in the rest of the year.

One study has been at variance with these others, that of Baron and Gruen (1988) who reported no difference in season of birth between familial and nonfamilial schizophrenics. Indeed, when they evaluated familial morbid risk of schizophrenia, they found this to be higher in the relatives of winter and spring born schizophrenics. However, there are difficulties in making such a calculation in

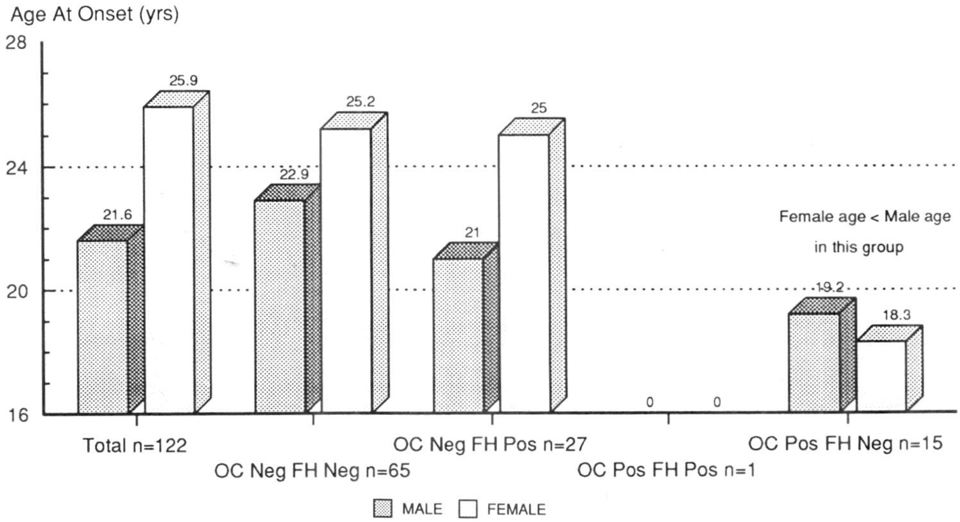

Figure 2. Age at onset by risk factors and sex.

a small series (with only 15 familial schizophrenics) where a few multiply affected families may have a profound effect on morbidity risks.

Fortunately, a more definitive study has now been carried out by O'Callaghan et al. (1990). These authors took a population of Irish schizophrenics known to have a 9% excess of births in the January-March period, and then compared the 161 familial and 185 non-familial cases; the latter were significantly more likely to be born in January-March. When compared with the control population, the non-familial schizophrenics showed a 34% excess of births in the January-March period.

Many environmental factors have been considered as instruments of the seasonal of birth effect (Torrey, 1987) but infections appear the most likely candidates at present as their incidence and neurological consequences most clearly vary with the seasons. For example, there are seasonal variations in births of individuals with congenital rubella (Peckham, 1978) and febrile convulsions (Sunderland, 1982). Watson et al. (1984) claimed that the winter birth excess of schizophrenia was greatest following those years marked by high levels of infectious diseases, particularly dyphtheria, pneumonia and influenza.

Machon et al. (1983) tested the hypothesis that schizophrenia would be more common in urban, winter-born than rural, summer-born subjects in a Danish high genetic risk sample; they assumed that viral infections are more common in urban populations. Their results indicated an interaction between place and season of birth in this singular sample, and they considered viral infection to be a possible mediator. Torrey et al. (1988) report a significant correlation between schizophrenic births and population rates of measles, varicella-zoster and polio infections in Connecticut and Massachussets. In Finland, Mednick et al. (1988) found that a significantly higher than expected number of psychiatric patients diagnosed as schizophrenic had been in the second trimester of gestation during the 1957 type A2 influenza epidemic. Further analysis indicated the sixth month of pregnancy as the period of maximum risk (LaFosse & Mednick, 1990). This epidemic was linked independently (Coffey & Jessup, 1959) to excess congenital central nervous system abnormalities. Although the results of Mednick's study are intuitively appealing, Kendell and Kemp (1989) failed to find a similar effect on rates of schizophrenia of the same epidemic in Scotland and the UK.

SEASON OF BIRTH AND STRUCTURAL BRAIN ABNORMALITIES

If the winter-birth excess of schizophrenics is a consequence of neurological damage to the developing brain, those patients forming the excess should show greater abnormalities on CT scan than other schizophrenic subjects. Once again, the difficulty is that those forming the excess cannot be identified and studied alone. Nevertheless, three studies have examined season of birth and CT scan findings.

Zipursky and Schulz (1987) examined a small series of schizophrenics and found that the mean ventriculo-brain ratio (VBR) was significantly lower in those born in the summer than those born in the four month period, either beginning or ending with December. As they point out, this result is heavily influenced by one patient with ventriculomegaly born in this month. A larger series was studied by Sacchetti et al. (1987) who compared 155 schizophrenics and 57 controls. Forty schizophrenics had VBR greater than two standard deviations above the mean for the control group; they were significantly more likely to have been born during the 5 month period December to April than in the rest of the year. Degreef et al. (1988) assessed both VBR and cortical sulcal markings in 65 chronic schizophrenics. They used yet another method of dividing the year and found significantly more prominent cortical sulci in those born between January to March compared to those born in August to October. There was also a trend for the winter-born subjects to have larger VBR.

We attempted to replicate these findings in the sample of 123 Maudsley Hospital schizophrenics described earlier and examined season of birth, VBR, cortical sulcal widening, and presence of severe obstetric complications (see Owen et al., 1988 for details of ratings). We divided the series into family history (FH) positive (n=35) and negative (n=88) individuals on the basis of a history of inpatient psychiatric care in a first degree relative. The seasons were defined as four periods of three months with winter beginning in December. This is a

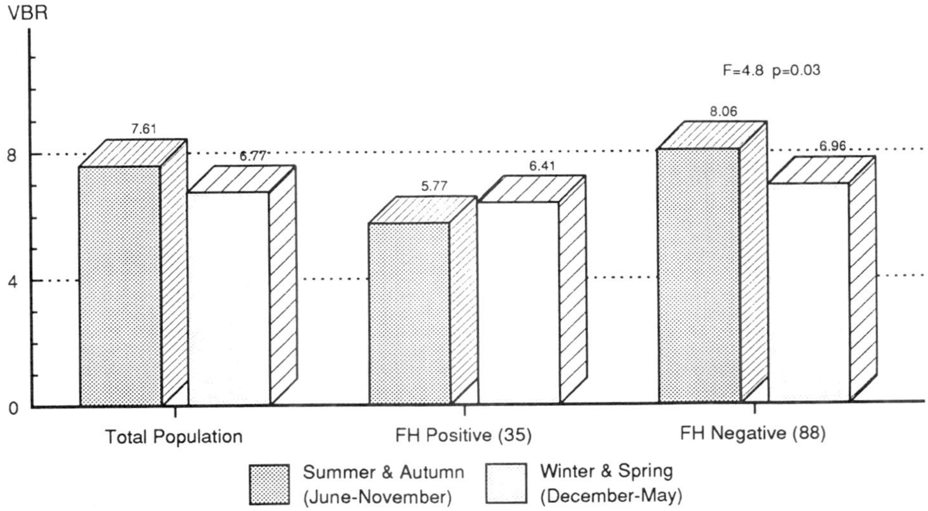

Figure 3. VBR by season of birth. Season of birth effect seen only in FH negatives.

definition which has been used in previous studies (Bradbury & Miller, 1985) and is that employed by the meteorological profession (Meteorological Office, London, personal communication). Analysis of the two periods winter-spring and summer-autumn helps to minimise the effects of cyclic trends. The series as a whole showed no significant seasonality, 67 being born in the winter and spring (p=0.08 n.s.); 24 FH positive and 43 FH negative subjects were born in this period.

Family history positive individuals showed no season of birth effect on CT measures. However, in the 88 family history negative individuals, there was a significant not only for VBR (Figure 3), but also for cortical sulcal ratings (Figure 4) and severe obstetric complications (Figure 5). Contrary to our expectations, it was those low genetic risk subjects born in the summer and autumm who experienced the excess of obstetric complications and who in adult life had high VBR and high scores of cortical sulcal markings on their CT scans. Such seasonality was not observed in the group with a positive family history.

The most likely reason for the odd findings is that our patients as a whole showed no significant seasonality. This is consistent with other evidence (A. MacDonald, unpublished observations) that Maudsley Hospital schizophrenics no longer show a season of birth effect. This may be because many Maudsley patients -- approximately one quarter of our sample -- are of Afro-Carribean origin, and thus born in a region without marked seasonal variation in temperature.

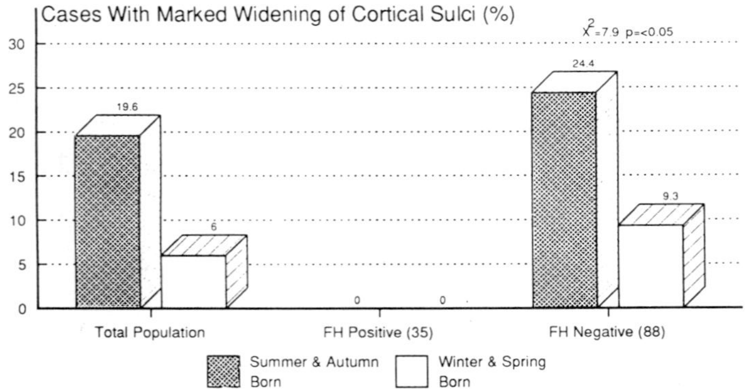

Figure 4. Marked widening of cortical suici occurred only in FH negatives and appears seasonal.

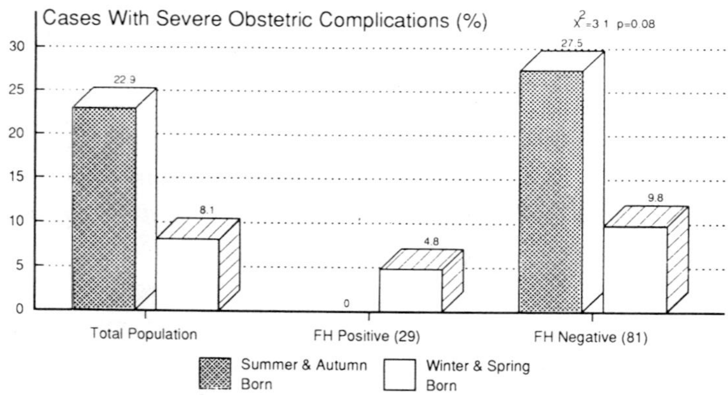

Figure 5. Obstetric complications tended to occur seasonally and almost exclusively in FH negative.

POSSIBLE MECHANISMS OF A DEVELOPMENTAL LESION

We have argued that some of the features of schizophrenia originally thought of as chronological curiosities in fact presaged the conclusions from recent direct studies of the brains of schizophrenics, namely, that an early developmental brain lesion underlies the neuropathology of the illness (Jacob & Beckman, 1986; Falkai & Bogerts, 1986; Roberts et al., 1987). It is most unlikely that the factors suggested by consideration of each epiphenomenon are of equal importance in all people with schizophrenia, which is, of course, characterised by its clinical heterogeneity. Perhaps there are different routes to the neurobiological predisposition to the disorder. How might diverse early influences such as mutant genes, viral infection, hypoxia and head trauma lead to similar psychological sequelae decades later?

A possible explanation has been provided by new ideas on the way in which the brain responds to developmental aberrations or injury. Even in adults, sprouting from transected axons can result in new connections, and axons in areas adjacent to necrosis can produce collateral sprouts which terminate on the vacated synaptic sites. The immature brain has greater powers of regeneration in such situations than the mature brain, and this process may produce synaptic misconnections (Schneider, 1979; Janowsky & Findlay, 1986). When the brain is already rendered abnormal, whether for genetic or environmental reasons, before the developing axons have reached their normal targets, then some of those axons will proceed to alternative destinations instead. Furthermore, the fetal brain consists of a large excess of neurons with very many interconnections not found in the normal adult brain. These "exuberant" connections are lost during normal development due to three types of regressive process (i) many brain and spinal cord neurons die in the course of development (Cowan et al., 1984; Land-messer & Pilar, 1974) and both (ii) axon collaterals (O'Leary & Stanfield, 1985) and (iii) synaptic or dendritic arborizations are "pruned" (Wiesel, 1982). This complex process is almost certainly determined by both genetic (Nowakowski, 1987) and environmental influences (Greenough et al., 1987). Aberrant genes or early brain damage could attenuate these regressive processes causing immature patterns of cells and their projections to persist, thus leading to abnormal functioning in an otherwise mature nervous system. Perhaps this represents the mechanisms whereby diverse abnormal influences on the developing brain result in a vulnerability to later psychosis.

To our knowledge the first person to suggest that such early anomalous neuronal connections play a role in schizophrenia was Randall (1983) who wrote, "input that would usually be destined for a particular neural substrate would become relayed by abnormally connected fibres into another area with which the integration of function did not normally occur. Since the recipient neural substrate would not usually receive and synthesize the input that would be connected in such a manner, the output result from the different area would appear as an aberrant and extraneous variation in the function it subserves." In addition to generating aberrant responses, misconnections could also reduce general cognitive efficiency (Goodman, 1989) as regions of the brain not normally connected would exchange irrelevant information or "noise." Such a poor signal to "noise" ratio could plausibly contribute to inattention and the impairments in problem-solving ability which are seen in schizophrenia. Randall's hypothesis implies that the brain is a hard-wired apparatus acting rather like a telephone exchange. The reality is almost certainly more complex with minor misconnec-tions leading to a cascade of developmental and functional errors as the ensuing receptor, neurotransmitter and neuromodulator anomalies amplify the original faults.

Further support for the importance of misconnections comes from studies of epiletic patients who have undergone temporal lobectomy (Taylor, 1975). Of epiletics with temporal lobe "hamartomas," 23% had concurrent psychosis compared to only 5% of those with mesial temporal sclerosis. Taylor believed that the reason for the difference was the greater likelihood of the epilepsy secondary to hamartomas beginning in adolescence, a period of vulnerability to psychosis. However, Goodman (1989a,b) considers that it is the time of origin of the lesion that is crucial. Hamartomas represent a type of "architectural folly" that appears in some instances to be an exaggerated form of the developmental abnormalities described earlier; the ganglioglial type contains wildly abnormal nerve cells (Taylor, 1975). These structures arise very early in development and are already present when axonal connections are first forming and throughout the phase of selective axonal loss. By contrast, mesial temporal sclerosis occurs significantly later in brain development, almost certainly post-dating the phase when axonal connections first form. Goodman argues that hamartomas may be more likely than mesial temporal sclerosis to initiate widespread misconnections within the limbic system or perhaps to be manifestations of some basic developmental abnormality also causing misconnections. Evidence for this notion is provided by both Bruton (1988) and Stevens (1988) who have shown that the removal of hamartomas by temporal lobectomy may actually induce psychosis, perhaps as a consequence of leaving similar aberrant lesions in the remaining temporal lobe, or alternatively through terminal regeneration and aberrant sprouting in projection sites.

Associations between schizophrenia and other conditions also imply some common abnormality of neurodevelopment. Thus, neuroradiological case studies of schizophrenic patients have reported associations between the disorder and aqueduct stenosis (Reveley & Reveley, 1983), porencephalic and arachnoid cysts (Blackshaw & Bowen, 1987), cavities of the septum pellucidum (Lewis & Mezey, 1985) and agenesis of the corpus callosum (Lewis et al., 1989; Andreasen, 1988). These associations have generally been interpreted in terms of a straightforward, neuropsychological structure-function relationship. However, they may be related by some underlying neurodevelopmental abnormality, the radiological signs merely being markers of this defect. Barth (1987) has pointed out that the abnormalities of the corpus callosum and septum pellucidum are manifestations of defective neuronal migration and are usually accompanied by pervasive neuronal abnormalities. A similar situation of widespread disarray has been demonstrated in mice with genetically determined neuronal migration disorders (Nowakowski, 1987) and may occur in autism where cerebellar and temporal lobe abnormalities have been reported in radiological studies (Jones & Kerwin, 1990). The heterotopic neurones noted in neuropathological studies of schizophrenic brains have been explained in terms of abnormalities of neurone migration (Jacob & Beckman, 1986). However, it is possible that the primary defect may not even be in the neurone but rather in the glial cells which play a vital role in orchestrating early brain development (Rakic, 1971). For instance, formation of the corpus callosum is dependent upon the pre-existence of a transitory glial "sling" between the primitive hemispheres (Silver et al., 1982).

One would anticipate that any such neurodevelopmental damage would manifest itself in some way in childhood long before the onset of positive symptoms of psychosis. Indeed, both Bleuler (1911; Trans. 1950) and Kraepelin (1919, Trans. 1971) emphasised the frequency of premorbid behavioural abnormalities in schizophrenia. More recent objective studies confirm these early observations (Parnas & Jorgensen, 1989; Foerster et al., 1990). We have suggested elsewhere (Murray et al., 1988) that neural dysplasia consequent on mutant genes or early brain insult is one route to the so-called type II syndrome of schizophrenia (Crow, 1980) with premorbid cognitive deficits and abnormal personality, as well as the negative symptoms and soft neurological signs which augur a poor prognosis. The explanation for the delayed onset of positive psychotic phenomena in the type I syndrome is as yet unclear. However, these may be expressed when a brain containing the early anomalous connections undergoes the normal maturational changes of adolescence and young adulthood.

CONCLUSIONS

Consideration of some of the puzzling chronological epiphenomena of schizophrenia reveals that several of them are explicable in terms of a neurodevelopmental origin for the condition, a conclusion which is echoed by the results of recent neuroimaging and post mortem studies of schizophrenic patients. It is our contention that schizophrenia is aetiologically heterogeneous and that the type which most closely approximates to Kraepelin's original concept of dementia praecox is a result of deviant development of the brain in fetal or neonatal life. This neuronal dysplasia may result from either mutant gene(s) and/or adverse fetal and neonatal circumstances and produces many of the negative signs of schizophrenia in childhood, thus antedating the positive syndrome by many years. Thus, we believe poor outcome schizophrenia to be congenital in origin.

REFERENCES

Achte, K.A., Hillbrom, E. & Aalberg, V. (1969) Psychosis following war brain injuries. Acta Psychiat. Scand., 45, 1-18.

Amato, M., Howald, H., Von Muralt, G. (1987) Fetal sex distribution of peri-intraventricular haemorrhage in preterm infants. Eur. Neurol., 27(1), 20-23.

Andreasen, N. (1988) Paper presented at the 4th Biennial Winter Workshop on Schizophrenia, Badgastein.

Aylward, E., Walker, E. & Bettes, B. (1984) Intelligence in schizophrenia. Schiz. Bull., 10, 430-459.

Baron, M. & Gruen, R. (1988) Risk factors in schizophrenia: Season of birth and family history. Brit. J. Psychiat., 152, 460-465.

Barth, P.G. (1987) Disorders of neuronal migration. Can. J. Neurol. Sci., 14, 1.

Blackshaw, S. & Bowen, R.C. (1987) A case of atypical psychosis associated with alexithymia and a left fronto-temporal lesion. Can. J. Psychiat., 32, 688-692.

Bleuler, E. (1950) Dementia Praecox or the Group of Schizophrenias. New York. I.U.P.

Bradbury, T.N. & Miller, A. (1985) Season of birth in schizophrenia. Psychol. Bull., 98, 569-594.

Bruton, C. (1988) A Neuropathological Study of Temporal Lobe Epilepsy. Maudsley Monograph, O.U.P.

Castle, D., & Murray, R.M. (1990) The neurodevelopmental basis of sex differences in schizophrenia. Psychol. Med. (submitted).

Coffey, V.P. & Jessop, W.J.E. (1959) Maternal influenza and congenital deformities: A prospective study. Lancet, ii, 935-938.

Cowan, L.M., Fawcett, J.W., O'Leary, D.D. & Stanfield, B.B. (1984) Regressive events in neurogenesis. Science, 225, 1258-1265.

Critchton-Browne, J. (1862) Psychical diseases of early life. J. Mental Science, 6, 284-320.

Crow, T.J. (1980) Molecular pathology of schizophrenia: More than one disease process? Brit. Med. J., 280, 66-8.

Davison, K. & Bagley, C.R. (1969) Schizophrenia-like Psychoses Associated with Organic Disorder of the CNS. R.N. Herrington (Ed.) Current Problems in Neuropsychiatry. Headley, Kent.

Degreef, G., Mukherjee, S., Bilder, R. & Schnur, D. (1988) Season of birth and CT scan findings in schizophrenic patients. Biol. Psychiat., 24, 461-464.

Falkai, P. & Bogerts B. (1986) Cell loss in the hippocampus of schizophrenics. Eur. Arch. Psychiat. Neurol. Sci., 236, 154-161.

Feuchtwanger, E. & Maver-Gross, W. (1938) Hirnverletzung und Schizophrenie. Schweizer Archiv fur Neurologie und Psychiatrie, 41, 17-99.

Flor-Henry, P. (1978) Gender, hemispheric specialisation and psychopathology, Soc. Sci. & Med., 12b, 155.

Foerster, A., Lewis, S.W., Owen, M.J. & Murray, R.M. (1990) Premorbid adjustment and personality in psychosis: Effects of sex and diagnosis. Brit. J. Psychiat (in press).

Goodman, R. (1988) Are complications of pregnancy and birth causes of schizophrenia? Dev. Med. Child Neurol., 30, 391-406.

Goodman, R. (1989a) Neuronal misconnections and psychiatric disorder. Is there a link? Brit. J. Psychiat., 154, 292-299.

Goodman, R. (1989b) Limits to Cerebral Plasticity. In: Johnson, D.A., Utley, D., Wyke, M. (Eds.) Children's Head Injury: Who Cares? Falmer, Basingstoke.

Green, M.F., Satz, P., Soper, H.V. & Kharabi, F. (1987) Relationship between physical anomalies and age at onset of schizophrenia. Amer. J. Psychiat., 144, 666-667.

Greenough, W.T., Black, J.E., Wallace, C.S. (1987) Experience and brain development. Child Dev., 58, 539-559.

Guy, J.D., Majorski, L.V., Wallace, C.J. & Guy, M.P. (1983) The incidence of minor physical anomalies in adult male schizophrenics. Schiz. Bull., 9, 571.

Hafner, H., Reicher, A., Maurer, K., Loffler, W., Munk-Jorgensen, P. & Stromgren, E. (1989) How does gender influence age at first hospitalisation for schizophrenia? A transnational case register study. Psychol. Med., 19, 903-918.

Jacob, H. & Beckman, H. (1986) Prenatal development disturbances in the limbic allocortex in schizophrenics. J. Neural. Transmiss., 65, 303-326.

Janowsky, R.T. (1972) Effects of viral infection on the developing nervous system. N. Eng. J. Med., 287, 599-604.

Janowsky, J.S. & Findlay, B.L. (1986) The outcome of perinatal brain damage. Devel. Med. Child Neurol., 28, 375-389.

Jones, P.B. & Kerwin, R.W. (1990) Left temporal lobe damage in Asperger's syndrome. Brit. J. Psychiat., 136, 570-572.

Kendell, R.E. & Kemp, I.W. (1989) Maternal influenza in the etiology of schizophrenia. Arch. Gen. Psych., 46, 878-882.

Kinney, D.K. & Jacobsen, B. (1978) Environmental Factors in Schizophrenia. Wynne, L.C., Cromwell, R.L. & Matthysse, S. (Eds.) The Nature of Schizophrenia. p.38-51. Wiley, New York.

Kokes, R., Strauss, J.S. & Klorman, R. (1977) Measuring premorbid adjustment. Schiz. Bull., 3, 186.

Kraepelin, E. (1971) Dementia Praecox and Paraphrenia. New York, Robert E. Krieger Publishing Corporation.

Kringlen, E. (1967) Heredity and Environment in the Functional Psychoses. London, William Heinemann.

Kringlen, E. (1987) Contributions of Genetic Studies on Schizophrenia. Hafner, H., Gattaz, W. & Janzarik, W. (Eds.) The Search for the Causes of Schizophrenia, p.123. Springer-Verlag, Berlin.

LaFosse, J.M. & Mednick, S.A. (1990) This volume.

Lancet, (1989) Editorial: Cerebral palsy, intrapartum care and a shot in the foot. Lancet, ii, 1251-1252.

Landmesser, L. & Pilar, G. (1974) Synaptic transmission and cell death during normal ganglionic development. J. Physiol., 241, 737-749.

Lewine, R. (1981) Sex differences in schizophrenia. Psychol. Bull, 90, 432.

Lewine, R., Burbach, D. & Meltzer, H. (1984) Effects of diagnostic criteria on the ratio of male to female schizophrenic patients. Am. J. Psychiat., 141, 84.

Lewis, S.W. & Mezey, G.C. (1985) Clinical correlates of septum pellucidum cavities. Psychol. Med., 15, 43.

Lewis, S.W., Chitkara, B., Reveley, A.M. & Murray, R.M. (1987) Family history and birthweight in MZ twins concordant and discordant for psychosis. Acta Genet. Med. Gemellol., 36, 267.

Lewis, S.W., Reveley, M.A., David, A.S. & Ron, M.A. (1989) Agenesis of the corpus callosum and schizophrenia: A case report. Psychol. Med., 18, 341-347.

Lewis, M.S. (1989) Age incidence and schizophrenia, Parts I and II. Schiz. Bull., 15, 1, 59-80.

Lewis, M.S. (1990) Res ipsa Laquitor: The author replies. Schiz. Bull., 16(1), 17-28.

Loranger, A.W. (1984) Sex differences in age of onset of schizophrenia. Arch. Gen. Psychiat., 41, 157.

Lyon, M., Barr, C.E., Cannon, T.D., Mednick, S.A. & Shore, D. (1989) Fetal neural development and schizophrenia. Schiz. Bull., 15(1), 149-161.

Machon, R.A., Mednick, S.A. & Schulsinger, F. (1983) The interaction, seasonality, place of birth, genetic risk and subsequent schizophrenia in a high risk sample. Brit. J. Psychiat., 143, 383-388.

McNeill, T.F. (1987) Perinatal influences in the development of schizophrenia. In: Biological Perspectives of Schizophrenia. Helmechen & Henn (Eds.), pp. 125-138. John Wiley & Sons, Ltd.

McNeill, T.F. (1988) Paper presented at the 4th Biennial Winter Workshop of Schizophrenia, Badgastein.

McNeill, T.F. & Kaij, L. (1978) Obstetric Factors in the Development of Schizophrenia. Wynne, L.C., Cromwell, R.L. & Matthysse, S. (Eds.) The Nature of Schizophrenia. p. 401, Wiley, New York.

Mednick, S.A., Machon, R.A., Huttenen, M.O. & Bonnett, D. (1988) Adult schizophrenia following prenatal exposure to an influenza epidemic. Arch. Gen. Psychiat., 45, 189-192.

Mosher, L.R., Pollin, W. & Stabenau, J.R. (1971) Identical twins discordant for schizophrenia. Arch. Gen. Psychiat., 24, 422.

Murray, R.M., Lewis, S.W. & Reveley, A.M. (1985) Towards an aetiological classification of schizophrenia. Lancet, i, 1023.

Murray, R.M. & Lewis, S.W. (1987) Is schizophrenia a neurodevelopmental disorder? Brit. Med. J., 295, 681-682.

Murray, R.M., Lewis, S.W., Owen, M.J., & Foerster, A. (1988) The Neurodevelopmental Origins of Dementia Praecox. In: McGuffin, P. & Bebbington, P. (Eds.) Schizophrenia: The Major Issues. Heinemann, London.

Nelson, K.B. & Ellenberg, J.H. (1986) Antecedents of cerebral palsy: Multivariate analysis of risk. New Engl. J. Med., 315, 81-86.

Nowakowski, R.S. (1987) Basic concepts of CNS development. Child Devel., 58, 568-595.

O'Callaghan, E., Larkin, C. & Waddington, J. (1988) Clinical correlates of obstetric complications in schizophrenia. Schiz. Res., 1, 125.

O'Callaghan, E., Gibson, R., Colohon, H., Walshe, D., Buckley, P.,Larkin, C. & Waddington, J.L. (1990) Season of birth effect in schizophrenia: Environmental damage or genetic morphism? Paper presented to the 5th Biennial Workshop on Schizophrenia, Badgastein.

O'Leary, D.D. & Stanfield, B.B. (1985) Occipital cortical neurons with transient pyramidal tract axons extend and maintain collaterals to subcortical but not intracortical targets. Brain Res., 336, 326-333.

Owen, M.J., Lewis, S.W. & Murray, R.M. (1988) Obstetric complications and schizophrenia: A computed tomographic study. Psychol. Med., 18, 331-339.

Owen, M.J., Lewis, S.W., & Murray, R.M. (1989) Family history and cerebral ventricular enlargement in schizophrenia: A case control study. Brit. J. Psychiat., 154, 629-634.

Parnas, J. & Jorgensen, A. (1989) Pre-morbid psychopathology in schizophrenia spectrum. Brit. J. Psychiat., 155, 623-627.

Pearlson, G.D., Kim, W.S., Kubos, K.L., Moberg, P.J., Jayaram, G., Bascom, M.J., Chase, G.A., Goldfinger, A.D., & Tune, L.E. (1989) Ventricle-brain ratio, computed tomographic density and brain area in 50 schizophrenics. Arch. Gen. Psychiat., 46, 690-697.

Peckham, C.S. (1978) Congenital rubella surveillance. J. Roy. Coll. Physicians, 12, 250-255.

Pollack, M., Levenstein, S. & Klein, D.F. (1968) A three year post-hospital follow up of adolescent and adult schizophrenics. Am. J. Orthopsychiat., 38, 94.

Randall, P.L. (1983) Schizophrenia, abnormal connection and brain evolution. Med. Hyothesis, 10, 247-280.

Rakic, P. (1971) Neuron-glia relationship during granule cell migration in developing cerebellar cortex: A Golgi and electron microscopic study in macacus rhesus. J. Comp. Neurol., 141, 283-312.

Reveley, A.M., & Reveley, M.A. (1983) Aqueduct stenosis and schizophrenia. J. Neurol. Neursurg. Psychiat., 46, 18.

Roberts, G.W., Colter, N., Lofthouse, R., Johnstone, E.C., Crow, T.J. (1987) Is there gliosis in schizophrenia? Investigation in the temporal lobe. Biol. Psychiat., 22, 1459-1468.

Rosanoff, A., Handy, L., Plesset, I. & Brusch, S. (1934) The etiology of so-called schizophrenic psychoses. Amer. J. Psychiat., 91, 247.

Rosenthal, D. (1962) Familial concordance by sex with respect to schizophrenia. Psychol. Bull., 59, 401.

Rosenthal, D. (1971) Genetics of Psychopathology. McGraw-Hill: New York.

Sacchetti, E., Vita, A., Battaglia, M., Calzeroni, A., Conte, T., Invernizzi, G. & Cazullo, C.L. (1987) Season of Birth and Cerebral Ventricular Enlargement in Schizophrenia. In: Cazullo et al. (eds.), Etiopathogenetic Hypothesis of Schizophrenia. MTP Press: Lancaster.

Sacchetti, E., Vita, A., Giobbio, G.M. (1989) Risk factors in schizophrenia. Brit. J. Psychiat., 155, 266-267.

Schulsinger, F., Mednick, S.A., Walker, E.F., Cudeck, R. & Moffitt, T. (1980) Biosocial implications growing from high-risk research. Acta Psychiat. Scand. Suppl., 285, 62, 112.

Schneider, G.E. (1979) Is it really better to have your brain lesioned early? A revision of the "Kennard Principle". Neuropsychologica, 17, 557-583.

Seeman, M.V. (1982) Gender differences in schizophrenia. Can. J. Psychiat., 27, 107.

Shur, E. (1982) Season of birth in high and low genetic risk schizophrenics. Brit. J. Psychiat., 140, 410.

Silver, J., Lorenz, S., Wahlsten, S. & Coughlin, J. (1982) Axonal guidance during development of the great cerebral commisures, descriptive and experimental studies, in vivo, on the role of preformed glial pathways. J. Comp. Neurol., 210, 10-29.

Stevens, J. (1982) Neuropathology of schizophrenia. Arch. Gen. Psychiat., 39, 1131-1139.

Stevens, J. (1988) Paper presented at the 4th Biennial Winter Workshop on Schizophrenia, Badgastein.

Sunderland, R., Carpenter, R.G. & Gardner, A. (1982) Are all born equal? Brit. Med. J., 284, 624.

Taylor, D.C. (1975) Factors influencing the occurrence of schizophrenia-like psychosis in patients with TLE. Psychol. Med., 5, 249-254.

Tennent, T. (1937) Discussion on mental disorder following head injury. Proceedings of the Royal Society of Medicine, 30, 1092-1093.

Torrey, E.F. (1987) Hypotheses on the seasonality of schizophrenic births. In: Etiopathogenic Hypotheses of Schizophrenia. pp. 41-48. Lancaster: MTP Press Ltd.

Torrey, E.F., Rawlings, R. & Waldman, I.N. (1988) Schizophrenic births and viral diseases in two states. Schiz. Res., 1, 73-77.

Tramer, T. (1929) Uber die biologische Bedeutung des Geburtesmonnates fur die Psychogerkrankung. Schweizer. Archiv fur Neurologie und Psychiatrie, 24, 17-24.

Turner, S.W., Toone, B.K. & Brett-Jones, J.R. (1986) Computerised tomographic scan changes in early schizophrenia - preliminary findings. Psychol. Med., 16, 219-225.

Watson, C.G., Kucala, T., Tilleskjor, C. & Jacobs, L. (1984) Schizophrenic birth seasonality in relation to the incidence of infectious diseases. Arch. Gen. Psychiat., 41, 85-90.

Weinberger, D.R. (1987) Implications of normal brain development for the pathogenesis of schizophrenia. Arch. Gen. Psychiat., 44, 660-669.

Wiesel, T.N. (1982) Postnatal development of the visual cortex and the influence of environment. Nature, 299, 583-591.

Wilcox, J.A. & Nasrallah, H.A. (1987) Childhood head trauma and psychosis. Psychiat. Res., 21, 303.

A NEURODEVELOPMENTAL APPROACH TO SCHIZOPHRENIA RESEARCH

Jose M. LaFosse and Sarnoff A. Mednick

Center for Longitudinal Studies
Social Science Research Institute
University of Southern California
Los Angeles, California

INTRODUCTION

Emil Kraepelin and, to a lesser extent, Eugen Bleuler both considered that a disease of the frontal lobes may be responsible for the clinical manifestation of schizophrenia (Kraepelin, 1919; Bleuler, 1911, trans. 1950). At the time of these formulations in the early part of this century, however, researchers did not have the technological capability to pursue this line of investigation. Perhaps as a result, those looking for the cause of schizophrenia turned their attention to a host of environmental factors presumed to be important for the onset of schizophrenia (Fromm-Reichmann, 1948; Bateson et al., 1956). Although these investigations have in some cases enlightened us to the impact of family variables (Brown et al., 1986; Leff, 1976), they have for the most part not proven sufficient to explain the development of the disorder.

With the advent of modern technologies that allow in vivo examination of the schizophrenic brain reliably and non-invasively, researchers have turned back to the brain in search of the neural substrate proposed when the disorder of schizophrenia was first systematically described. In the fifteen years since the first computed tomography (CT) study found that schizophrenics showed enlarged ventricles relative to age-matched normal controls (Johnstone et al., 1976), and after many additional CT and magnetic resonance imaging (MRI) studies (see Raz & Raz, 1990; Cannon, 1991 for recent reviews), there is widespread support for the hypothesis than an important part of the etiology of schizophrenia involves structural and/or functional brain deficits.

The continual development and refinement of neuroimaging technologies has

Developmental Neuropathology of Schizophrenia
Edited by S.A. Mednick *et al.*, Plenum Press, New York, 1991

allowed us to ascertain with increasing precision the nature of the brain anomalies found in schizophrenics. CT findings of ventricular enlargement and sulcal widening, while interesting and robust (Shelton & Weinberger, 1986), only indicated that there was a pathogenic process occurring somewhere in the brain. MRI studies have provided evidence of more specific structural abnormalities (Suddath et al., 1989, 1990; Rossi et al., 1990; Bogerts et al., 1990). Cerebral blood flow and positron emission tomography (PET) studies have also contributed to our understanding of functional brain deficits (Buchsbaum and Haier, 1987). While neuroimaging studies do not directly address the issue of the time at which these deficits appeared, there is a growing belief that at least some of the deficits may have a perinatal or prenatal origin.

To our knowledge the notion that perinatal factors may be important in schizophrenia received its first empirical support over 50 years ago when Katz (1939) found that schizophrenics suffered significantly more obstetric complications than normal controls. Perinatal factors have continued to play an important role in etiological formulations of schizophrenia (Mednick, 1970; see Dykes et al., this volume). Prenatal origins of brain abnormalities associated with schizophrenia have recently started to be thought of in terms of neurodevelopmental disturbances (Weinberger, 1987; Lewis and Murray, 1987). This new trend represents a refinement of the old idea that schizophrenia involves a disease process in the brain. The neurodevelopmental hypothesis gained real momentum after the influenza epidemic study in Helsinki (Mednick et al., 1988). The rest of this chapter will briefly review the details of that study, then highlight further evidence that implicates a disturbance in fetal neural development in the later onset of adult schizophrenia.

THE HELSINKI STUDY

From October 8 to November 14, 1957, the citizens of Helsinki experienced a severe type A2 influenza epidemic. Previous research led Mednick and colleagues to hypothesize that those exposed to the virus during their second or third trimester of fetal gestation would have an increased risk for developing schizophrenia as adults (Mednick et al., 1988). The index cohort was made up of children born in Helsinki from November 15, 1957 to August 14, 1958 who had been admitted as inpatients to one or more of eight area psychiatric hospitals before the age of 26 years. Results of this study demonstrated that those exposed during the second trimester had a significantly higher rate of schizophrenia admissions than control subjects and those exposed during the first or third trimester. Although this effect was strongest for the sixth month of gestation, the schizophrenic sample was not sufficiently large to conduct an adequate statistical test of this more limited time period. The second-trimester effect was also seen in higher rates of schizophrenia per 1000 Helsinki live births. No such second-trimester effect was seen for any other diagnosis. These results held independently for males and females and for the eight psychiatric hospitals in greater Helsinki.

Mednick and collaborators proposed that the type of environmental stress may not be as critical in determining the risk for schizophrenia as the timing of the stress. In other words, there is something critical about the process of fetal neural development during the second trimester of gestation that, when subjected to severe environmental stress, increases the risk for schizophrenia. Stressors such as viral infections may interfere with the generation of late-developing cortical neurons, destroy already existing neurons, and/or disrupt the migration of young postmitotic neurons from the ventricular zone in which they proliferate to cortical areas, all of which can occur during the second trimester.

Although provocative, the Helsinki study had a number of limitations including a relatively small sample of diagnosed schizophrenics, the emphasis on a single epidemic in only one city, and a lack of explicit controls for climate-related variables. Barr and coworkers (1990) overcame these limitations in a much larger study conducted in Denmark that aimed to replicate the Helsinki findings.

THE DANISH STUDY

The original Helsinki study was extended in the following four ways: 1) A different country (Denmark) was used; 2) The study examined an entire national population of hospitalized schizophrenics; 3) The effects of influenza epidemics were evaluated over a 40 year period; 4) The potential confounding effect of climatic variables was evaluated. The number of live births, of births of future schizophrenics, and of cases of influenza reported to the Ministry of Health in Denmark was obtained by month from 1911 to 1950. Results of this study indicated that influenza rates higher than seasonally expected, occurring in the sixth month of gestation, were associated with a greater number of schizophrenic births than seasonally expected (Barr et al., 1990). This association was not attributable to a winter-related third factor or to climatic variables.

FURTHER VIRAL STUDIES

A successful replication of the Mednick et al. Helsinki (1988) findings has recently been reported by O'Callaghan and colleagues (1991). This replication study examined the effects of the 1957 type A2 influenza epidemic in England and Wales on subsequent schizophrenia. The results demonstrated that those exposed to the epidemic during their fifth month of gestation had an 88% increase in risk for schizophrenia relative to those born during the same period from four non-epidemic control years. The apparent one month discrepancy between the Mednick et al.

(1988) and O'Callaghan et al. (1991) critical month of gestation (6th vs. 5th respectively) may in large part be attributed to slightly different methods of calculating the month of gestation during which the fetus was exposed to the influenza epidemic. When the Helsinki study method is employed for the UK data, it seems very likely that the critical month is actually the sixth month of gestation (LaFosse & Mednick, 1991).

Murray and his associates have recently completed a replication of the Danish findings in a study of the effects of influenza epidemics between 1939-1960 on later schizophrenia in England and Wales (personal communication, June 1991). They have found a strong association between adult schizophrenia diagnoses and exposure to influenza epidemics between the fifth and seventh month of fetal development, centering on the sixth month. In a different study, Torrey and coworkers (1988) failed to find an association between prenatal viral exposure and later schizophrenia (Torrey et al., 1988). Barr et al. (1990) have suggested that this failure to replicate may be due to methodological problems. Kendell and Kemp (1989) found an association between exposure to the 1957 influenza epidemic during the 6th month of gestation and increased schizophrenia in the city of Edinburgh. They also reported an absence of this relationship when examining data for all of Scotland. Mednick et al. (1990), in a reanalysis of the Kendell and Kemp data, have pointed out that a significant second trimester effect does appear in the Scotland data.

SIGNIFICANCE OF THE VIRAL STUDIES

The importance of neuronal migration in the second trimester and its possible relationship to schizophrenia has been articulated by Mednick and his collaborators (Mednick et al., 1988). They have suggested three possibilities that may account for disturbances of fetal neural development: 1) genetic predisposition; 2) pathogenic environmental factors during a critical period of development (which may simply mimic the genetic effect); 3) the interaction of these two factors.

A recent study explored the question of whether exposure to diseases other than influenza during the second trimester would lead to an increased risk for schizophrenia (Barr et al., 1991). The number of live births, births of future schizophrenics, and the number of cases of 25 diseases including influenza reported to the Ministry of Health in Denmark was obtained by month from 1911 to 1950. The relationship between fetal exposure to each of these 29 diseases and adult schizophrenia was examined. The results demonstrated an association between high levels of influenza, especially during the sixth month of gestation, and high rates of schizophrenic births. No such association was found for any other disease or combination of diseases. The results of this study suggest that there may be an influenza-specific pathogen which increases the risk of schizophrenia.

A number of mechanisms have been proposed to explain this relationship (DeLisi & Crow, 1986; Torrey, 1991). For example, Conrad and Scheibel (1987) hypothesize that a specific protein on the jacket of the influenza virus interferes with the adhesive behavior of migrating neurons. Although there is growing evidence that influenza may be a unique schizophrenogenic agent, it is difficult to ascertain whether it is mimicking a more prevalent genetic effect or exerting a unique environmental effect. It is important to note, however, that there seems to be something critical about the sixth month of gestation that is specifically involved with the etiology of schizophrenia. This period is marked by three important developmental events that may be related to neuropathological findings reported in many schizophrenics: neuronal migration, an increase in the risk of hemorrhage due to the dissolution of the germinal matrix, and an explosive increase in brain growth.

NEUROPATHOLOGICAL EVIDENCE FOR THE NEURODEVELOPMENTAL HYPOTHESIS

A number of post-mortem studies have reported neuropathological alterations in the brains of schizophrenics that are consistent with a neurodevelopmental disturbance. These anomalies include reduced temporolimbic and thalamic structure volumes and nerve cell numbers, cytoarchitectural anomalies in the hippocampal formation, frontal cortex, cingulate gyrus, and entorhinal cortex, and left lateralized temporal horn enlargement (for discussion and references, see Bogerts & Falkai, this volume). The neurodevelopmental disturbance most often posited by the authors of these studies involves neuronal migration.

Gliosis, which refers to greater densities or absolute numbers of reactive glial cells, is indicative of a progressive degenerative or inflammatory brain disease. Evidence of gliosis is associated with pathological events that occur only after birth (Larroche, 1984). Six controlled quantitative studies failed to find evidence of gliosis (Falkai & Bogerts, 1986; Roberts et al., 1986, 1987; Benes, 1987; Falkai et al., 1988; Stevens, 1988). The lack of gliosis in these studies strongly supports the hypothesis that structural changes occur in the brain during fetal development.

It is interesting to note that most post-mortem studies which have focused on medial temporal lobe structures (ie, hippocampal formation including the dentate gyrus, parahippocampal gyrus including part of the entorhinal cortex, amygdala) and the cingulate gyrus found structural abnormalities in one or more of these limbic areas among schizophrenics. Although similar findings have been reported in other regions such as the diencephalic periventricular grey matter (Lesch & Bogerts, 1984), globus pallidus (Stevens, 1982; Bogerts et al., 1985), corpus callosum (Nasrallah, 1983, Bigelow, 1983), prefrontal cortex (Benes, 1986), and catecholaminergic brainstem systems (Bogerts et al., 1983; Lohr & Jeste, 1988), limbic system pathology is a robust finding in the brains of schizophrenics. This suggests that MRI findings of limbic pathology might be interpretable as indications of a disruption occurring during fetal development. A number of investigators have recently reported MRI evidence of temporal lobe and hippocampal abnormalities (DeLisi et al, 1988a, 1988b; Johnstone et al., 1989; Rossi et al., 1989; Bogerts et al., 1990; Rossi et al., 1990; Suddath et al., 1990; Dauphinais et al., 1990), with many of them attributing their findings to a neurodevelopmental disturbance.

Also of interest are the increasing indications that structural abnormalities of the limbic structures are more common in anterior and middle regions. Kovelman and Scheibel (1984) reported alterations of pyramidal cell orientation in anterior and middle hippocampal regions. Bogerts and colleagues (1985) found tissue loss restricted to the anterior hippocampus. Falkai and Bogerts (1991) reported more heterotopic clusters in the anterior entorhinal cortex. These findings are of note since the anterior regions of these areas develop in the latter part of fetal development (Carpenter & Sutin, 1983), possibly near the end of the second trimester.

THE POSSIBLE CLINICAL SIGNIFICANCE OF NEUROPATHOLOGICAL FINDINGS

As indicated above, most findings of cytoarchitectonic anomalies in limbic structures are not believed to be the result of a progressive degenerative process. Rather, they are suggestive of a disturbance that occurred during early brain development. How might these brain abnormalities be related to the clinical presentation of schizophrenia? Bogerts (1991) has described a model of information processing that may explain how limbic anomalies are associated with schizophrenic symptoms. Visual, auditory, and somatosensory information is sent from the sensory organs to unimodal association areas surrounding the primary sensory cortical areas via a number of sensory pathways. After initial analysis in the unimodal association cortex, sensory information is transferred to polymodal association areas where it is integrated with information from other sensory modalities. This information is then transferred to the supramodal association cortex where all sensory modalities are integrated. Paralimbic brain regions such as the cingulate gyrus, parahippocampal gyrus, temporal pole, and orbital cortex are regarded as highly organized supramodal association and integration areas (Jones & Powell, 1970; Swanson, 1983; Mesulam, 1986; Schmajuk, 1987).

The hippocampus and amygdala, which are central limbic structures, are anatomically and functionally interposed between the supramodal sensory association areas and the septum-hypothalamus complex. All sensory information eventually converges on the hippocampus and amygdala, both of which are key structures in sensory information processing (Jones & Powell, 1970; Mesulam, 1986). Thus, it is reasonable to assume that structural and functional deficits of paralimbic and limbic areas are associated with defective integrative and associative brain functions, resulting in distorted interpretations of external reality, and an inability to filter out irrelevant sensory information, ie, poor "sensory gating" (Bogerts, 1991).

ADDITIONAL EVIDENCE FOR THE NEURODEVELOPMENTAL PERSPECTIVE

Impressive support for the importance of the second trimester in neural development has been presented in a preliminary study that ties together findings from both viral and neuropathological studies (Scheibel et al., 1991). Scheibel and colleagues exposed pregnant mice (Balb-C) to the WSN strain of influenza virus during the equivalent of their second trimester of pregnancy (about day 14). The mothers were allowed to come to term and their pups were followed for about three weeks. The pups were then sacrificed and their hippocampi were studied with routine histological techniques. The investigators found some degree of disorganization in the anterior two-thirds of the hippocampus, especially in the CA 2-3 area, and a very significant degree of neuronal disorientation ($p=.002$) in comparison to hippocampi of pups from non-virus infected mothers. Pups from mothers who were exposed to both influenza virus and cold shock (the latter to simulate the lowered immunocompetence they suspect is contributed by the genetic component of schizophrenia) showed more disorganization.

Further evidence for the neurodevelopmental perspective is provided by studies examining dysmorphological hand development and fingertip ectodermal ridge count (Bracha et al., 1991a, 1991b). Development of the distal upper limb and migration of fingertip ectodermal cells that form ridges both occur during the second trimester of fetal development. In studies of monozygotic twins discordant for schizophrenia, Bracha and collaborators reported that the affected co-twins had significantly higher dysmorphological hand anomalies and reduced ectodermal ridge counts than their healthy co-twins, again attesting to the importance of the second trimester of fetal development.

THE IMPORTANCE OF GENDER

While the evidence presented thus far in this chapter clearly supports the neurodevelopmental hypothesis of schizophrenia, further elaboration of this perspective will need to take into account the effects of gender. Previous research has consistently demonstrated that an earlier age of onset, a poorer premorbid history and subsequent course of illness, more negative symptoms, and a poorer response to neuroleptics is more characteristic of schizophrenic males than schizophrenic females (Goldstein & Tsuang, 1990).

Previous literature also suggests that schizophrenic males may have more structural brain abnormalities than schizophrenic females (Nasrallah et al., 1986; Lewine et al., 1990; Flaum et al., 1990). In a recent CT study, schizophrenics showed significantly greater ventricular enlargement than a group of healthy normal volunteers (Andreasen et al., 1990). However, it was found that the statistically significant difference was accounted for primarily by the schizophrenic males. Andreasen and coworkers noted that similar reports of gender effects have not frequently been reported, probably owing to the fact that investigators have not regularly described the sexual composition of their samples, broken their data down by gender, or used sufficiently large sample sizes to adequately evaluate gender effects.

Some investigators have suggested that certain brain areas may be more vulnerable to damage in men than in women (Kopala & Clark, 1990). Others have proposed that men are at greater risk for left hemisphere abnormalities whereas women are at greater risk for right hemisphere abnormalities (Flor-Henry, 1990). It is possible that some of these issues may be clarified by a better understanding of the sequence of normal fetal brain development. For example, the left hemisphere develops more slowly than the right hemisphere so that by the end of the second trimester, the right hemisphere has achieved almost full term size while the left hemisphere has not (Chi et al., 1977). Although the significance of this for gender differences in schizophrenia is not directly clear, it has been proposed that the indications of greater left hemisphere damage in schizophrenia can be explained by prenatal injury during the second trimester of gestation (Bracha, 1991).

FETAL NEURAL DEVELOPMENT AND SCHIZOPHRENIA ONSET: WHY THE LONG LATENCY?

The focus of this chapter has been on the effects of a disturbance in fetal neural development during the second trimester and its relationship to schizophrenia. If such a theory is to be plausible, then it must account for the long latency between the early developmental disturbance and the onset of schizophrenic symptoms.

Weinberger (1987) has proposed that a neurodevelopmental disturbance interacts with normal brain maturational events that do not occur until late adolescence or early adulthood, the reason being that effects of brain abnormalities associated with the disturbance would not become apparent until the brain areas involved reach functional maturity. Two such maturational events that continue through puberty are myelination (Benes, 1989) and synaptic pruning (Huttenlocher, 1979). Weinberger (1987) also mentions human and animal research which suggests that early adulthood is the time of maximum dopaminergic activity in cortical and subcortical areas.

A different maturational theory has focused on the role of hormonal factors during puberty (Bogerts, 1989). During puberty, limbic structures become the main targets of age- and stress-related hormones such as gonadosteroids and corticosteroids. The suggestion is made that abnormal limbic structures decompensate under the influence of such hormones, resulting in the onset of psychotic symptoms.

An alternative position is that subtle premorbid signs are evident during childhood and adolescence as early as infancy (Parnas et al., 1982). Strong empirical support for such a position has been found in a recent report of the Copenhagen high-risk project. Cannon and colleagues (1990), using prospectively-obtained scales of adolescent school behavior, demonstrated that high-risk subjects who succumbed to schizophrenia marked by predominantly negative symptoms had evidenced more negative-type premorbid school behavior disturbance (ie, passivity, lack of spontaneity, social unresponsiveness); those who developed schizophrenia marked by predominantly positive symptoms had exhibited more positive-type premorbid school behavior disturbance (i.e., overactivity, irritability, aggression).

What the results of this study suggest is that there is not necessarily a long latency between neurodevelopmental disturbance and the onset of schizophrenia, but that associated premorbid behaviors are already evident by adolescence. Moreover, this study found evidence relating two independent sets of antecedent factors to two longitudinal syndromes of schizophrenia. Predominantly negative-symptom schizophrenics were characterized by elevated genetic risk, a high number of delivery complications, and ANS non-responsiveness. Predominantly positive-symptom schizophrenics were characterized by genetic risk, severe disruptions of the early family rearing environment, and high ANS responsiveness. Thus, it is proposed that the type of schizophrenia one develops depends on the interaction between genetic risk (possibly manifested as a neurodevelopmental disruption during the second trimester of pregnancy) and differential life experiences and individual characteristics.

SUMMARY

This chapter has given a brief overview of the new neurodevelopmental trend in schizophrenia research, based on the old idea that the brain is somehow involved in the manifestation of the disorder. Lest this new trend suffer the fate of old ones that failed to adequately explain the actual development of schizophrenia, it should be stressed that consideration of the <u>interaction</u> between a neurodevelopmental disturbance and environmental stressors holds the most promise for the eventual understanding of this extremely debilitating disorder.

To conclude, this chapter will close with a summary of the information presented herein.

1. Some form of disturbance during the second trimester of fetal neural development, particularly the sixth month of gestation, seems to be of critical importance for determining the risk of adult schizophrenia.

2. Neurodevelopmental disruption during the second trimester seems to especially involve defective neuronal migration and positioning.

3. Although an influenza infection during gestation appears to increase the risk of adult schizophrenia, it is unclear as to whether it is mimicking a genetic effect or exerting a unique environmental effect.

4. Limbic system pathology is a robust finding in schizophrenia, and may be related to the clinical symptoms of the disorder.

5. The time is ripe for animal models to assume an important role in elucidating the nature of the neurodevelopmental perspective in schizophrenia.

6. Gender should be given prominent status as an independent variable in future research, necessitating the collection of larger patient samples.

7. Environmental experiences may interact with genetic risk to produce schizophrenia marked either by predominantly negative symptoms or predominantly positive symptoms.

8. Predominantly negative- and predominantly positive-symptom schizophrenia are longitudinal syndromes, with associated premorbid behaviors already evident by adolescence.

ACKNOWLEDGEMENTS

Preparation of this chapter was supported by a Social Science Merit Fellowship from the University of Southern California and a Minority Fellowship from the American Psychological Association to J. M. LaFosse, and a Research Scientist Award from the National Institute of Mental Health to S. A. Mednick.

REFERENCES

Andreasen, N. C., Swayze, V. W., Flaum, M., Yates, W. R., Arndt, S., & McChesney, C. (1990). Ventricular enlargement in schizophrenia evaluated with computed tomographic scanning. Archives of General Psychiatry, 47: 1008-1015.

Barr, C. E., Mednick, S. A., & Munk-Jorgensen, P. Exposure to influenza epidemics during gestation and adult schizophrenia: A 40-year study. Archives of General Psychiatry, 47: 869-874.

Barr, C. E., Mednick, S. A., & Munk-Jorgensen, P. (1991, April). Prenatal infection and schizophrenia in the offspring: A survey of 25 diseases. Paper presented at the third International Congress on Schizophrenia Research, Tucson, AZ.

Bateson, G., Jackson, D. D., Haley, J., & Weakland, J. (1956). Toward a theory of schizophrenia. Behavioral Science, 1: 251-264.

Benes, F. M., Davidson, B., Bird, E. D. (1986). Quantitative cytoarchitectural studies of the cerebral cortex of schizophrenics. Archives of General Psychiatry, 43: 31-35.

Benes, F. M. (1987). An analysis of the arrangement of neurons in the cingulate cortex of schizophrenic patients. Archives of General Psychiatry, 44: 608-616.

Benes, F. M. (1989). Myelination of cortical-hippocampal relays during late adolescence. Schizophrenia Bulletin, 15: 585-593.

Bigelow, L. B., Nasrallah, H. A., Rauscher, F. P. (1983). Corpus callosum thickness in chronic schizophrenia. British Journal of Psychiatry, 142: 282-287.

Bleuler, E. (1911, trans. 1950). Dementia Praecox or the Group of Schizophrenias. New York: International Universities Press.

Bogerts, B., Hantsch, J., & Herzer, M. (1983). A morphometric study of the dopamine containing cell groups in the mesencephalon of normals, Parkinson patients and schizophrenics. Biological Psychiatry, 18: 951-960.

Bogerts, B., Meertz, E., & Schonfeld-Bausch, R. (1985). Basal ganglia and limbic system pathology in schizophrenia. Archives of General Psychiatry, 42: 784-791.

Bogerts, B. (1989). Limbic and paralimbic pathology in schizophrenia: Interaction with age and stress related factors. In S. C. Schulz & C. A. Tamminga (Eds.), Schizophrenia: Scientific Progress (pp. 216-226). Oxford, England: Oxford University Press.

Bogerts, B., Ashtari, M., Degreef, G., Alvir, J. Ma.J., Bilder, R. M., & Lieberman, J. A. (1990). Reduced temporal limbic structure volumes on magnetic resonance images in first episode schizophrenia. Psychiatry Research: Neuroimaging, 35: 1-13.

Bogerts, B. (1991). The neuropathology of schizophrenia: Pathophysiological and neurodevelopmental implications. In S. A. Mednick, T. D. Cannon, C. E. Barr, & M. Lyon (Eds.), Fetal Neural Development and Adult Schizophrenia (pp. 153-173). Cambridge, England: Cambridge University Press.

Bracha, H. S., Torrey, E. F., & Bigelow, L. B. (1991a). Prenatal maldevelopment of the palm/thumb in schizophrenia: A monozygotic twins study. Schizophrenia Research, 4: 274.

Bracha, H. S., Torrey, E. F., Karson, C. N., & Bigelow, L. B. (1991b). A twin study of prenatal injury markers in psychosis: Timing the insult. Schizophrenia Research, 4: 250.

Bracha, H. S. (1991c). Implications of normal fetal brain development for the pathogenesis of structural brain asymmetry in schizophrenia. Schizophrenia Bulletin, (in press).

Brown, G. W., Bone, M., Dalison, B., & Wing, J. K. (1966). Schizophrenia and Social Care. London: Oxford University Press.

Buchsbaum, M. S., & Haier, R. J. (1987). Functional and anatomical brain imaging: Impact on schizophrenia research. Special Report: Schizophrenia 1987, 129-146. (Schizophrenia Bulletin, Vol. 13, No. 1, 1987).

Cannon, T. D., Mednick, S. A., & Parnas, J. (1990). Antecedents of predominantly negative- and predominantly positive-symptom schizophrenia in a high-risk population. Archives of General Psychiatry, 47: 622-632.

Cannon, T. D. (1991). Sources and correlates of structural brain abnormalities in schizophrenia. In S. A. Mednick, T. D. Cannon, C. E. Barr, & M. Lyon (Eds.), Fetal Neural Development and Adult Schizophrenia (pp. 174-198). Cambridge, England: Cambridge University Press.

Carpenter, M. B., & Sutin, J. (1983). Human Neuroanatomy. Baltimore: Williams & Wilkins.

Chi, J. G., Dooling, E. C., & Gilles, F. H. (1977). Gyral development of the human brain. Annals of Neurology, 1: 86-93.

Conrad, A. J., & Scheibel, A. B. (1987). Schizophrenia and the hippocampus: The embryological hypothesis extended. Schizophrenia Bulletin, 4: 577-587.

Dauphinais, D., DeLisi, L. E., Crow, T. J., Alexandropolous, K., Colter, N., Tuma, I., & Gershon, E. S. (1990). Reduction in temporal lobe size in siblings with schizophrenia: A magnetic resonance imaging study. Psychiatry Research, 35: 137-147.

DeLisi, L. E., & Crow, T. J. (1986). Is schizophrenia a viral or immunologic disorder? Psychiatric Clinics of North America, 9: 115-132.

DeLisi, L. E., Alexandropolous, A., Colter, N. et al. (1988a). Reduced temporal lobe area: A study of siblings with schizophrenia. Schizophrenia Research, 1: 169-170.

DeLisi, L. E., Dauphinais, I. D., & Gershon, E. S. (1988b). Perinatal complications and reduced size of brain limbic structures in familial schizophrenia. Schizophrenia Bulletin, 14: 185-191.

Falkai, P., & Bogerts, B. (1986). Cell loss in the hippocampus of schizophrenics. European Archives of Psychiatry and Neurological Science, 236: 154-161.

Falkai, P., Bogerts, B., & Rozumek, M. (1988). Cell loss and volume reduction in the entorhinal cortex of schizophrenics. Biological Psychiatry, 24: 515-521.

Falkai, P., & Bogerts, B. (1991, April). Qualitative and Quantitative Assessment of Pre-Alpha-Cell Clusters in the Entorhinal Cortex of Schizophrenics. A Neurodevelopmental Model of Schizophrenia? Paper presented at the third International Congress on Schizophrenia Research, Tucson, AZ.

Flaum, M., Arndt, S., & Andreasen, N. C. (1990). The role of gender in studies of ventricular enlargement in schizophrenia: A predominantly male effect. American Journal of Psychiatry, 147: 1327-1332.

Flor-Henry, P. (1990). Influence of gender in schizophrenia as related to other psychopathological syndromes. Schizophrenia Bulletin, 16: 211-227.

Fromm-Reichmann, F. (1948). Notes on the development of treatment ofschizophrenics by psychoanalytic psychotherapy. Psychiatry, 11: 263-273.

Goldstein, J. M., & Tsuang, M. T. (1990). Gender and schizophrenia: An introduction and synthesis of findings. Schizophrenia Bulletin, 16: 179-183.

Huttenlocher, P. R. (1979). Synaptic density in human frontal cortex: Developmental changes and effects of aging. Brain Research, 163: 195-205.

Johnstone, E. C., Crow, T. J., Frith, C. D., Husband, J., & Kreel, L. (1976). Cerebral ventricular size and cognitive impairment in chronic schizophrenia. Lancet, 2: 924-926.

Johnstone, E. C., Owens, D. G. C., Crow, T. J., Frith, C. D., Alexandropolous, K., Bydder, G., and Colter, N. (1989). Temporal lobe structure as determined by nuclear magnetic resonance in schizophrenia and bipolar affective disorder. Journal of Neurology, Neurosurgery, and Psychiatry, 52: 736-741.

Jones, E. G., & Powell, T. P. S. (1970). An anatomical study of converging sensory pathways within the cerebral cortex of the monkey. Brain, 93: 793-820.

Kendell, R. E. & Kemp, I. W. (1989). Maternal influenza in the etiology of schizophrenia. Archives of General Psychiatry, 46: 878-882.

Kopala, L., & Clark, C. Implications of olfactory agnosia for understanding sex differences in schizophrenia. Schizophrenia Bulletin, 16: 255-261.

Kovelman, J. A., & Scheibel, A. B. (1984). A neurohistological correlate of schizophrenia. Biological Psychiatry, 19: 1601-1621.

Kraepelin, E. (1919). Dementia Praecox and Paraphrenia. Edinburgh, Scotland: Livingston.

LaFosse, J. M., & Mednick, S. A. (1991). Critical month of prenatal exposure to influenza and subsequent schizophrenia. The Lancet, 338:118.

Larroche, J. L. (1984). Malformations of the nervous system. In J. M. Adams et al. (Eds.), Greenfield's Neuropathology (pp. 385-403). London: Edward Arnold.

Leff, J. P. (1976). Schizophrenia and sensitivity to the family environment. Schizophrenia Bulletin, 2: 566-574.

Lesch, A., & Bogerts, B. (1984). The diencephalon in schizophrenia: Evidence for reduced thickness of the periventricular grey matter. European Archives of Psychiatry and Neurological Science, 234: 212-219.

Lohr, J. B., & Jeste, D. V. (1988). Locus ceruleus morphometry in aging and schizophrenia. Acta Psychiatrica Scandanavica, 77: 689-697.

Mednick, S. A. (1970). Breakdown in individuals at high risk for schizophrenia: possible predispositional perinatal factors. Mental Hygiene, 54: 50-63.

Mednick, S. A., Machon, R. A., Huttunen, M. O., & Bonett, D. (1988). Adult schizophrenia following prenatal exposure to an influenza epidemic. Archives of General Psychiatry, 45: 189-192.

Mednick, S. A., Machon, R. A., Huttunen, M. O., & Barr, C. E. (1990). Influenza and schizophrenia: Helsinki vs. Edinburgh. Archives of General Psychiatry, 47: 875-876.

Mesulam, M. M. (1986). Patterns in behavioral neuroanatomy: Association areas, the limbic system, and hemispheric specialization. In M. M. Mesulam (Hrsg.), *Principles of Behavioral Neurology* (pp. 1-70). Philadelphia: Davis.

Nasrallah, H. A., McCalley-Whitters, M., Rauscher, F. P., et al. (1983). A histological study of the corpus callosum in chronic schizophrenia. *Psychiatry Research*, 8: 151-160.

Nowakowski, R. S. (1991). Some basic concepts of the development of the CNS. In S. A. Mednick, T. D. Cannon, C. E. Barr, & M. Lyon (Eds.), *Fetal Neural Development and Adult Schizophrenia* (pp. 17-39). Cambridge, England: Cambridge University Press.

O'Callaghan, E., Sham, P., Takei, N., Glover, G., & Murray, R. M. (1991). Schizophrenia after prenatal exposure to 1957 A2 influenza epidemic. *Lancet*, 337: 1248-1250.

Parnas, J., Schulsinger, F., Schulsinger, H., Teasdale, T. W., & Mednick, S. A. (1982). Behavioral precursors of the schizophrenia spectrum: A prospective study. *Archives of General Psychiatry*, 39: 658-664.

Raz, S. & Raz, N. (1990). Structural brain abnormalities in the major psychoses: A quantitative review of the evidence from computerized imaging. *Psychological Bulletin*, 108: 93-108.

Roberts, G. W., Colter, N., Lofthouse, R., Bogerts, B., Zech, M., & Crow, T. J. (1986). Gliosis in schizophrenia: A survey. *Biological Psychiatry*, 21: 10431050.

Roberts, G. W., Colter, N., Lofthouse, R., Johnstone, E. C., & Crow, T. J. (1987). Is there gliosis in schizophrenia? Investigation of the temporal lobe. *Biological Psychiatry*, 22: 1459-1468.

Rossi, A., Stratta, P., D'Albenzio, L., Tartaro, A., Schiazza, G., DiMichele, V., Ceccoli, S., & Casacchia, M. Reduced temporal lobe area in schizophrenia by magnetic resonance imaging: Preliminary evidence. *Psychiatry Research*, 29: 261-263.

Rossi, A., Stratta, P., D'Albenzio, L., Tartaro, A., Schiazza, G., di Michele, V., Bolino, F., & Casacchia, M. (1990). Reduced temporal lobe areas in schizophrenia: Preliminary evidence from a controlled multiplanar magnetic resonance imaging study. *Biological Psychiatry*, 27: 61-68.

Scheibel, A. B., Conrad, A., & Sanders, V. (1991, April). *An Animal Model of the Schizophrenic Hippocampus: An Attempt to Influence Fetal Hippocampal Development by Means of Maternal Viral Infection*. Paper presented at the third International Congress on Schizophrenia Research, Tucson, AZ.

Schmajuk, N. A. (1987). Animal models for schizophrenia: the hippocampally lesioned animal. *Schizophrenia Bulletin*, 13: 317-327.

Shelton, R. C. & Weinberger, D. R. (1986). X-Ray computerized tomography studies of schizophrenia: A review and synthesis. In H. A. Nasrallah & D. R. Weinberger (Eds.), *The Neurology of Schizophrenia* (pp. 207-250). Amsterdam: Elsevier Science Publishers.

Stevens, J. R. (1982). Neuropathology of schizophrenia. *Archives of General Psychiatry*, 39: 1131-1139.

Stevens, C. D., Altshuler, L. L., Bogerts, B., & Falkai, P. (1988). Quantitative study of gliosis in schizophrenia and Huntington's chorea. Biological Psychiatry, 24: 697-700.

Suddath, R. L., Casanova, M. F., Goldberg, T. E., Daniel, D. G., Kelsoe, Jr., J. R., & Weinberger, D. R. (1989). Temporal lobe pathology in schizophrenia: A quantitative magnetic resonance imaging study. American Journal of Psychiatry, 146: 464-472.

Suddath, R. L., Christison, G. W., Torrey, E. F., Casanova, M. F., & Weinberger, D. R. (1990). Anatomical abnormalities in the brains of monozygotic twins discordant for schizophrenia. The New England Journal of Medicine, 322: 789-794.

Swanson, L. W. (1983). The hippocampus and the concept of limbic system. In W. Seifert (Ed.), Neurobiology of the Hippocampus (pp. 3-19). London: Academic Press.

Torrey, E. F. (1991). A viral-anatomical explanation of schizophrenia. Schizophrenia Bulletin, 17: 15-18.

Torrey, E. F., Rawlings, R., & Waldman, I. N. (1988). Schizophrenic births and viral diseases in two states. Schizophrenia Research, 1: 73-77.

Weinberger, D. R. (1987). Implications of normal brain development for the pathogenesis of schizophrenia. Archives of General Psychiatry, 44: 660-669.

PARTICIPANTS

Christopher E. Barr
Social Science Research Institute
University of Southern California
Los Angeles, California 90089-1111
USA

Brigitte Berger
I.N.S.E.R.M. U-106
Histologie Normale et Pathologique Du Systeme Nerveux
Hopital de la Salpetriere
47, Boulevard De L'Hopital
75651 Paris Cedex 13
France

Bernard Bogerts
Department of Psychiatry
University of Dusseldorf
Postfach 12 05 10
W-4000 Dusseldorf 12
Germany

Robert M. Bilder
Hillside Hospital, Long Island Jewish Medical Center
Albert Einstein College of Medicine
Glen Oaks, New York 11004
USA

Tyronne D. Cannon
Social Science Research Institute
University of Southern California
Los Angeles, California 90089-1111
USA

Gustav Degreef
Hillside Hospital, Long Island Jewish Medical Center
Albert Einstein College of Medicine
Glen Oaks, New York 11004
USA

Karen L. Dykes
Social Science Research Institute
University of Southern California
Los Angeles, California 90089-1111
USA

Katarzyna M. Dziegielewska
Department of Physiology and Pharmacology
The University of Southampton
Bassett Crescent East
Southampton, Hants SO9 3TU
England

Peter Falkai
Department of Psychiatry
University of Dusseldorf
Postfach 12 05 10
W-4000 Dusseldorf 12
Germany

R. Goodman
University Department of Child and
Adolescent Psychiatry
Institute of Psychiatry
De Crespigny Park
Denmark Hill
London SE5 8AF
England

Mette Stagaard Janas
Institute of Medical Anatomy, Dept. A
The Panum Institute
University of Copenhagen
Blegdamsvej 3, DK-2200
Copenhagen N.
Denmark

Edward G. Jones
Department of Anatomy and Neurobiology
317 Med. Surg. II
University of California at Irvine
Irvine, California 92717
USA

Peter B. Jones
Genetics Section
Institute of Psychiatry
De Crespigny Park
Denmark Hill
London SE5 8AF
England

Jose M. LaFosse
Social Science Research Institute
University of Southern California
Los Angeles, California 90089-1111
USA

S.W. Lewis
Department of Psychiatry
Charing Cross and Westminster Medical
Fulham Palace Road
London W6 8RF
England

Sarnoff Mednick
Social Science Research Institute
University of Southern California
Los Angeles, California 90089-1111
USA

Kjeld Mollgard
Institute of Medical Anatomy, Dept. A
The Panum Institute
University of Copenhagen
Blegdamsvej 3, DK-2200
Copenhagen N.
Denmark

Torbin Moos
Institute of Medical Anatomy, Dept. A
The Panum Institute
University of Copenhagen
Blegdamsvej 3, DK-2200
Copenhagen N.
Denmark

Richard S. Nowakowski
Department of Neuroscience
and Cell Biology
University of Medicine and Dentistry
of New Jersey
Robert Wood Johnson Medical School
675 Hoes Lane
Piscataway, New Jersey 08884
USA

Robin Murray
Kings College Hospital and Institute of Psychiatry
De Crespigny Park
Denmark Hill
London, SE5 8AF
England

Henry A. Nasrallah
Department of Psychiatry
Room 071, Upham Hall
The Ohio State University
473 West 12th Avenue
Columbus, Ohio 43210-1228
USA

Steven C. Olson
Department of Psychiatry
The Ohio State University
473 West 12th Avenue
Columbus, Ohio 43210-1228
USA

M.J. Owen
Department of Psychological Medicine
University of Wales College of Medicine
Heath Park, Cardiff, CF4 4XN
Wales

Pasko Rakic
Section of Neuroanatomy
Yale University School of Medicine
333 Cedar Street
New Haven, Connecticut 06510
USA

Norman R. Saunders
Clinical Neurological Sciences
Room LF73B, Level F, South Block
Southampton General Hospital
Tremona Road
Southampton, Hants, SO9 4XY
England

Fini Schulsinger
Psykologisk Institut
Dommunehospitalet
Psykiatrisk Afdeling
1399 Copenhagen
Denmark

Steven B. Schwarzkopf
Department of Psychiatry
Room 071, Upham Hall
The Ohio State University
473 West 12th Avenue
Columbus, Ohio 43210-1228
USA

AUTHOR INDEX

SUBJECT INDEX